ADVENTURES IN PSYCHIATRY

The Scientific Memoirs of
Dr. Abram Hoffer

KOS Publishing Inc.

Dedication

When I applied for a job with the Department of Public Health, I had no idea it would lead to these adventures. Tommy created the unusual set of circumstances which made our research possible. I dedicate this book to Tommy Douglas, Premier of Saskatchewan. He inherited a Psychiatric Division that was totally dysfunctional, that had two of the three worst mental hospitals in the world, that had too few doctors and nurses and where, because there was no treatment, an admission was a real life sentence. Under his direction he swung the resources of government behind what we were doing and brought us together: especially Dr. H. Osmond, Dr. D.G. McKerracher and many others who conceived and nurtured the research. He never wavered in his support. Thank you Tommy.

A. Hoffer, M.D., Ph.D., FRCP(C)

Copyright © 2005 by Dr. Abram Hoffer

National Library of Canada Cataloguing in Publication

Hoffer, Abram, 1917–

ISBN 0-9731945-6-1

1. Psychiatry. 2. Nutritional medicine. 3. Orthomolecular medicine. 4. Autobiography

Cover and text design/layout: Heidy Lawrance Associates
Printed in Canada

Published and distributed by

KOS Publishing Inc.
Caledon, Ontario Canada L7K 0N3
Tel: (519) 927-1049 • Fax: (519) 927-9542
Email: info@kospublishing.com

Contents

PREFACE

A memoir is a personal history, and the lesson in all histories is the same: if we do not learn from history, we are doomed to repeat it.

This book contains Dr. Abram Hoffer's recollections of and observations from his "adventures" in the often dysfunctional field of psychiatry. Dr. Hoffer is distinguished as an original and rational thinker in medicine and, more specifically, a pioneer in orthomolecular medicine—what many people have come to call vitamin therapy.

"Orthomolecular", a word coined by Nobel laureate Linus Pauling, means "to correct the molecules" of the body. Using nutrients in this way makes sense because they serve as the basic chemical building blocks of our bodies, our biochemistries, and even our DNA. Good nutrition creates a solid foundation for health, whereas poor nutrition provides a flimsy one. Although the use of nutrients may at first seem too simplistic, the underlying biochemistry can be complex.

But this is a memoir, not a biochemistry book. And there are two historical lessons for the reader to appreciate. One is that the "cures" for most of what ail us exist already, are inexpensive, and highly effective. The other lesson is that if conventional medicine cannot rise above its arrogance and internal politics, patients will continue to suffer instead of being helped.

Although the United States and Canadian medical establishments generally frown on nutritional therapies, they are evidence-based treatments that take both a fundamental and a conservative approach. Unlike conventional drug therapy, orthomolecular medicine embodies Hippocrates' medical advice of "first do not harm." In fact, orthomolecular medicine could almost be called "fundamental medicine." It should be the first line of treatment, not an alternative treatment.

I first met Dr. Hoffer in 1976, and I have learned something new every time I have talked with him or heard him speak. He possesses a rare humility and has a knack for instantly seeing through the nonsense and contradictions of modern medicine. He looks at the world with an almost childlike honesty and directness, and I am always amazed by his insights and clarity of thought.

Like all pioneers, Dr. Hoffer has faced a variety of obstacles—in this case, from more conventional and less imaginative researchers and physicians. I think a pioneering spirit runs in his blood. He was the son of immigrant pioneers who settled on the Canadian prairie and farmed the land. Dr. Hoffer still retains the humility of a person born of the land.

His medical contributions are many and profound. By earning his Ph.D. degree as a cereal chemist, he gained a clear understanding of the B-complex vitamins. When he returned to school to obtain his M.D. degree, he was lucky enough to avoid being indoctrinated in psychoanalysis, then the prevailing theology of psychiatry. This combination of training, plus the serendipity of working with the right professional collaborators, led to a series of remarkable discoveries. With a scientific mind, he followed the research to a biochemical understanding of mental illness, though he has always acknowledged the psychosocial influences on disease as well.

Beginning in the early 1950s, Dr. Hoffer codeveloped:
- the first biochemical theory to explain schizophrenia (a mental illness characterized by delusions and hallucinations);
- the adrenochrome hypothesis; that is, that some people, under stress, produce their own hallucinogen as a byproduct of adrenaline, resulting in schizophrenia;
- the first nutritional/biochemical treatment for schizophrenia, namely high doses of vitamins B3 and C, which doubled the recovery rate in recent-onset schizophrenia;
- the first double-blind studies conducted in the field of psychiatry;
- one simple and accurate question-and-answer diagnostic test for schizophrenia, the Hoffer-Osmond Diagnostic test;

- the concept of orthomolecular psychiatry and orthomolecular medicine, and the creation of a new paradigm that uses vitamins to treat disease, not just to cure classical deficiency states;
- the theory behind and the discovery of kryptopyrrole, also known as the mauve factor, a marker of free-radical stress and the possible presence of mental illness; and
- the safe treatment of elevated cholesterol using vitamin B3, which was approved by the Food and Drug Administration in 1955.

In a little-known but fascinating chapter of Dr. Hoffer's professional life, he also codeveloped psychedelic therapy for the treatment of alcoholism. Anything but an advocate of recreational drug use, Hoffer and his colleagues discovered that hallucinogens could trigger profound insights in alcoholics that led to their recovery. This innovative research came to a halt when LSD and mescaline were banned in Canada and the United States, but Harvard University-affiliated physicians are now planning follow-up studies on this very work.

Honest, idealistic, and ethical, Dr. Hoffer's discoveries were confronted by people with petty jealousies, those who wanted to steal his ideas, and a general resistance to new ways of treating mental illnesses. Only the naïve would now believe that such events are rare in medicine. After all, medicine rejected for one hundred years Simmelweiss's advice that doctors wash their hands before surgery. Today, much of the resistance to orthomolecular medicine comes from deeply vested interests in medical academia and the pharmaceutical industry. Yet to his great credit, Dr. Hoffer has remained steadfast.

Why has conventional medicine resisted so many of his ideas? I believe there are several reasons. First, medicine had always been ambivalent about nutritional therapies. Although medicine celebrated many of the discoveries about vitamins during the first half of the twentieth century, the field later developed the attitude that treating serious diseases could never be quite as simple as just taking large amounts of certain micronutrients. Second, nutrients could never be as profitable as drugs, so the powerful pharmaceutical industry never embraced nutritional therapies. And third, nutrients are part of foods, and I believe that a built-in sexism has tended to denigrate nutrition to the level of dietetics, a field dominated by women. Nutrition was not the stuff of physicians working heroically to save their patients' lives.

Dr. Hoffer has been blessed, though some would say cursed, to have outlived all of the other pioneers in orthomolecular medicine and most of his harshest critics as well. Approaching ninety years of age, Dr. Hoffer possesses a rare historical perspective of medicine. And remarkably, he has the energy of a much younger man and still works full time.

I was honored when Dr. Hoffer asked me to write this preface. Although I am only in my mid-fifties, I have been around long enough to appreciate the value of history. Over the years, I have known many of the other pioneers in orthomolecular medicine and heard their stories of being attacked when they simply wanted to treat their patients in the safest and most straightforward ways. Some of these remarkable physicians were beaten down, but Dr. Hoffer is clearly one of the survivors.

This memoir is an important part of the historical record of orthomolecular medicine and the experiences that shaped one of the most remarkable men of medicine and science. His recollections and reflections add to an already significant legacy. There are lessons here in integrity, courage, and perseverance in the face of overwhelming odds. All people, especially medical professionals, must learn from what Dr. Hoffer relates. This is the only way to avoid the mistakes of the past and to create a healthier future.

Jack Challem
Author, *Feed Your Genes Right*
Tucson, Arizona

I

Chemistry Studies

I was born on a Canadian prairie farm, in southern Saskatchewan, towards the end of World War I on November 11, 1917 to Israel and Clara Hoffer, Jewish-Hungarian immigrants attracted to Canada's west by the promise of affordable land. I was welcomed into the family by three older siblings, Esther, Stanley, and Marion, and my father's brother and business partner, Meyer, and his wife, Rose.

Mother and Father valued education. They were determined that their children would have the best then available. I liked school and took enthusiastic part in all its activities, even in the school plays put on every Christmas. My teachers considered me to be intelligent, but I cannot recall why. On the academic side, I was an average student who received Cs without having to work too hard. I remember that in the sixth grade, I was given a simple IQ test consisting of 80 questions. I found the test very straightforward, and I answered every question correctly, to my teacher's surprise. A year later he gave our class exactly the same test and, remembering how I had answered the questions before, I did so again. Since then I have been very skeptical of intelligence tests.

My scholastic career suddenly improved in my 15th year when Mr. Reid Purdie arrived in our area to teach grades 11 and 12. He had had one or two years study at the University of Saskatchewan in sciences and had hoped to become a chemist, but the Great Depression of the 1930's was in full swing and suddenly straitened circumstances had forced him to take a teaching job.

Mr. Reid Purdie was a very good teacher with a sunny personality and a great flair for inspiring his students. He aroused my interest in chemistry, and before I had completed grade 11, I had decided I would take a university degree in the subject. There was no question in my family, despite the challenges we faced during the Depression years, that I would go to university. I believe my mother was the most determined about this. She felt that I ought not to remain on the farm, whereas my father wanted me to follow in his footsteps, as he expected my older brother to do. In grades 11 and 12 our final exams were set by a central provincial government agency and distributed to all students in the province. I did not find these exams particularly difficult and, after completing them, fully expected I would easily get my usual C average. The final results of my Grade 11 exams surprised me more than anyone else. I had received As in every subject. Even then I was cynical about exams and their grades. I concluded that the general ability for the whole province must have been considered so low by the exam writers that it would require little skill to surpass the provincial average.

I had the greatest difficulty with English literature, and the next year I decided I would concentrate on that and improve my performance. Indeed, in my final exams in grade 12, I performed as well in English as in the other subjects, achieving a grade of 97 percent. (I believe this result was a fluke, because the next year at the University of Saskatchewan, I would achieve only a C in English and that was the only C I ever received during my university years.) Overall, I passed grade 12 with a high A average and now looked forward with anticipation to beginning my chemistry studies at the University of Saskatchewan in Saskatoon. I eventually studied there from 1934 to 1940, first taking a four-year course in agricultural chemistry leading to a Bachelor of Science in Agriculture (BSA) degree.

Going to Saskatoon and back home was in those days a major undertaking, but I always came home for Christmas holidays between 1934 and 1938. However, in 1939 and 1940 I stayed at the university over the break, analyzing wheat from different parts of the province for protein content in the chemistry laboratory because I needed the money so badly. In 1933 I met and befriended Max Milner, another chemistry student. He would later become Professor and Head of Cereal Chemistry at a midwestern university in the United States, and after that, head of one of the sections of the World Health Organization. His family's house had the advantage of being close to the buildings where my classes were held, so I moved in with the Milners. I was determined to live on $30 per month and even that was an enormous hardship for my parents. Room and board with the Milners, including laundry, cost $25 per month. That left me $5 per month for all other expenses, including recreation. Movies cost 15 cents and one could take a date for an additional penny.

In those days I always knew exactly how much money I had in my pocket, down to the last penny. I still remember what it meant to be short of money. Once I had to see the campus doctor about a minor skin irritation. As he was the University physician we could see him for free. He gave me a prescription which cost 15 cents to fill. But I only had ten cents since it was close to the end of the month and my cheque for $30 had not yet arrived. I remember how embarrassed I was because I had to borrow twenty-five cents from my closest friend, another student from a farming family. But this was not poverty. There were many who were much worse off than me.

Many years later, my friend's son began developing schizophrenia. I treated the youth and he had a full recovery. The treatment was continued by Dr. Glen Green of Prince Albert who did an excellent job. My friend's son is still well and I am glad to this day that I was able to repay my friend for helping me out so many years ago. I stayed with the Milners for one year and through them, met Jack Wilner. Jack, after graduation, married Pearl Miller, cousin to Rose— who later became my wife.

All BSA students took the same courses in their first two years. These covered the subjects considered essential for success in modern farming and included studies of grains, animals, poultry, first year biochemistry, some biology, English, and so on. One took one's specialty courses during the last two years of the degree; in my case, these were my chemistry studies. I had long ago decided to become a chemist. The agricultural chemistry program represented a compromise between my wish and my father's desire that I remain on the farm. The last two years were heavily loaded, and included much laboratory work and physics. I also took a course in Agricultural Economics which I particularly enjoyed. Our professor was a strict disciplinarian and would not even tolerate anyone chewing gum in his class. The last assignment of the year was an essay in which we were asked to predict what would happen to rural agriculture, if we assumed that rubber-tired tractors would replace horses. In 1930 very few tractors had rubber tires. Most had heavy steel wheels. They were very uncomfortable to ride and could not go very fast. Around this time, trucks were also coming into more general use. With horses one could haul grain up to three miles. With trucks one could travel many more miles with the same load. Thus, in my essay, I predicted the demise of the small hamlets, each with its grain elevator, dotting the western prairie, and an increase in the size of the typical farm. My argument was based on the assumption that with increased mobility it would no longer be necessary for farmers to remain close to their land; with rubber-tired tractors they would be able to travel many miles to and from work. By contrast, with horses one had to be within a mile of the farm, and with steel-wheeled tractors perhaps within two or three miles. The professor gave me the highest mark in the class, 81 out of 100, and apparently he had never given anyone else a higher mark. I was delighted, of course. I believe his response increased my confidence that, provided the assumptions were correct, one might be able to reasonably assess the future. This growth in my sense of confidence would prove very helpful to me when years later I began to work on the adrenochrome hypothesis of schizophrenia (to be discussed in detail as this book proceeds).

I found my third and fourth years at the University much more interesting than the first two. By this time our classes had become very small and we got to know our professors very well. Roger

Manning gave us our biochemistry lectures. While methodical, he also livened up his lectures by telling us stories about his graduate years at the University of Toronto. He had been a classmate of Dr. Best in the graduate school. He told us that when Charles Banting had needed an assistant for his work on diabetes in dogs, volunteers were called for. No one volunteered, so the head of the department designated Best to be that assistant. According to Manning, Best took the post very reluctantly. Thus was one of Canada's Nobel Prize winners launched on his path to scientific acclaim. (Banting and Best discovered insulin and its ability to control Type I diabetes, a previously fatal disease.)

Manning also spoke to us about adrenochrome, the red coloured oxidized derivative of adrenaline. He had done some research investigating it. Manning was also responsible, indirectly, for resurrecting the term vitamin B-3 for niacin and niacinamide. Many years later, Bill Wilson, co-founder of Alcoholics Anonymous, was searching for a better term to use than "niacin" when talking about this vitamin, and decided to use vitamin B-3 after I told him about Roger Manning's lectures. The usual trend in naming vitamins was to drop the letters and use the chemical name of the vitamin instead. With B-3 this trend was reversed, and today even the most conservative chemical texts use the term. Thus I trace the origins of my later investigation into adrenochrome's possible role in causing schizophrenia and my interest in the medical use of vitamin B-3 to their earliest exact roots, the lectures in Biochemistry One, attended in my third year of agricultural chemistry studies in 1937 at the University of Saskatchewan.

Medical students also had to take this course. We chemists looked upon them with some disdain because they were so slow to grasp any of the principles of biochemistry. I understood why they were not interested after I began to work as a physician in 1950. They could see no direct relevance between chemistry and what they expected to be doing as doctors later on. If Dr. Manning had been a medical doctor and had been able to talk to them about the way nutrition was useful in treating patients, they might have been much more interested. I believe we need to turn nutritional biochemistry into a popular subject amongst prospective doctors, taught by clinical nutritionists and doctors able to make these classes relevant.

During my fourth year I became a demonstrator in chemistry. This meant that I wandered about the laboratories where junior students were doing their laboratory work, assisted when asked and generally made myself useful. This job paid $40 per month, marking my first move upward on the economic scale and proving to me that education was useful. Academically I did very well throughout my first four years of study, earning almost all As, and I fully expected to be awarded Great Distinction when I received my degree. After I wrote the last exam, I returned home and eagerly awaited the publication of the results. I could not afford to stay in Saskatoon for graduation because I was needed at home to work on the farm. When the letter from the registrar finally arrived I was horrified to find that I had been given only Distinction. I calculated and recalculated my grades, and every time the results indicated that my point average was sufficient for a *Great* Distinction. I concluded that a simple error had been made, and would be corrected when I contacted the University again. The following fall, I arranged an interview with the Dean of Agriculture. I showed him my calculations and found to my surprise that he was very annoyed by what I was able to prove to him. Yet he had to agree with me, and my degree was amended to show that I had received Great Distinction after all. I have never been paranoid, except for two weeks when I took adrenochrome (an event also to be discussed later), nor have I ever been sensitive to anti-semitism, but his odd reaction made me wonder if the error had come more easily to him because I was the only Jewish student in that graduating class. As the dean of a major college he knew full well how important such matters were to students whose entire future depended largely upon the grades they earned.

Now that I had my BSA with Great Distinction, I was able to fully focus my attention on the next phase of my studies, a Master's degree in Agricultural Biochemistry, which I worked on between 1938 and 1940. I took the few compulsory courses and was given a position as a teaching assistant. The problem I was assigned as the subject of my Master's thesis was a disease of wheat popularly called root rot. Root rot is caused by a fungus which attacks the roots of seedling wheat plants, and it appeared to occur at random. Many parts of an affected crop remained healthy. But because the rootlets of the affected wheat were killed by the fungus, the field's overall yield would be reduced. One of my supervisors was Professor T.C. Vanterpool, in the department of biology, who had been investigating this problem for many years and was the recognized expert. He demonstrated to me more than once that he could spot infected plants at a distance if the light was just right. I concluded that it might be possible to find something unique in the soil around affected plants that made them more vulnerable; I thought that perhaps a vitamin was missing. My hypothesis was that if a nutritional factor was missing, the fungus (*Pythium arrhenomanes*) would leave behind peaceful co-existence with the wheat and become a parasite in its search for the vitamin, which would be present in the rootlets of the wheat plants.

My research was also directed by Professor T.T. Thorvaldson, Head of Chemistry and the Professor of Bacteriology, V. Graham, whose participation was considered important since he was also an expert in the study of fungi. Thus I had three supervisors.

My research plan called for me to make extracts of soil samples and determine if these extracts had an effect on the fungus, which I cultured in two laboratories. I worked on this problem for nearly two years and eventually wrote my Master's thesis on it. I did not make any great contribution, but I did learn a little about research methodology and I also began to learn how to write, a skill I have tried to improve on ever since. In the course of my research, I also spent many hours in the library reading the latest articles in the chemical and biological journals. My reading eventually convinced me that the probable reason the fungus attacked the wheat plants was that it found itself in soil not containing enough thiamin (vitamin B-1). But the results in my lab provided no clear proof for this conviction. I have never followed this matter up and do not know what has happened to my favourite fungus, *Pythium arrhenomanes,* since.

I was awarded my Master's Degree in 1940 and won a graduate scholarship worth $800 a year for two years. Only one of these was given each year and the money permitted the winner to study toward their PhD at any US university. The scholarship was very valuable to me, as no Canadian university provided the specialized education I wanted. However, in this particular year the university split the scholarship and gave it to two students, myself and Eric Putt. After obtaining his PhD, Dr. Putt worked at the Swift Current Experimental Farm until he retired several years ago. Being forced to share the scholarship meant I was given only enough money for one year, which was disappointing, but did not deter me from starting my doctoral studies in chemistry at the University of Minnesota in the autumn of 1941.

The year went by quickly and I passed with an A average. Then it was back to the farm again for the summer's work, and since I had no more money, a decision with respect to my future became difficult. World War II was still in progress. I had been trained in the Canadian Officers Training Course, compulsory for all students, but I did not want to volunteer. Farmers were exempt from going to war because the Allies desperately needed the food they produced, but I did not want to stay on the farm either. During this time I received a note from A.W. Alcock, Chief Chemist at Purity Flour Mills in Winnipeg, the capital city of the more easterly prairie province of Manitoba. He needed a chemist to set up a laboratory that would measure thiamin (vitamin B-1) levels in grain products. He offered me $125 a month. Dr. Geddes, Chairman of the Chemistry Department at the University of Minnesota, had recommended me to him without my knowledge. I later learned that Geddes and Alcock were close friends. I was delighted to receive this offer.

II

PURITY FLOUR MILLS, WINNIPEG, 1941 TO 1945

My two younger sisters, Lilly and Fannie, moved to Winnipeg at the same time I did. We three rented a two-bedroom apartment in the city's downtown. Lilly took courses in art and Fannie obtained a job with the *Winnipeg Free Press* as a reporter. The flour mill where I would work, then called Purity Flour Mills, was in St. Boniface, across the Red River from Winnipeg. My laboratory was a small room. The work benches were new and had not yet been varnished dark black, as most laboratory furniture was then. My first job was to obtain the glassware and other equipment that would be needed and to rub onto the benches the chemicals that would make them black, shiny, and resistant to chemical spills. I also soon settled into family life in Winnipeg.

As mentioned earlier, I had met Rose Miller in 1936. We had maintained our relationship mostly by mail after I had completed my Master's degree and left Saskatoon, and in 1940, we decided to marry. In 1941 I suggested that we marry in Winnipeg. Neither Rose nor I wanted a formal wedding and we decided that by marrying quietly in Winnipeg, both our families (mine in Hoffer, hers in Saskatoon), would be treated equally and we could avoid the fuss, cost, and bother of a regular wedding. So, in February, 1942, Rose came to Winnipeg. We contacted the chief rabbi of the city and had our wedding at his home. Rose and I then moved into new quarters.

Our first child, Bill, was born in 1944. While Rose attended to our home and children, as was customary at that time, my work brought me into greater and greater familiarity with the vitamins that would one day be so important in my medical practice.

The Canadian government had decided to enrich all flour shipped to Canadian and British armed forces based in England. Prior to this, the US government had become concerned over the poor state of health of their new army recruits. They were advised by a small group of nutritionists that they should add various vitamins to the white flour to prevent the usual deficiency diseases, such as pellagra. The Americans had recently had to deal with widespread pellagra in the southeast and were sensitive to the need for improvement in their soldiers' diets.

They introduced an enrichment program. This meant that millers were obligated to add thiamin (vitamin B-1), riboflavin (vitamin B-2), niacinamide (vitamin B-3), and iron to white flour. A smaller group of nutritionists in Canada had recommended against implementing this program in the country. They reasoned that it was illogical to remove these and other nutrients from the wheat by milling, to use only the white centre of the wheat (the endosperm) to make bread, and then to replace only a few of the many vitamins and nutrients lost in the process. But Canadian millers were convinced that whole wheat products would not sell. They took the position that if Canada wanted to improve the quality of its white flour products, the country should follow the American plan. But in Canada, adding any number of substances to white flour was considered adulteration. Oddly, vitamins were classified as adulterants, but not chemicals such as potassium bromate and the gases used to bleach and improve the baking qualities of the product. At the same time, the Canadian army wanted the enriched flour. The Department of Indian Affairs also wanted it, so that Canada's native peoples could bake with it their wheat bannock, a staple food since contact with Europeans. As a result, the anomalous situation developed that only servicemen based overseas and native Canadians were permitted to buy and use enriched flour. When the decision to ship enriched flour overseas was made, it became necessary to establish standards for the product. Thus Purity Mills found themselves requiring a laboratory for measuring the amounts of vitamin that had been added. Thanks to this development, they hired me. The method then in use for measuring the amount of thiamin in flour products involved the addition of enzymes to the flour, which released the bonds between thiamin and wheat protein. This method revealed the levels of both naturally occurring and added thiamin in the flour, but it took eight hours to complete one test. I was able to run only four samples each day, two duplicates of each one. Its slowness made the test almost valueless.

The flour mill could make 20,000 100-pound sacks of flour each day. But only a small fraction of the workers' time was used to produce enriched flour, which was made by adding a vitamin mixture to the mill streams. If too much or too little of this vitamin mixture was added it would take over eight hours to determine that this had happened. If the values came in and were way out of line, every sack would have to be opened and the flour reworked. What we needed was a technique that could sample the stream of flour and let the millers know as soon as possible that they were adding too little or too much.

It occurred to me that to measure the amount of thiamin added to the flour did not actually require the use of enzymes since the synthetic vitamins were already free. A simple extraction procedure would do. The new procedure would not measure naturally occurring thiamin, but this was not of great importance, since so little of it remained in the milled flour. I tested my idea by mixing some flour with a strong potassium chloride solution, removing the resulting liquid and then analyzing it for its thiamin content. (Other vitamins in addition to thiamin were added, but it was not necessary to measure them all. If too little of one was added it meant that there would be too little of all of them.) I checked my results against those I obtained via the old laborious method and the correlation was good. I therefore began to use the new method. It required only one hour to complete one test and I could run up to 60 samples per day with little effort. It thus became possible to sample the mill stream regularly. Using the old method, I had been completely occupied every day. Using the new method, I had only enough work to fill about two days of a five-day week.

I soon realized that I now had so much free time that it might be possible to do my doctoral research and obtain my PhD where I was without compromising the work I had to do for the flour mill. I discussed this with my supervisor, Mr. Alcock, who talked to Dr. Geddes at the University of Minnesota. Dr. Alcock then informed me that the University would accept a dissertation based upon research carried on in my laboratory at Purity Mills under Mr. Alcock's supervision. Mr. Alcock generously offered to buy any extra equipment that I would need.

Since the laboratory was equipped only to do thiamin assays, I decided to investigate the distribution of thiamin in the various components of the wheat kernel. This had not been done before. It meant analyzing numerous samples of bran, of other layers of the wheat kernel that lie close to the bran, and of various grades of flour. Until then I had been very bored at work because there was nothing I could do when I was not analyzing flour for the mill. But as it turned out, the new rapid-assay method for detecting thiamin that I had developed made my PhD possible. I worked under the supervision of Dr. Geddes and Mr. Alcock to prepare my thesis. Finally I had to pass my oral PhD examination—the final hurdle to obtaining the degree.

The examination would be conducted by Dr. Geddes and other scientists, including one from another university; he would chair. Geddes sent me an outline of the work I should be familiar with. I studied and prepared for the final day, then went to Minneapolis by overnight train from Winnipeg. The first round of questions had to do with my general knowledge of the field of cereal chemistry. The second round considered details of the thesis that the examining committee thought I should change or enlarge. I stumbled through my answers until the professor from another university asked me to define oxidation. This is a very simple question for a chemist to answer. But the questioner, a biologist, was not familiar with the chemical definition. Like many people, he thought the word refers to an addition of oxygen to a substance. Chemists, however, define oxidation as a loss of electrons to oxygen. For example when a cut apple turns brown (oxidizes), what is happening is that the sugars in the apple are losing electrons to oxygen. This process creates a new compound that is a combination of what was previously sugar and oxygen. In the process, the apple also slowly turns brown. But when I gave my examiner this answer, he told me it was wrong. I argued with him and he insisted that oxidation meant only the addition of oxygen to a substance. Finally the other examiners broke in and pointed out to him that he was in the wrong. In the view of those trained in biochemistry, such as myself, this scientist had made a serious error. Many years later, several of my associates, including Linus Pauling, were involved in a confrontational meeting with some psychiatrists from the National Institute for Mental Health in Washington. Dr. Morris Lipton, PhD, MD and chairman of the committee which produced the dismissive American Psychiatric Association report on megavitamins was present. During the heated discussion he made the same error and was promptly chastised by Pauling for his lack of knowledge of chemistry. Lipton had a PhD from the University of Wisconsin and he should have known better.

The examiner who had just embarrassed himself then asked me about Professor Elvehjem, then working at the University of Iowa, who had shown that niacin was vitamin B-3. As the vitamins were isolated, and before their chemical structure was known, they were given capital letters, eg. A, and if related, numbers as well, eg. B-1 and B-2. The anti-pellagra vitamin was the third water-soluble vitamin in the B series to be identified, and so was called B-3. The term applies to both common forms, niacin and niacinamide. I was very familiar with Elvehjem's work and described it with precision. Then he asked me what I thought of the Professor and I replied that he had done excellent and important work. To my surprise, my questioner disagreed with me. Later I found that this scientist and Elvehjem did not get on with each other. The other examiners then asked more along the usual line of questions. Dr. Geddes finally took his turn and the examination was over. I was sent out of the room to await the outcome of the exercise. About an hour later Dr. Geddes came to me and said, "Congratulations, Dr. Hoffer!" That was the usual greeting for a PhD candidate who had passed the examination. Nonetheless, the committee recommended that I make a few changes in my manuscript, which I was happy to do. I rewrote the thesis and in due course was awarded my PhD. My work had established that the concentration of vitamins in the kernel is lowest in the center (the endosperm, from which white flour is made) and richest in the outer layers of the wheat kernel, in the bran and wheat germ. My study was not important but it did sensitize me to the importance of knowing where the vitamins are. In 1942 most Canadians ate white bread. The wheat was ground, passed through fine silk sieves and the pure white flour sold for bread and pastry making. The bran and germ were fed to livestock. This year (2005) in a book Professor Harry Foster and I are writing, we discuss the implications of the discovery of silk sieves in about 1800; with the introduction of very pure white flour, an enormous decrease in the amount of vitamins consumed by the public ensued. In our book we present the argument that this is one of the factors which has led to the major increase in the incidence of psychosis which we are witnessing now.

I completed two other studies while working for Purity Flour Mills. The same equipment I had used to measure thiamin in wheat kernels could be used to determine the amount of riboflavin (vitamin B-2) in plant products. I undertook a joint study with Dr. Geddes in which we examined a large number of different fractions of seedlings that he had collected. The idea was to determine what happened to vitamins during the growth of these plants from germination to the seedling phase. I agreed to do one of the riboflavin studies, and the appropriate samples were sent to me for analysis.[1] In the second study I examined why oatmeal went rancid so quickly. I concluded that the problem was due to rapid oxidation sparked by

---

1. This work led to the publication: Hoffer, A., Levine, M.N. & Geddes, W.F.: Effect of leaf and stem rust on the content and distribution of riboflavin in hard red spring wheats at successive stages of kernel development. *Cereal Chemistry*, 32, 347-355, 1955.

enzymatic activity in the ground grain. My equipment was very crude and I am still not certain that I drew the right conclusion. Nevertheless, based upon this work, millers began heating oatmeal to a higher temperature during its preparation and this seems to have solved the problem.

My work with Dr. Geddes also introduced me to vitamin C. In preparation for the riboflavin research, I obtained all the information I could about all the vitamins. Merck and Co., then the main manufacturers of vitamins, had prepared a series of excellent brochures describing the then-known vitamins and listing the relevant literature references. I became intrigued with vitamin C's antioxidant capabilities. The idea of antioxidants appears new and exciting to some people today in medicine, but it was old stuff to chemists even fifty years ago. I purchased some vitamin C in bulk and used it in the laboratory. I also began to take it myself, I believe at the dose of one gram each day. After some time, I realized that I was not getting as many colds as I used to. I became so convinced that the vitamin C was helping me resist infection that I sent a letter to *Science* magazine describing my idea in some detail. It was rejected and I did not keep a copy. I look back now and think that if I had pursued my observations more tenaciously, I might have pushed forward the use of this vitamin by several decades.

III

MEDICAL SCHOOL, SASKATOON AND TORONTO, 1945 TO 1949

After I was awarded my PhD in Agricultural Biochemistry, I found my job at Purity Flour Mills boring. I realized I really enjoyed planning and doing research and had developed a powerful interest in nutritional research. Rose suggested that I become a medical doctor. We discussed this possibility at length and eventually concluded that this course of action would be feasible because of financial support offered by her father, Frank Miller. I could not expect any help from my father, as he was just barely beginning to recover financially from the Depression. I planned on working on the farm in the summers to earn further money that way.

I resigned from the flour mill in 1945. I was content that I had made the right decision, but sorry to leave the company. I remain grateful to Purity Mills and to Chauncey Alcock, the chief chemist, for being so helpful and gracious and for allowing me, indeed encouraging me, to obtain my PhD and pursue further research with the help of their laboratory. We came to Saskatoon early in the summer of 1945, Rose, our first child Bill, and I, and soon settled with Rose's parents. Here I would begin my medical studies at my *alma mater*, the University of Saskatchewan.

I did not enjoy being a medical student. It was very hard work and took every free moment. Also, I had to adjust to a huge philo-sophical gap between the education I had received toward my PhD and my medical education. In my PhD program I had had to learn a large number of facts, principles, and hypotheses, from which it was possible to deduce other ideas that could be confirmed or disproven through research. My learning had been heavy on reasoning and relatively light on memorizing. In sharp contrast, the medical curriculum placed its major emphasis on memorization, and very little attention was paid to teaching us how to reason out medical problems. We had to master a huge volume of facts, for example, the course that would be taken by an artery down the leg. There was no reason given why that artery would be near a nerve or another vessel on one side of the body and not on the other. To help me retain everything, I developed a pattern of going over the material as frequently as possible, depending mostly on the textbooks and using the lectures as a guide.

I survived my first year with a reasonably good record, mostly As, a few Bs. The summer was much more interesting. I was offered a summer job working in the cereal chemistry department on some baking research funded by a grant from the National Research Council of Canada. The problem posed was why wheat flour was the only flour that could make a good looking, upstanding loaf of bread, compared to the results obtained when oat, rye, or barley flour were used. The other flours could be baked, but the loaves were more like heavy cake when the product came out of the oven. Only wheat flour had enough tenacity to retain the bubbles of gas, formed by fermentation with yeast, long enough during the baking process that they would be set by the heat. What was unique about wheat flour?

By the end of the summer I had developed a hypothesis to account for its unusual properties. During the mixing and kneading of the dough, protein was pulled out from its protein-containing globules normally present, into long fibrous chains. These chains interacted with each other to form sheets of tough planar protein. The gas formed by the fermentation with yeast would be released into little pockets within these sheets and would gradually distend these pockets to form gas cells. Baking rigidified these gas cells and so the final loaf would maintain its risen state. The baking quality of flour thus depended upon the ability of its proteins to change from a globular to a fibrous state and to remain firmly anchored in that fibrous state. Barley flour did not contain the right type of protein nor did oat, rice, or corn flour. Further, the fibrous protein molecules had to become anchored to each other. This process was facilitated in wheat by naturally occurring oxidizing molecules that cross-linked the protein molecules, much as sulfur does when it is added to latex to produce rubber. If there were too few of these anchoring molecules, the flour was green, i.e. it would not rise enough; if there were too many, the flour would be too tough and would not rise. There had to be just the correct amount. The right levels of oxidizing molecules used to be achieved by allowing the flour to rest for several months. But this practice exposed the flour to possible pest infestation or deterioration.

Over the course of this summer's work, I collected enough data to allow me to write four reports which I hoped would be published in cereal chemistry journals. In these papers, completed during my second year of medical school, I presented my hypothesis, planning to leave it to the world of cereal chemistry to support or rebut my findings. The first three described my literature search, the methods I used, and the data I had collected; the fourth paper outlined my hypothesis regarding the role oxidant molecules played in producing desirable loaves of bread. I submitted the papers to Dr. W.F. Geddes, the man who had supervised my PhD research and who remained a friend. He was then editor of the journal *Cereal Chemistry*. Dr. Geddes accepted them for publication. A few weeks later, Dr. Geddes wrote to tell me that it had occurred to him that since my summer's research had been paid for by the National Research Council of Canada, I should, as a courtesy to this body, show my papers to one of its members. With their approval I could give credit to the Council for having supported the research when it was published. He thought this step would be a formality only. I thought so too and agreed. I sent the manuscripts to a Dr. A. Anderson who was working in Winnipeg for the Wheat Board as head of their research and control laboratory and was a member of the Council. I had met

Dr. Anderson while I was working at Purity Flour Mills in Winnipeg. I was not close to him, but I was friendly with some of his staff. From what they had told me, I had felt glad not to be in any close connection with him. He was apparently obsessive about minute details. For example, if his secretary misplaced one comma in a page of manuscript he would make her type out the whole page again without allowing her to correct the minor error. However, as Dr. Geddes had already accepted my papers, I did not foresee any difficulty with Dr. Anderson. I was delighted to imagine I would have this work behind me and could get on with my studies in medicine without distraction.

But to my amazement, all my papers came back from Dr. Anderson with a large number of suggestions for change. He had assumed it was his job not just to approve their publication but to edit them. Since I had already spent so much time on them and was now heavily involved in my medical studies, I was most reluctant to rewrite these papers—but I did so anyway, after I had overcome my anger. Most of the changes involved matters of style, which in my opinion were none of his business. He was to give his opinion about the quality of the research and the conclusions drawn from it. I sent them all back once more to Dr. Anderson after having rewritten them. Three months later they returned and this time he had made an entire new set of recommendations for changes. I proceeded to make these changes also. But the papers came back a third time with yet another set of recommendations. I now realized that if I had to depend upon Dr. Anderson's opinion they would never be published. If I had been a Professor of Cereal Chemistry at that time, there is no doubt that these papers would have been published as they had originally been written. But clearly, I was unable to continue this game. I wrote to Dr. Anderson and gave him my opinion of his behaviour, then withdrew the papers from Dr. Geddes. I then sent the manuscripts to the University of Saskatchewan for their Graduate Library. Many years later they were referred to by a Professor of Cereal Chemistry, but I do not recall in what sense. Looking at this episode now, I realize I was naïve. I could have appealed to the National Research Council as a whole. I could also have asked that Dr. Geddes publish them without the Council's blessing, as he had already accepted them. But these options never occurred to me.

For a long time I was puzzled by Dr. Anderson's behaviour. Then I wondered if he had wanted to kill my hypothesis so that he could later on use the same ideas. This is a too-common tactic in science. And he knew that in my new profession, as a doctor, I would be in no position to follow the cereal chemistry literature and would not know what he might publish later on. Later I learned that, in fact, he did eventually publish material based on my ideas. For many years now I have been editor of a journal, now called the *Journal of Ortho-molecular Medicine*. It has been my firm policy never to impose my style or my ideas on any of the manuscripts I receive. I consider papers to be either good enough to be published (though they usually require minor changes to clarify certain items) or too weak for acceptance. After my experience with Dr. Anderson, I would not have it any other way.

Second year medicine was similar to the first year. We attended our first clinics at the bedsides of patients in Saskatoon's two small hospitals, City Hospital and St. Paul's Hospital. Halfway through this year we all had to decide to which medical school we wanted to go to complete our medical training, since the University of Saskatchewan offered only the first two years. By agreement with four other Canadian schools, our 24 students were absorbed into third year classes and so could complete our studies.

A month or so later, I was called to the dean's office. The University of Toronto had rejected me, they said, because I was a resident of Manitoba, which did have a medical school. The dean had failed to change my address from Winnipeg to Saskatoon, my actual official place of residence. Later, I discovered that Toronto had wanted to reject me for other reasons—mainly because I had a PhD and therefore was believed to want to do research. The Toronto school felt it their function to train doctors to go into practice, not to do research. They also considered me to be too old—I was 30. But they did not want to use either of these reasons officially, and when they were informed (incorrectly) that I was a Manitoba resident, they felt fully justified in turning me down. The dean happily wrote them that he had made an error and that I was really a Saskatchewan resident. So I was finally accepted.

The two preclinical years in Saskatoon had given me a solid grounding in what were then considered the basics in medicine: anatomy, histology, physiology. But much more helpful to my future research would be the relationships I established while there with some of the medical faculty, including Professor of Physiology L. Jaques and Professor of Anatomy R. Altshul. As a biochemist, I also enjoyed a close relationship with the Department of Biochemistry.

The last two years in medicine were difficult for me and my family. I went to Toronto in the fall, came home for the Christmas holidays and returned to Toronto again until spring. Rose stayed in Saskatoon with our growing family.

I found it difficult to become involved in my studies and always felt somewhat out of place. I found the work and the classes dull. I can still recall with something close to horror the many hours when it was almost impossible for me to stay awake during the lectures, especially the ones just before lunch. It occurred to me many years later that there might have been another factor responsible: hypoglycemia.

Perhaps the lectures were not as boring as I thought and the reason I could not stay awake was that my blood sugar was dropping too low due to my poor diet. I developed a pattern of dealing with my lectures which allowed me to survive medicine. I simply missed most of those classes where I could reasonably do so and attended only those where attendance was actually taken. I also made sure to attend enough lectures in each subject to allow me to understand the continuity of the course. After classes I would read the textbooks to cover the lectures I had missed. Since I was alone, with no family members present to distract me, I was able to spend a lot of time studying.

The dullest and most boring course, in my opinion, was psychiatry. We were given instruction by Dr. J. Dewan, a former PhD in biochemistry who, after a distinguished career in that field, went into psychiatry. In his first lecture he patiently outlined the material we would cover in his classes. In the second lecture, he spent the first ten to fifteen minutes reviewing what he had given us in the first hour. This pattern went on lecture after lecture. His approach was so uninspiring and boring that my friends and I would often discuss why he acted as he did as we walked home. We eventually concluded that he made his lectures *intentionally* intolerably boring in order to discourage us from going into psychiatry! We decided that it could not be possible that he himself did not realize how consistently dull his course was.

I cannot remember any of the content of my initial psychiatry studies, but I do remember one clinic vividly. A man and wife came to the outpatient department. The husband complained bitterly about his wife's behaviour until I was convinced that she must be mentally ill. But after talking to her and learning about her husband's hallucinations it became clear that he was schizophrenic and she was normal. I have never forgotten this experience and later, when I actually became a psychiatrist (a development I would not have predicted in medical school!), the incident served to remind me to talk to as many members of the family as possible in difficult cases before accepting the facts as related by the patient. My learning in this instance was reinforced by my memories of a similar episode I had witnessed many years earlier, when I was very young. My father was then Justice of the Peace for our district in Saskatchewan. That meant that if the RCMP suspected a person of being mentally ill and wanted to take them to a mental hospital, they had to bring the individual to our house for a hearing. If Dad was convinced of the person's illness, he would issue a committal paper. These hearings were held in our kitchen. We children were not allowed to be present but we often would peek in through the door of our living room. Our parents surely were aware we were there but did not drive us away. On this particular day, the RCMP officer brought in two men, farmers. One was dressed neatly, in suit and tie. He was quiet and well behaved. The other was a gruffer individual dressed in ordinary pants and shirt, and no tie. We immediately assumed that the man in the suit was normal and the man without the tie was ill. To our surprise, it was the man in the suit who had developed the delusion that he was the Prince of Wales. He was committed to the mental hospital in Weyburn, Saskatchewan. I doubt he was ever released, for in those days an admission to a mental hospital was a life sentence. The doctors had no effective drugs and megavitamin treatments would be discovered only several decades into the future.

I successfully completed my courses and examinations in the spring of 1949. We had to write two sets of examinations, one for the University of Toronto and one for the Canadian Medical Council. The latter exams qualified new doctors to practise anywhere in Canada. I returned to Saskatoon and had a few weeks to rest before starting my internship at City Hospital in Saskatoon. Miriam had been born on May 15, a few days before I returned home, joining her two older brothers, Bill and John.

IV

CITY HOSPITAL INTERNSHIP, SASKATOON, 1949 TO 1950

On July 1, 1949, I went on duty for the first time as an intern at City Hospital, Saskatoon, along with four other interns. We began our day at 8 am and worked until 5 pm unless we were on 24-hour duty, which occurred every five days. While on duty, we were responsible for the entire hospital—the emergency service, the isolation wards, all the medical and surgical wards, and the obstetrical wards. We had a little room with a cot and a telephone just outside the door where we would try and get some sleep on our 24-hour shifts. Almost every problem was referred to us, unless the nurse on duty called the patient's doctor. This did not happen frequently. Often, when the doctor was called, he would ask the intern to handle the problem anyway.

I was much more interested in medicine as an intern than I had been as a student, although I still found it difficult to become very interested in any particular disease unless I had a patient with that condition. Then I would read as much as I could about it and was able to remember the information fairly easily. I had no natural aptitude for nor interest in surgery and quickly determined that I would never become a surgeon.

We were rotated through various wards about every three months. As soon as I went onto a new ward I would make the rounds, get to know each patient, and review each one's chart. Their orders were written by their own doctors, but in an emergency we were expected to write the correct orders as required. In most cases the physicians did not want to come back to the hospital after hours, unless it was a dire emergency. We were expected to cover for them. I depended heavily on the knowledge and skill of the head nurses on each ward. I learned much from them and I am still grateful to the nurses who were so helpful to me during my training.

On one occasion I was called to see a diabetic who had fallen into a coma. Glucose is the main source of energy for the brain and it must have a continuous supply. When the blood glucose levels drop too far, brain function slows and may stop, and the person will become unconscious or fall into a coma. We could not locate this patient's own doctor (always the first thing we tried to do). It was clear he had taken too much insulin and as a result his blood sugar had plummeted. We called this condition insulin shock. Our patient needed intravenous glucose immediately. I began to inject him. After a few seconds I could see that he was beginning to respond and I continued. Suddenly, without warning, and with a crafty look on his face, he hit me with his free arm. I continued the injection and a few minutes later he was back to normal—and had no recollection at all of having hit me. This was one of the first clear demonstrations to me of the importance of blood sugar in determining the ability to reason. He had been paranoid simply because the sugar in his brain had not yet returned to its normal level.

Another case was equally interesting and renewed my acquaintance with adrenaline, a substance that would play a central role in my later schizophrenia research: one evening a young woman came to the emergency complaining of severe abdominal pain. A physical examination gave no clues. I had recently read that an injection of a tiny dose of adrenaline had helped similar cases. I therefore gave her an intramuscular injection. Within a few minutes she was free of pain. Was this a placebo reaction, which I had read about by that time, or had she had a type of severe allergic reaction which the adrenaline relieved, much as it relieves acute allergic shock reactions (anaphylaxis)?

Overall, I had little opportunity in the City Hospital setting to conduct research. However, when a new antibiotic, aureomycin, became available in an ointment form, I decided to test it on a few children with chickenpox. I wondered whether the antibiotic could protect against residual scarring. I applied the ointment on half the face and body of a few children, leaving the other half as a control. When they were well there were no residual scars on the treated side and a few on the untreated side. I wondered then—and still do—whether the pocks left behind by chickenpox (usually very few) and the pocks from small pox are due to an infection of the erupted vesicles by bacteria responsive to antibiotics.

As interns we were very critical of some of the doctors. A few were above average in diagnostic and treatment skills. A few we considered to be surgical butchers. One had such a bad reputation for removing healthy organs, such as gall bladders, uteruses, etc. that whenever we saw that he had booked an operation, we guessed that he was short of money or had planned a holiday trip. This surgeon prided himself on the speed with which he could complete an operation. Of course, it is much easier to be fast if there is no underlying pathology. He also had a reputation for not operating on patients who really needed surgery, that is, where serious pathology was present. Fortunately today's interns will not see this kind of surgery or medicine practised.

The best examples of surgical incompetence were provided by a well-respected general surgeon who became a brain surgeon after a few months' training at a neurological institute. Among other operations, he performed lobotomies on schizophrenic patients brought from the nearest mental hospital. These patients were then returned to their home or the hospital. The soap with which he should have scrubbed before an operation irritated him. He would therefore wear fairly thick gloves instead of washing; over these he would place his surgical gloves. Since he had thick fingers this arrangement greatly decreased his sensitivity to touch and made him more awkward in surgery. These facts did not inhibit him in any way, but could explain why one-third of his patients developed infections after their operation. He also did not always depend upon the original psychiatric diagnosis before doing his surgeries. One young man with catatonic schizophrenia was referred to this doctor by his family and was booked for a lobotomy. During my examination of his mental state he told me about his bizarre delusional thought system. I did not think he should have a lobotomy. After discussing the case, my colleagues and I decided to talk to this doctor about our views. I told him that this patient had had intercourse with an animal. This was true. Bestiality does occur rarely. The doctor was horrified and promptly cancelled the operation.

One positive memory I have of this doctor is that he had a curious interest in vitamins; I call it curious in that he was the only one in the whole hospital with this interest. His favorite treatment for multiple sclerosis was to administer large amounts of vitamins, especially thiamin, using every possible route: oral, parenteral, and intrathecal. An injection directly into the fluid surrounding the spinal cord in the spinal canal is called an intrathecal injection. All other injectable treatments are called parenteral. He had so many MS patients on the ward that I became an expert in doing intrathecal injections of vitamin B-1. At that time I did not agree with the doctor about the use of thiamin for MS and I do not recall that any of these patients got any better. Now, in hindsight, I see he was far ahead of the rest of us in this area. He was following up on the report of a Canadian physician who had found this vitamin useful. He was not aware of the work of Fred Klenner from Reidsville, North Carolina, who had restored a large number of MS patients to good health using nutrients. I know some of them. I have since treated over 60 patients using Klenner's program with good success.

When I first began to work in his ward I became familiar with all the patients. Many of them were on a wide variety of vitamin preparations. I saw no good reason why one vitamin should be given by so many different routes. I therefore went through the orders and cancelled the ones that I thought redundant. The patients still got the vitamins he had ordered, but in more rational form. Within a week he had gradually built up the entire program again. However, we got along well in spite of these differences. Many years later his son became mentally ill and came under my care.

I think I infected my intern colleagues with my love of research. That year a book appeared called *Natural Childbirth* by Dr. Dick Grantly Reed. We read it with great interest because it promised so much relief to patients in labor and during childbirth. Dr. Harvey Gurion and I decided to try out Dr. Reed's technique when an opportunity arose. The book maintained that women in labor need not suffer undue pain if they are treated with kindness and patience and if they are informed of the progress they are making while giving birth. One afternoon I was called to the delivery room. The woman was going to give birth and her doctor could not be located. I asked Harvey to come with me and we decided to deliver her ourselves before he got there. This in itself was a breach of etiquette, since the patient's doctor wanted to be there and it was our job to slow down the delivery to give him more time. I decided to become the anesthetist and Harvey decided to be the gynecologist. I immediately began to talk gently to the patient explaining what was going on and asking her to relax. Within a few minutes she was free of pain and the child's head began to show. Everything was going along very smoothly when suddenly the doctor breezed in and began to scrub for the delivery. As he entered he remarked to the woman casually, "How are the pains?" She replied, "Doctor, I do not have any pain." He promptly retorted, "Nonsense, of course you have pain!" Suddenly her pains returned and the progress of the delivery stopped. He ordered me to start the anesthetic which then consisted of an ether drip over a gauze mask. I had to take her down to third stage anesthesia and he had to use forceps to extract the baby. Before my eyes, a simple delivery, going very well, with little pain, was converted into a complicated operation requiring anesthetics and surgical delivery (forceps). Had this doctor arrived five minutes later, the baby would have been born with no damage to mother or child. Here I was given a most dramatic demonstration of the relationship between mind and body and of the need to have a proper understanding of the doctor-patient relationship. We interns were impressed with *Natural Childbirth* thereafter but did not have any further opportunity to try out the ideas it expressed. The doctor did not know the drama that had just been played out and we did not dare tell him. He assumed that we had merely been doing our job as interns, in waiting for him to arrive.

After a few months I had mastered the routine and was comfortable as an intern. I found myself increasingly interested in psychosomatic medicine, a new branch of medicine which seemed to me to show a lot of promise, especially after my experience with attempted natural childbirth. I also became aware that there were two types of patients admitted to our hospital. The first had acute surgical emergencies, such as acute appendicitis. They had to be diagnosed quickly and treated vigorously and rapidly if they were to be saved. The second were patients with chronic complaints which had not yielded to treatment in the past. I became much more interested in the second group because I could not understand why they came to hospital. These patients were sick with pain, nausea, and a number of symptoms for which no physical explanation could be found. Psychosomatic medicine was just beginning to be developed and as medical students we were not taught any. Fifty years ago patients had either entirely physical (organic) complaints, or their problems were psychological. There appeared to be nothing tying body and mind together. I became adept therefore, at taking two kinds of histories: a brief one for the first group, and a more thoughtful and thorough one for the second group.

In clear appendicitis cases, the chief complaint would generally be severe pain in the right lower quadrant of the abdomen. The history of the illness would show that this patient had developed pain in this area the previous night, that the region was tender to the touch, and that the pain had become more severe since its beginning. The final tentative diagnosis would be acute appendicitis. The surgeon, of course, would have known this all along and probably have already booked the operating room.

The people with chronic complaints would present a very long history of illness, with myriad symptoms. I would attempt to find out what other factors could be involved. I would spend a lot of time with the second type of patient and very little with the first. As I continued on this road, my interest in psychosomatic medicine increased. Eventually, I bought a book by English and Pearson, the first volume ever entitled *Psychosomatic Medicine,* and I read it carefully, over and over again, my past distaste for all things psychiatric forgotten.

Early in 1950, John Cumming, the hospital's senior intern, told me that a Dr. McKerracher was going to lecture to the Saskatchewan branch of the newly formed Canadian Mental Health Association (CMHA); John was going to this meeting. By then, he was also thinking about going into psychiatry. Dr. McKerracher had been instrumental in establishing the Saskatchewan chapter of the CMHA and was director of Psychiatric Services Branch in the Department of Public Health for the province of Saskatchewan. My going to that lecture marked a major change in my life. I found McKerracher's talk fascinating. During that presentation and the social hour afterward I finally gained a clear view of what I wanted to do. I was certain that I would never be a surgeon and dreaded the idea that I might have to go into general practice. I knew now that I wanted to combine my knowledge of chemistry, medicine, and psychiatry and start a career in psychiatric research. I spoke to Dr. McKerracher about my new-found inspiration. He listened with interest and asked me to send him a letter outlining my experience and ideas. This I did. He then invited me to Regina, Saskatchewan's capital city, the seat of the provincial government, to discuss the matter further.

I was attracted by the field of psychiatric research because it was wide open—hardly anything was known about useful treatments for mental illness. There were no tranquilizers; the first one was just being investigated in France. I recall that one report I read as an intern claimed that a combination of benadril, the first antihistamine discovered, and one gram of vitamin C daily had cured a few cases of schizophrenia. This news was very exciting. But when I tried the treatment later, I saw no response. Still, this report may have been one of the pieces of information I put to use when later on I decided to give schizophrenic patients *megadoses* of vitamin C—my minimum dose was 3 grams per day in three divided doses. I must credit this early paper for anticipating the most effective current therapy for schizophrenia, the use of nutrients in large doses. Further all modern tranquilizers are good antihistamines which do not cause as much sedation as the early ones did when they came onto the market.

V

The Munroe Wing, General Hospital, Regina, 1950 to 1955

In 1950, I passed my internship and was able to move on to my newly chosen career in psychiatry. In the spring of 1950 I went to Regina at Dr. McKerracher's invitation to continue my talks with him about my idea of starting a psychiatric research program. After our first meeting in Saskatoon following his lecture, he had discussed my proposal with the University of Toronto Department of Psychiatry and they had agreed that it would be a good idea to set up such an enterprise. During my visit he showed me around Regina's General Hospital and the Munroe Wing, the hospital's psychiatric ward. Soon after, he offered me a job. In point of fact, I was given three positions. I became a psychiatric resident as I needed to learn psychiatry. My residency at the Munroe Wing lasted four years. My second position was consultant in biochemistry to the Pathology Department of the General Hospital. My third was Director of Psychiatric Research. In this position my employer was the provincial government, specifically the Department of Public Health. These three jobs paid me my total salary of $15,000 per year, an enormous sum in those days, more than the premier of Saskatchewan made.

I and my family moved to Regina. Most of my time was spent pursuing my duties as a resident at the Munroe Wing. The director of the wing was responsible to Dr. McKerracher. Dr. McKerracher also led the training program for the residents. Every type of psychiatric patient was admitted to the 37 beds on our two floors. Some came voluntarily, others were committed on the basis of two certificates to be prepared by two physicians. On their first admission patients were assigned according to a rotational system to the next resident on the list, meaning patients had no choice of doctor and the residents had no choice about their patients. Patients who had to be readmitted usually went back to the same resident who had treated them previously, and patients and doctors alike found the system fair. The average stay was about one month. Patients with chronic illness, those likely to need long-term treatment, were quickly sent on to the Saskatchewan Hospital in Weyburn, 70 miles southeast of Regina. There they might have been kept forever, but under the new, more enlightened policies being introduced by Dr. McKerracher, they were discharged much earlier than they would have been under the older system. We no longer considered mental hospitals to be depositories where patients would be kept for the rest of their lives.

Dr. William Hanley, the Clinical Director of the Munroe Wing, was the only fully-trained psychiatrist on staff. The rest of us were recent graduates, namely Dr. Harvey Gurian, Dr. John Cumming, two or three doctors who were refugees from Europe (they were only allowed to come to Saskatchewan if they went into one of the mental hospitals) and myself. The refugee doctors had to learn English and then psychiatry.

We examined all patients within a couple of days of admission. The case and treatment were then discussed with Dr. Hanley. In addition, major clinical diagnostic and teaching seminars were held each week. Cases would be gone over in detail and the treatment determined. All the residents, the director, often Dr. McKerracher himself, and the wing's nurses, psychologists, and social workers would be present also; all were allowed to participate freely. These meetings were vigorous and sometimes even argumentative, but we learned much from them.

Schizophrenia was our major problem. Over half of the 5,000 patients in the Saskatchewan mental hospitals had the condition. The most effective treatments then available for mental illness were insulin coma and electroconvulsive therapy (ECT). Insulin coma had been developed in response to the observation that epileptics and convulsive patients had less schizophrenia. This observation somehow inspired European doctors to give schizophrenics large doses of insulin, causing blood sugar to plummet and coma to set in. The treatment was helpful to some patients, but always very dangerous, as it could easily cause death. ECT, used for depression and schizophrenia, had been introduced in Saskatchewan shortly after its discovery in Italy some years before. In those days, it was given without anesthetic or muscle relaxants. Patients hated the treatment, unless they were so desperately depressed that they were prepared to do anything. About six years after my arrival, the present ECT protocol was introduced, which includes a general anesthetic combined with a muscle relaxant. Since then, patients have had very little fear of the treatment and the incidence of fractures, always low, dwindled to almost zero. ECT is still one of the more reliable treatments in psychiatry, but is used much less than it used to be due to the introduction of modern tranquilizers and antidepressants. The major outcry against its use in recent years has come from a few psychiatrists who appear never to have used it and have not seen the remarkable recoveries it has brought about. In my view, the many patients who also advocate against ECT appear to have forgotten what they were like before they were given it, and now believe that all their continuing difficulties have arisen from its use. Unfortunately, ECT did not cure schizophrenic patients. Relapse usually occurred within a year of treatment, and after five or more years the prognosis for schizophrenic patients with or without ECT was about the same. My research would come to indicate that a biochemical defect leads to schizophrenia. It is highly unlikely that a treatment given over a period of several weeks could control such a defect over the long term.

The most recent treatment that had been introduced at the Munro Wing was psychotherapy, an offshoot of psychoanalysis, a treatment modality and school of thought which was becoming very powerful and influential in the US. It was the ambition of several of the young psychiatrists I knew to become psychoanalysts. But there was no one in Saskatchewan who could train us. We approached psychoanalysis as closely as we could by practising what was called dynamic psychotherapy. We spent about three hours per week with each patient reviewing their past, trying to determine what had gone wrong and caused their present condition. Due to time constraints I decided to combine group and individual therapy for all my patients.

After two years, I was expert in both individual and group psychotherapy. My clinical experience led me to the opinion—which I still hold—that so-called dynamic psychotherapy, as well as group therapy, are quite useless modalities for treating mentally ill patients, although they may have other uses, especially for people who are not ill and wish to undergo the experience.

Overall, considering that we had no modern drugs, only ECT as an effective treatment, I think the Wing did a creditable job of helping patients. Of course, the first use of megavitamin therapy later started there and this greatly improved the prognosis for the schizophrenic patients. Morale was high and the Wing had a very fine record in terms of its psychiatric residents passing their specialty examinations after four years. I was content that I would build my career there, and undertake to organize a course of research at the Wing.

In January 1951, as part of my preparation for beginning that research program, Rose and I started a six-week tour of Canadian and American psychiatric research centres. My parents made Rose's travel possible by leaving their farm to look after our three children for the duration of our trip. This tour, I hoped, would give me an overview of the progress being made in the field. I also hoped to gain inspiration for my own scientific direction.

First, we visited Toronto, where Professor A. Stokes, Chairman, Department of Psychiatry, had started a biochemical research program on a form of schizophrenia called periodic catatonia. This particular type appears to have vanished today, unless it is now called manic-depressive psychosis or bipolar psychosis. The original studies that inspired Stokes' work had been done in Norway by a

Professor Gjessing. Gjessing had carefully measured changes in blood and urine chemistry and correlated them to patients' clinically observable fluctuations. His data suggested that the blood and urine changes were related to thyroid function. But in order to establish these relationships beyond doubt required very careful control of the patients and their nutrition. Patients might have to remain in the research setting for many months while their condition oscillated from psychosis back to normality and back again into psychosis. Partly because of this difficulty, Stokes' research did not lead anywhere and eventually was dropped.

Next we went to Montreal to visit Professor Ewen Cameron at the Allan Memorial Hospital. He had established a very substantial investigative group based there which probably spent as much money on psychiatric research as all the other Canadian research centres put together. Cameron's projects included a psychosomatic unit, which sought to examine the connection between psychodynamics and certain diseases then considered to be psychosomatic in origin: peptic ulcer, ulcerative colitis, rheumatoid arthritis, and several others.

Cameron's group also included a small biochemical division, a psychological group, and one unique study being done by Dr. Lovett Doust. He studied the structure of the capillaries in the fingernail beds of patients. He asserted that the capillary structure in schizophrenics was different from that in other patients. I found his studies the most interesting of those being carried out at Allan Memorial but later, when I tried to repeat his work, was not able to do so. It requires special skill to "read" the capillaries the way he could and although I sought out personal instruction from Dr. Doust, I was not able to master the technique. I do not know of any research group that followed up this lead with any success.

During that first visit in 1951, I did not learn from Dr. Cameron anything about his clinical research. Margaret Callbeck, a psychiatric nurse working at the Munroe Wing, had trained in psychiatric nursing at the Allan Memorial Hospital and I had seen notes she had been given containing the gist of Dr. Cameron's lectures. I was intrigued by several of his studies. One was based upon his theory that he could desensitize patients to anxiety by giving them increasing quantities of adrenalin by injection. I cannot recall seeing publications arising from this research. It is impossible to guess what theory he based these experiments on. Perhaps he considered this treatment approach similar to desensitizing patients against allergens by giving them very tiny amounts of what they are allergic to and gradually increasing the dose. In any case, his was an odd idea; I heard from those who worked with him that most of the patients treated this way became worse or were not helped. A second study was based on his theory that one could regress patients back to their infancy, psychologically speaking, and then help them mature again, but with a different set of attitudes and values. He was also giving some patients, as I recall, up to several ECT treatments per day, a massive intervention. A further refinement was to make patients listen to tapes on which certain messages were repeated over and over. A few years later, when lysergic acid diethylamide (LSD) became a popular subject for investigators, he also began to use it. But in my opinion he did not use it properly. In time I saw a few patients he had treated. I recall a very disturbed and anxious young man. He had graduated with a medical degree, but he sought help from Dr. Cameron because he was very anxious. Dr. Cameron gave him 100 micrograms of LSD intravenously the first day, 200 micrograms the second day, and 300 micrograms the third day. Following that experience, this young man became psychotic and was still suffering from residual effects six months later, when I saw him. I advised him to start treatment with large doses of nicotinic acid (vitamin B-3), because by then I was familiar with this vitamin as a treatment for schizophrenia and for prolonged LSD reactions. This treatment helped him recover. These severe reactions, in my opinion, are in reality manifestations of schizophrenia stirred up in a person who is potentially schizophrenic anyway. I have seen several other patients who suffered ill effects from Dr. Cameron's LSD prescriptions as well, the last as recently as 1985. Eventually a number of former patients sued him. Many years later the damaging impact of Cameron's LSD treatments was described in many newspaper accounts of his work and in several books detailing his connection with the US Central Intelligence Agency. His "treatments" had in many cases been attempts to establish protocols for mind control.

While in Montreal, I also visited the Verdun Protestant Hospital, later renamed Douglas Hospital, where Dr. H. Lehmann was clinical director. This hospital was the mental health hospital for the English-speaking population of Montreal, a bilingual city. The French-speaking patients went to their own hospital, the much larger Hotel Dieu. I had seen films made by Dr. Lehmann showing patients exhibiting various types of psychiatric disorders. While we had a pleasant visit with Dr. Lehmann and his wife, this particular visit did not give me any leads I found useful when I eventually established my own research program. Dr. Lehmann had not yet started his research with chlorpromazine on manic-depressive patients. This drug is an antihistamine and was the first one in this class to have major tranquilizing properties. It was discovered in France by a surgeon, was taken on by psychiatry, and later found its way to Canada via Dr. Lehmann. He was the first to publish the results of his treatment of manic depressive patients, now called bipolar, with chlorpromazine and he became known as the father of tranquilizer therapy. Unfortunately, several years later, when my group at the Munroe Wing began to publicize our research with vitamins and schizophrenia, my relationship with him soured and eventually he became very hostile toward me, a development that surprised me.

From Montreal we went to Boston, where I visited Dr. Harry Solomon at the Psychopathic Hospital. Dr. Solomon was one of the leaders in American psychiatry and had not succumbed to the lure of psychoanalysis. I found Dr. Solomon interesting and friendly and walked through the ward with him, but I did not learn anything which later proved valuable to me. A few years later this hospital became one of the first places where Dr. Max Rinkel began to examine the effects of LSD. But the last time I visited this hospital in the 1960s, its name had been changed to the Massachusetts Mental Health Center, and it had become totally converted to psychoanalysis. In their library, a small bookcase containing Freud's complete works stood free from each wall, so they had four copies of the man's entire *oeuvre!*

We then visited the Worcester Foundation, a few miles west of Boston, then under Dr. Hudson Hoagland's leadership. His research group was looking at the relationship between schizophrenia and steroid hormones. In their large laboratory, they analyzed urine samples and tried to correlate them to the diagnosis they had for each patient. At first this research program looked to be very promising, but in the end it did not yield useful results.

In Boston I also met Professor Mark Altschule, who was working at the McLean Hospital on the city's outskirts. He was investigating the biochemical correlates of schizophrenia. He had looked at the connection between schizophrenia and steroid hormones and had come to the conclusion that there was no significant relationship. This opinion was contrary to the views of Dr. Hoagland and his group, but Dr. Altschule was later shown to be correct. Many years later Altschule and I co-operated in joint studies of adrenochrome. He told me later that as our adrenochrome hypothesis emerged, he had been convinced that his work of that time would eventually destroy ours. However, the more he studied the underlying phenomena, the more convinced he was that we were on the correct path, and he joined our efforts as a result. Professor Altschule also did some of the basic research involving the pineal gland and endured his share of ridicule because of it. Yet, melatonin, that gland's hormone, is now the latest rage in *avant garde* medicine.

In New York City, my most memorable visit was with Dr. Nolan D.C. Lewis, of the Psychiatric Institute at Columbia University. Dr. Lewis had the best psychiatric research group in North America, probably in the world. He had brought in a very eclectic group of scientists who later became world famous for their work. Dr. H. Waelsch headed biochemistry, Dr. F. Kallmann, human genetics[2], Dr.

---

2. Dr. Kallman was subjected to enormous criticism by analysts because he had found a high degree of genetic similarity between schizophrenic identical twins. His twin studies paved the way for all the subsequent genetic studies. This supercritical attitude toward all genetic research, characteristic of that era, was only dispelled twenty years later when an enormous amount of money was spent in trying to prove that Dr. Kallmann was wrong.

Pietrowski, psychology. He also had a psychoanalyst on staff. Dr. Lewis had a distinguished background in pathology and biochemistry and was the first American psychiatrist to become interested in psychoanalysis. He visited Dr. Freud in Austria personally. During their conversation Lewis asked Freud whether he himself ought to undergo a personal psychoanalysis before practicing the technique. In response Dr. Freud asked him how many of his patients had committed suicide. When hearing that none of Lewis' patients had done so, Freud said that it would be all right for Dr. Lewis to practise psychoanalysis. Lewis never did become a fanatical psychoanalyst. On the contrary, he became a thorn in the side of the psychoanalytic movement, which was then quickly gathering momentum in the United States. Lewis was irritated by the rapid fossilization of this school of thought. He told me about a meeting he had attended where a senior analyst had severely castigated a younger analyst for questioning some of the basic Freudian principles and for offering a different interpretation. At the end of this attack, Dr. Lewis had remarked that perhaps each meeting by analysts ought to be started by reverentially reading excerpts from Freud.

I asked Dr. Lewis about Dr. H. Rosen, a resident at Brooklyn State Hospital, and what he thought of Rosen's claims that he was able to cure chronic schizophrenics by what he called "direct psychoanalysis." In this work, Rosen sought to enter the world of his psychotic patients by spending hours and days with them, conversing with them in their psychotic language and actually trying to act as psychotic as they did. He claimed that with this technique he was able to bring his patients back to normal in a few days. His first reports aroused huge general interest among analysts, who began to hold meetings to discuss and interpret his work. Rosen became the darling of the psychoanalytic movement and on one occasion, even addressed the New York Academy of Science. In those heady days of psychoanalysis, the idea that schizophrenia was a biochemical (biological) disease was anathema. This attitude totally ignored Freud's own recommendation that psychoanalysts should leave schizophrenics alone because such patients could not, in Freud's opinion, respond to the technique.

Dr. Lewis informed me that a committee had been created in New York to examine Dr. Rosen's claims and he was acting as its head. He told me that none of Dr. Rosen's claims could be confirmed and his examination of the evidence suggested that some of them may have been fraudulent at worst, grossly exaggerated at best, and it was doubtful that any patients had really benefited. He described one patient Rosen had treated. She was a chronic schizophrenic from one of the New York mental hospitals. Dr. Rosen installed her in one of the New York hotels with a nurse who was to help out. He gave the woman "direct analysis" for a couple of days, pronounced her cured, then sailed off to England to give a lecture or two. He did not bother to tell the nurse that he was leaving, nor the patient's family. Nurse and woman were later discovered in the hotel and the patient returned to the mental hospital just as sick as she had been before. This failure to help one patient, asserted Lewis, did not seriously undermine Rosen's theory, since no treatment can help every patient. But it was a serious breach of medical ethics to state she was cured and later use her case history to bolster his claims.

Lewis' committee eventually presented a critical report to the American Psychiatric Association's annual meeting in 1957. Dr. Rosen had claimed that his method of "conversing with the patient in the language of the unconscious" and interpreting that unconscious to him while spending 1 to 3 hours daily with him, had led to the recovery of all 37 cases cited in one of his reports, following treatment of anything from 3 days to 11 months. But the New York Psychiatric Institute had located 12 of the Rosen patients who were schizophrenics. Not one was any better and all had required continuous and active treatment since their encounter with Rosen.

Later, Dr. Rosen moved to Philadelphia where he began a private practice in direct psychoanalysis. Several years after that he was awarded a large research grant from the Rockefeller Brothers' Fund (not the Rockefeller Foundation). This fund represented the Rockefellers' way of giving to charity. Each of the brothers would donate money to the fund, which was administered by a permanent management group. Final decisions on the money's destination were made by the brothers. I became familiar with this fund in later years because I visited the director several times to attempt to obtain more money for our research in Saskatchewan. Families who wanted their children treated by Dr. Rosen as part of his so-called study had to move them into a special house and provide round the clock nursing services for the duration of the treatment. When I first visited the director of the Rockefeller Brothers' Fund I discovered that Rosen's "research" had been monitored by the University of Pittsburgh, as one of the conditions of the grant. The director told me that one of the Rockefellers had allocated this grant to Dr. Rosen. I replied that this act indicated a remarkable degree of broadmindedness, but refrained from telling him what I really thought. Later, after the University carried out an investigation, the grant was discontinued and the money left over recaptured. Apparently, Dr. Rosen had included patients in his report who did not exist. I have never seen a final report on his "study." Gradually no more was heard about direct analysis.

Back to my visit with Dr. Lewis. It was one of the most memorable of that trip and it provided the greatest value to what would become my research. Dr. Lewis had been one of the first scientists to take mescaline, an extract of the peyote mushroom used in Native American religious rituals. He described his experience to me and later also to Dr. Humphry Osmond, the man who would one day be my main collaborator at the Munroe Wing. Mescaline, he said, caused a marked increase in auditory acuity. Under its influence he had been able to hear his cat walking across the rug. I was also impressed by a study he had published with Pietrowski.

In this study, Lewis and his colleagues discussed the re-examination of about 70 patients treated in their hospital who had been diagnosed as being manic-depressive following their first admission. They wanted to find out how many of these patients were re-diagnosed as schizophrenic on subsequent admissions and whether, in fact, this second assessment represented the correct diagnosis. In other words, the question was: were these patients manic-depressives who eventually became schizophrenic, or were they misdiagnosed during the first admission? And if they were actually schizophrenics, why was that diagnosis missed? This re-analysis found that about half of the studied patients first found to be manic-depressives had been re-diagnosed on subsequent admissions. They further found that had the original group of patients diagnosed as manic-depressive been examined for the presence of a specific group of ten diagnostic signs and symptoms, a positive finding for any five of these would have ferreted out those patients who were in reality schizophrenics.

What interested me was that five of these diagnostic criteria were concerned with perceptual capabilities, that is, they identified errors in perception, such as hearing voices and having visions. The originally diagnosed manic-depressive patients who also had reported perceptual changes were, therefore, in actuality schizophrenics, and this diagnosis had been missed. If all of the patients in this group had been examined more carefully, the original diagnosis would have remained stable over subsequent admissions. I consider this study one of the great classical works in diagnosis. Sadly, it has been totally ignored by the psychiatric profession, whose members remain in a perpetual muddle about diagnosis to this day. Today, diagnosis is far more dependent on the psychiatrist's orientation than it is on the objectively observable symptoms of the illness itself. Psychiatrists fearful of schizophrenia diagnose their patients as manic-depressive (in modern terminology, bipolar). They believe that lithium is a treatment specific to bipolar disorders and that any patient who responds to lithium must therefore have been bipolar.

This valuable research by Lewis and Pietrowski aroused my interest in the perceptual component of schizophrenia and later contributed to the development of the Hoffer Osmond Diagnostic (HOD) test for schizophrenia, described in detail in Chapter Eight. I later also repeated Lewis' and Pietrowski's original study several times and found that very seldom was a schizophrenic re-diagnosed as being manic-depressive on subsequent admissions, and that up to one-third of all depression cases were eventually re-diagnosed as schizophrenic. The subsequent diagnosis was forced by the clear development of perceptual changes which had not even been considered and asked for at the time of first admission. I have no doubt that the "schizophrenias," to use Carl Pfeiffer's term, are a group of perceptual disorders caused by a variety of biochemical abnormalities. Dr. John Conolly described insanity in about 1850 as a *disease of perception combined with an inability to tell whether these changes were real or not.* There has never been a better description, and probably will be none, until the biochemical laboratories are able to provide diagnostic tests not yet discovered that allow the medical profession to fully understand the biology of psychiatric disorders.

While in New York City I also visited the Sackler brothers, who were doing groundbreaking research on histamine as a schizophrenia treatment. Their work would inspire some of the initial biochemical research undertaken at the Munroe Wing; that story will be told in more detail in due course.

From New York, Rose and I went to Washington, D.C. I can only remember one episode from this part of our journey. I was taken to the site of the yet-to-be-built National Institute of Mental Health (NIMH) where the first sod had just been turned. (Little did I suspect that I was therefore present to witness the beginnings of an organization that would be part of the attempt to destroy my work.) After that, we traveled to Chicago, where I met Dr. H. Kluver at the University of Chicago and Dr. Franz Alexander at the Chicago Institute of Psychoanalysis.

Dr. Kluver was a most versatile scientist of the type rarely found today. The Kluver-Bucy syndrome is named after him. He was the first biochemist to prove the existence of porphyrins. Porphyrins are a class of compounds similar to hemoglobin, found throughout the body, and when produced in excess can cause psychosis. This condition is known as porphyrinurea. He had also studied the mescaline experience and written the first major American treatise on peyote.

He also did research with mescaline, and this proved very important to me, especially when later in 1951, Dr. Osmond came from England to become Clinical Director of the Saskatchewan Hospital at Weyburn. Fortunately, Dr. Kluver later became a very strong proponent of our research. Until his death, both Humphry and I visited him whenever we were in Chicago, and never did he waver in his support.

My meeting with Dr. Franz Alexander reinforced my growing doubts about the value of psychoanalysis. I was still very interested in psychosomatic medicine and Dr. Alexander, as head of the Chicago Institute of Psychoanalysis, was a leader in this field.

Dr. Alexander had been analyzed by Freud himself, which added to his prestige. At my first meeting with him, he told me about a study his research group had had underway for a year or more and invited me to have lunch with him and his staff the following day to learn more about it. His group was studying the hypothesis that, given the psychodynamics of a patient, one could diagnose the psychosomatic condition these had generated. To simplify the study, they had limited it to seven of the so-called psychosomatic diseases. I can remember only six of the diseases included: arthritis, peptic ulcer, ulcerative colitis, hyperthyroidism, hypertension, and asthma. Patients who had one of these diagnoses were interviewed and a transcript made of the entire conversation. Later, any statement in the interview which betrayed the diagnosis was carefully removed. The transcript was then circulated to all the residents and staff of the Institute, who had to study it carefully and deduce from what they read what the patient's disease was. At the lunch I attended, the meeting was chaired by Dr. French, an expert in Freudian dream interpretation. Only he knew the correct diagnosis in each case considered that day. He asked the resident to his left to begin. The man stood up, stated what he thought the diagnosis was and gave his reasons, using an interpretation based upon the written transcript and psychodynamic theory. Dr. Alexander had also given me a copy earlier and asked if I would like to participate. I had agreed, but then regretted my decision. No matter how often I read that transcript, I could come to no clarity with respect to the diagnosis. I therefore decided I would simply guess. Since there were only about half a dozen diseases to choose from, I had about a 14 percent chance of being correct. During the first half of the meeting everyone at the table hazarded his or her opinion and I did the same. When we were finished, the chairman announced what the disease was. To my delight, not a single one of the persons present, myself included, had hit upon the correct diagnosis. The second half of the meeting began with the resident next to the chairman outlining why he had made the incorrect diagnosis. Knowing the correct diagnosis made it so much easier to interpret the dynamics present in the interview properly. When it came to my turn, I passed.

I approved of that study, which must have cost a good deal of money, because it showed that the basic premise of psychosomatic medicine was flawed and that one could easily determine a patient's psychodynamics if one knew the disease, but that things did not work the other way around. In other words, there was very little substance to psychosomatic theory. As far as I know, the results of this experiment were never published. I believe that the Chicago School of Psychoanalysis never had the courage to do so. I also believe it would have been much better for the development of psychiatry had they published their findings, namely that one could not diagnose disease by studying a patient's psychodynamics.

After this visit with Dr. Alexander, Rose and I returned to Regina, glad to be home and back with our family. I was not fully satisfied with my North American tour because I had not yet found what I wanted, namely a sense of direction which I could use to shape the Wing's research program. I had become interested in the study of mescaline. I had learned the virtue of being eclectic from Dr. Lewis and his group, and I had confirmed serious and growing doubts about psychosomatic medicine and psychoanalysis. Looking back 50 years later, I feel I should be more grateful to my American colleagues because they did guide me in the right direction. I also realized after this journey that any research program I would design could not or would not follow any of the then existing Canadian or American models.

Back at work, I prepared a comprehensive report on my experiences for Dr. McKerracher. I continued to study psychiatry, decided to learn hypnosis, and initiated a simple psychosomatic study using a newly designed machine that could measure physiological variables such as blood pressure, respiratory rate, pulse, etc. I hoped to correlate increases and decreases in these physiological functions with anxiety, depression, and other emotional states. The machine was like a large radio console, and was fun to look at and play with. My plan was to take baseline measurements of bodily functions in those patients or volunteers who would be hooked up to the machine. I would then use hypnosis to control their level of anxiety or effect their mood and study the correlations between that mood and the hard data supplied by the machine. Through this work I did become a good hypnotist. I also made other studies of the impact of hypnosis, including the use of hypnosis to study dreams, but was never able to design a study which yielded any useful data. My work in this area represented an almost total waste of money. (I was able, however, to put my hypnotism skills to good use in 1960 when Dr. S. Fogel and I ran a large series of studies showing how various psychiatric syndromes could be elicited by giving the correct post-hypnotic suggestion.) Luckily, Dr. Osmond arrived later that year and shortly after that it was clear to me that there would be no more psychosomatic research under my direction. The new research pathway opened up by Dr. Osmond's interest took precedence.

Dr. Humphry Osmond arrived in the fall of 1951. On a hot, dry, dusty afternoon I went to Dr. McKerracher's office to meet him for the first time. He had just arrived in Regina from Toronto by a slow train with his wife Jane and his daughter Helen. I had first heard about Osmond after McKerracher came back from England earlier in 1951, where he had gone to recruit English psychiatrists for the Psychiatric Services Branch of the Saskatchewan Department of Public Health. The province was desperately short of psychiatrists and this fact prevented McKerracher from introducing some of his plans for improving psychiatric care in Saskatchewan. We especially needed a clinical director at Weyburn, one of the two large mental hospitals. The Saskatchewan government placed an advertisement in several United Kingdom papers, giving Saskatchewan House in London as the contact for interested psychiatrists. Candidates were to contact Mr. Graham Spry, the House's director and representative of the Saskatchewan government. Dr. McKerracher interviewed some 60 to 70 applicants while he was there and became thoroughly exhausted in the process. After he had interviewed the last applicant, Graham Spry came in and told him that one more psychiatrist had appeared and that he must interview him. Dr. McKerracher did not want to do so, but said he would see him for about ten minutes. Several hours later they were still talking. Dr. McKerracher promptly offered him the job as Clinical Director of the Saskatchewan Hospital at Weyburn. This choice I consider to be one of the best made during a long career of selecting and bringing psychiatrists to Saskatchewan. Now it would be Humphry's job to undertake the very difficult task of bringing one of the worst hospitals in the world into the twentieth century.

Back in the United Kingdom, Dr. Osmond and his colleague and friend Dr. John Smythies had investigated mescaline. They hoped it would help them develop a treatment for schizophrenia. But when they approached their superiors with this idea, they were rudely rebuffed. Dr. Osmond was so distressed by this experience that he decided not only to leave England, but to move as far away as possible. He wanted to come to a place where he would be free to pursue any investigation that he was interested in. His wife Jane had seen the ad in the *London Times* and told him about it. Canada seemed sufficiently far away and he thought it unlikely that he would be blocked by a lot of superiors here.

My first meeting with Humphry went very well. He knew that I was going to start a research program but did not know what I was interested in. He thought that I might react to his proposals in the same way as his English superiors. I, on the other hand, knew he was on his way, but did not know he was interested in research. After some initial conversation, Humphry brought out a manuscript he had written in England, outlining the work he had done with Dr. Smythies. They had studied the experiences induced in normal subjects who had taken mescaline and compared them with the experience induced in schizophrenics by their pathology. They found remarkable similarities between the two states when they systematically sorted out the various signs and symptoms. They knew the two conditions were not identical, yet they were similar enough that they believed the mescaline experience could be used as a model for the understanding of schizophrenia. This idea had been suggested earlier by Dr. T. Stockings, who had published his paper on the subject in the *Journal of Mental Science* in 1940. However, Osmond and Smythies had gone further than Stockings when they discovered that a few asthmatic subjects who had taken discolored, deteriorated adrenaline also had an experience similar to the mescaline experience. This fact led them to suggest that there might be a substance, an "M" substance (for mescaline) in the body that is somehow related to adrenaline, a hormone produced in response to stress, with properties similar to those of mescaline. They pointed out that mescaline and adrenaline are, chemically speaking, structurally similar compounds. (Indeed, the idea that schizophrenia might be caused by chemical toxins goes back many years, perhaps even further back than the late nineteenth century, when Carl Gustav Jung enunciated his "toxin X hypothesis" of schizophrenia. Dr. Jung had observed that the personalities of schizophrenics and hysterics were similar, yet in all other diagnostic respects these diseases were entirely different. He concluded there must be a second factor involved in schizophrenia and he called it toxin X.) The uniqueness of the Osmond-Smythies hypothesis was the combination of these two basic observations, namely the similarity between the psychological effect of mescaline and schizophrenia and mescaline's chemical similarity to adrenaline.

This hypothesis was very interesting to me and I thought that it might be used as a basis for the research I hoped we could start in Saskatchewan. I asked Humphry to leave a copy of the paper with me and at the same time urged him to have it published as quickly as possible so as to establish that he and Smythies were indeed the first to present these ideas. From the beginning, I had decided that there would be no plagiarism of ideas in any research I directed. I did not want anyone to think that I or anyone else had usurped his and Smythies' original insights.

A story will serve to illustrate why the paper Osmond shared with me so excited me. In 1957, after the first international congress on schizophrenia held in Zurich in honor of Eugene Bleuler, Humphry and I visited Arne Tiselius, who had been awarded the Nobel Prize for his discovery of chromatography, a new method of separating chemicals within the same solution from one another. We spent a pleasant afternoon with him telling him about our research on schizophrenia. Toward the end of the afternoon Dr. Tiselius told us that over the years many psychiatrists had come to him and asked him how they could go about finding this elusive schizophrenic toxin. They had suggested that he should undertake such research. After each doctor left, he would turn to his chief assistant and ask: "But where do we begin?" The beauty of the Osmond-Smythies hypothesis was that it provided a way to begin. We could search the schizophrenic's body for a substance related to adrenaline that also had certain key properties of mescaline. Adrenaline is derived from tyrosine, an essential amino acid (protein). We did not know how many compounds similar to tyrosine were present in the body, but we did know that it would be a very small fraction of all the possible chemicals present.

Humphry and I got along very well and would become close, lifelong friends and collaborators. From the beginning, I wanted our relationship to be open and honest at all times. I closed our first meeting by urging him again to submit his paper for publication to the *Journal of Mental Science*. He promised to consider this. Then he left for Weyburn and I went back to my duties at the Munroe Wing. I began to study his manuscript very carefully. I also began to search the literature for information on every compound known to cause similar reactions to those brought on by mescaline. Lysergic acid diethylamide (LSD) seemed most similar in its action. The first reports on its activity had been published and LSD was available from Sandoz, the company in Switzerland whose chemist Albert Hoffmann had first discovered its properties and effects. One of the first things Humphry and I did was adopt the word "hallucinogen" to characterize LSD, mescaline, and other such compounds. The word "hallucinogen" was first used by Dr. Donald Johnson, an English doctor who later became a Member of Parliament; he was also a book publisher. In my search of the literature I came across a monograph he had written called "Hallucinogens." I contacted him and this led to a research relationship that continued until he died. He would also eventually publish the book I co-authored with Dr. Osmond, *How To Live With Schizophrenia*. There are many chemicals that will poison the brain and cause strange reactions, including alcohol, narcotic drugs, atropine, heavy metals, insecticides, and so on. These compounds not only create changes in perception and thinking but also decrease the level of consciousness. The best examples of this effect are provided by the anesthetics. We, therefore, defined hallucinogens as compounds which caused changes in perception and in thinking with consequent changes in mood, but in the absence of a decrease in consciousness and without disorientation. We ruled out substances whose effects mimicked organic psychoses or deliria. These types of psychoses are caused by brain damage, or by powerful drugs like anesthetics and narcotics. Our definition narrowed the field considerably, but we thought it essential to do so. A well-known rule in biochemistry is that chemicals similar in structure also tend to have similar effects in the body, both chemically and psycho-biologically. We decided to search out all the hallucinogens that fitted our definition and investigate whether they had some common structural properties.

As our coming research began to take clearer and clearer shape in our minds, Humphry and I met as often as we could, either in Regina or in Weyburn. In between we called each other frequently for long telephone conversations about various points we had thought about or had read in the psychiatric literature. We also wrote frequently. These letters and the minutes of the meetings of the Saskatchewan Committee on Schizophrenia Research (which would be formed shortly) are now my main source of information on those years, combined with what I can remember of events. I sent my first letter to Humphry on Oct 12, 1951, to thank him for leaving with me his paper, "Schizophrenia—A New Approach." I told him that this work suggested many interesting research possibilities and that we should follow up on some of them. Humphry, in the meantime, prepared a working paper entitled "The Relationship Between Mescaline, Adrenaline, and Amphetamine, with Reference to the Etiology of Schizophrenia" with J. Smythies as co-author. Dr. Smythies was still in England at the time. In this paper he and Humphry referred to the similarity in structure of adrenaline and mescaline as well as to Kluver's work with mescaline. They quoted Kluver: *"Only by studying the whole complex of symptoms in mescaline intoxication, including the hallucinatory symptoms, has it become possible to recognize mescaline as an agent for the production of 'experimental psychoses,' and only in such a way have psychiatrists recognized the symptomatological similarity between mescaline intoxication and the acute phases of schizophrenia. No matter what the symptomatological relations may be, the 'mescal psychosis' is produced by a well-defined chemical substance and not by hypothetically assumed toxins, metatoxic intermediaries and the like. It seems that psychotic symptoms resembling those of mescaline intoxication appear not only in the course of the schizophrenic disease process, but also under other conditions. In view of these findings, it is unfortunate that at present so little is known about the biochemical processes involved in mescaline action."*[3]

This paper provided a complete review of what was known at the time about the chemistry, pharmacology, and physiology of mescaline, including its structural similarity to adrenaline. It also reviewed the biochemical and physiological findings recorded to date about schizophrenia. Humphry then recommended research that ought to be initiated, including a study of many mescaline-like compounds, a study of their metabolites in urine, mescaline metabolism in humans, a study of normal human fluids for the presence of similar compounds, and finally, a study searching for the compounds that would inhibit the enzymatic reactions leading to the formation of the postulated M substance or toxin. The last suggestion was the most important one to deal with. If it proved possible to block the formation of this

---

3. *Studies in Personality*. McGraw-Hill, New York, 1942.

postulated M substance, that would open the possibility of developing a new and effective therapy for schizophrenia.

It was my job as Director of Psychiatric Research to initiate studies and to obtain the money we needed to get started. With Dr. Osmond, a clear research direction had arrived. I asked Humphry to begin the costing process while I continued to explore the literature and ways and means of obtaining grant support. Humphry was full of enthusiasm and generated ideas at a great rate. It was obviously impossible to implement every one of them, and I had to decide what was practical for us to do, considering that we had no money yet, no research staff, and no place in which to do our work.

On November 14, 1951, Humphry and I met in Dr. McKerracher's office. The latter had arranged for us to meet Dr. Devries, head of the Connaught Laboratory at the University of Toronto, and a biochemist, Dr. Young. Dr. Young had been a classmate of mine during my PhD studies and was also a friend of Charles McArthur, the chairman of the department of biochemistry at the University of Saskatchewan, in Saskatoon. Humphry later sent me a copy of the notes he made immediately after this meeting. When we had begun to discuss the details of our biochemical theory, including the possible connection between mescaline and adrenaline, Dr. Young had become very interested. This ignited Dr. Devries' enthusiasm and he promised us advice and help, saying he would do all he could to secure funds. This meeting was another of those essential events which eventually made our research possible. As luck would have it, both Dr. Devries and Dr. Young were members of the federal government committee that evaluated psychiatric research grant proposals in Ottawa, Canada's capital, when our first grant request came up for approval. They both supported it, despite the opposition of the three psychiatric members of that committee.

By the end of December of 1951, after many further meetings and discussions, I finished a grant request which was approved by Dr. McKerracher and the Saskatchewan Deputy Minister of Health; it was then sent to Ottawa. We asked for $23,000 and planned on using the money to hire a psychologist and biochemist who would help us start our research into the biochemical basis of schizophrenia.

While we waited to hear from Ottawa, we decided to initiate some research on our own. I had proposed that one of our first therapeutic trials be to examine the use of histamine in schizophrenia treatment. The pioneers of this treatment were the Sackler brothers, who I had met on my first research excursion, during my time in New York City. At that point, Dr. Arthur Sackler and his two younger brothers had already published several papers in which they described the positive results they had been getting by treating schizophrenic patients with high doses of histamines injected under the skin. I had visited them in their brownstone offices in central Manhattan, and later toured Creedmoor State Hospital, a large psychiatric hospital on an island just east of Manhattan Island, where they were conducting their therapeutic trials. I had been very impressed with their dedication and zeal, and even more with the results they were seeing.

The Sackler histamine studies reinforced my belief that the biochemical approach to treatment was correct, as they were using large doses of a natural hormone already present in the body. I acknowledge them as truly the first practitioners of what would later be called orthomolecular psychiatry, namely, the supplemental use of molecules naturally present in the body to treat mental illness.

Now I decided to attempt to corroborate their findings at the Munroe Wing.

On December 28 I wrote to Humphry and sent him a copy of the research design I proposed to use at the Munroe Wing in testing histamine therapy. I suggested he might modify it to suit the special needs existing at Weyburn.

I should also note here that the Sacklers' work played an indirect role in our group's research of nicotinic acid, or niacin. Histamine produces a characteristic vasodilatation, that is, a dilation of the blood vessels. This, in turn, produces a flush that begins in the head and gradually travels down until the whole body is enveloped. This flush is associated with a sensation of heat and itching. From my work with vitamins in my cereal chemistry days, I knew that nicotinic acid produced similar effects. As I contemplated the Sacklers' histamine work, I was reminded of this fact and my interest in niacin was sparked. The very first written notation I have dealing with my thoughts about nicotinic acid as a possible treatment for schizophrenia is in a penciled notation written on the first page of a letter dated December 31, 1951, from Humphry.

I should also note that beyond this initial association between the two substances, the Sacklers' use of histamine did not further motivate our use of niacin. The two compounds have different biochemical actions against schizophrenia. The niacinamide form of the vitamin, for instance, is just as effective as niacin, but causes no flush.

On January 4, 1952, Humphry and I again met and discussed how the body might deal with excess production of adrenaline. We had previously discussed the possibility that schizophrenia might represent one of the body's defenses against excessive production of adrenaline. In effect, the body might convert the extra hormone to methylated amines (compounds similar in structure to mescaline). But this response, with its potentially perception-altering results, would increase anxiety levels even more and thus establish a vicious cycle as more adrenaline was produced in response to the anxiety. A biochemical process called transmethylation (which creates methylated amines) had been shown to exist in the body only within the previous year. I had at that time suggested that nicotinic acid might be used to block it. Humphry had given some nicotinamide to an acute young schizophrenic patient, but to no effect. The use of this form of vitamin B-3 was not continued on that patient. On January 10, 1952, Humphry wrote: *"I had a very acute young schizophrenic here and tried him for three days on large doses of niacinamide, about 500 milligrams per day. These did not have any special effect on him. You may remember we wondered if it might not help pick up a methoxyl group."* He also wrote: *"Dr. Jedwab has done extensive research of the literature and has produced an interesting observation that there is no special correlation between vitamin deficiency and the hallucinations which nicotinic acid are known to cure. Quite a number of people he says are reported to have recovered from hallucinations when given nicotinic acid in whom there has been no evidence whatever that there has been a deficiency of this stuff."*

At that time we still believed that vitamins were needed only in very small amounts to prevent deficiency states. Since 20 milligrams daily of vitamin B-3 prevented pellagra (the B-3 vitamin deficiency disease), 500 milligrams per day did seem an enormous amount. On January 25, 1952, I wrote a long letter to Humphry discussing 11 items that had come up for discussion between us. I included a discussion of histamine, niacin, and adrenaline, as outlined following. Histamine decreases blood pressure by opening up the capillaries; this action also produces a flush. In allergic shock reactions, the body produces copious quantities of histamine; adrenaline injections are used to counteract this dangerous effect. As these two natural compounds, histamine and adrenaline are antagonistic to each other, it was possible, I thought, that niacin, which also causes a flush, and can temporarily decrease blood pressure due to dilatation of the capillaries, might be antagonistic to adrenaline. Many years later it was found that niacin does protect the body against one of the toxic effects of adrenaline: the release of fatty acids from their storage sites. I also considered the dose of nicotinic acid which would be required. I wrote: *"I feel that if it is to be used at all, it must be given in such massive doses that there is a prolonged vasodilatation as shown by marked flushing. I think that something of the order of up to 5 grams per day should be investigated. The amide does not produce any flushing, therefore it might be preferable to use nicotinic acid. The toxic dose is approximately 4 grams per kg so we have a very safe therapeutic tool."*

I further discussed one of the first schizophrenic patients I treated using the Sackler histamine therapy. After four weeks of treatment she was taking 4 milligrams per day. Her psychiatrist found an amazing change in her personality. She had dropped her projected defenses and was discussing readily with him her previous need for them. There had also been a marked change in her behaviour on the ward. It appeared that we were able to claim some success with histamine.

On February 29, Humphry wrote: *"Dr. Coulter has been kind enough to say that we can buy a good quantity of nicotinic acid. I have asked for half a pound to begin with and Mr. Cathcart, our pharmacist, is going to make it up possibly in cachet or capsules and I think we will give it in thousand milligram doses. What do you think our limit should be? It seems to me that we want to really flood the CNS [central nervous system] with it and probably concentrations much higher than have ever been used before are indicated. Can you tell me of any possible danger? As far as I can make out in the past over a thousand milligrams have been thought a very large dose, but considering its extreme non-toxicity there is no reason whatever why it should be thought so large.*

Dr. Coulter was mentioned here because he, as the superintendent at the hospital where Humphry was clinical director, was the cause of much difficulty in Weyburn and tended to resist every move Humphry and McKerracher wanted to make to improve the hospital. But Humphry had requested a very small amount of nicotinic acid and perhaps that was why he had not encountered opposition in this case. We had to make up our own pills, as no tablets containing more than 50 milligrams were available on the market and these contained so much inert filler material that giving patients three grams per day of the actual vitamin would have necessitated filling them up with a prohibitive amount of inactive material which might have made them sick.

On March 14, I wrote Humphry that I had ordered two pounds of nicotinic acid from Fisher Scientific Co. I added that it would be safe to give up to 10 or even 15 grams each day. I also speculated that because of the similarity in structure between nicotinic acid and adrenaline, that nicotinic acid might be absorbed through the same cell receptor sites and thus prevent the absorption of adrenaline. When the body is flooded with nicotinic acid then, adrenaline would be prevented from accessing these receptors. However, after this initial flushing, the adrenaline secreted in the blood would gradually tend to be picked up again by these receptors, while at the same time the nicotinic acid would be rapidly excreted. Later, it was discovered that nicotinic acid does protect fat storage sites from the action of adrenaline, preventing the release of fatty acids under stress.

I continued to search the literature for drugs with properties similar to mescaline, and in addition to LSD, came across references to two more hallucinogenic alkaloids, harmine and ibogaine.

One evening in March 1952, after I had finished my day's work at the Munroe Wing, I sat down at my family's dinner table and wrote down the formulae of the few compounds then known to have hallucinogenic properties. Three of them had an indole nucleus: all chemicals that contain two rings of atoms attached to each other, the larger with six carbon atoms and the smaller one with two carbon and one nitrogen atom, are called indoles. Mescaline resembled adrenaline, but could theoretically be converted to an indole through the fusion of its side ring with its main benzene ring. Perhaps mescaline was converted to an indole in the body? We also knew that discolored adrenaline had hallucinogenic properties, though we did not yet know what caused the pink color in deteriorated adrenaline. Suddenly, on that one sheet of paper, I saw the entire new hypothesis taking shape. We would search for an indole derived from adrenaline—this might be the elusive schizophrenic toxin. At last we had a map to guide us in the search through unknown terrain. I still vividly remember the sudden surge of excitement as I realized we had hit upon a possible solution: *Look for an indole derivative of adrenaline which has the psychological properties of mescaline or LSD.*

My insight had just narrowed the field from thousands of chemicals present in the body to less than a dozen, derived from known precursors. I quickly shared my insight with Humphry by telephone. He was as excited and pleased as I was.

This main hypothesis suggested several sub-hypotheses which could be tested. The value of a hypothesis is determined by its refutability. If a hypothesis can be disproven by research, then it is a good hypothesis because it is testable and may lead to even better ones. We selected three of these testable sub-hypotheses: (1) the indole derivative should be present in the body; (2) it would be an hallucinogen comparable to the pink compound in discolored adrenaline; (3) decreasing the amount of this compound formed in the body would be therapeutic for schizophrenia. We now knew we needed a biochemistry group, a psychological group, and a team of research psychiatrists to help us test these sub-hypotheses.

It was also in March, 1952 that we learned of the progress of our grant request. Its fate in Ottawa foreshadowed a theme that would continue for years to come, to the detriment of many schizophrenics' health—the psychiatric profession's refusal to consider seriously a course of treatment based on biochemical rather than psychoanalytical principles. Indeed, we received our first Canadian federal government research grant early in 1952 only because Dr. Nolan Lewis, the aforementioned head of the Psychiatric Institute at Columbia University and one of my hosts on the research excursion I had made, interceded on our behalf.

We were supposed to be advised early in 1952 as to whether or not we were going to get the grant. When the deadline had passed, I approached my chief, Dr. McKerracher, about not having heard yet. He telephoned Ottawa. In those years seeing someone pick up the telephone and nonchalantly make a long-distance call was still very surprising to me. He spoke to Dr. C. Roberts, the psychiatrist with the federal government in charge of grants. Dr. Roberts told him that the committee which had vetted all the Canadian grant requests was split on our request and that he had sent it to Dr. Lewis for his opinion, which the committee had agreed to accept as binding. So Dr. McKerracher called New York. Dr. Lewis was away for the weekend on his farm, where he was working on breeding square tomatoes, so Dr. McKerracher was advised to call back early Monday morning. I went back to Dr. McKerracher's office on Monday and listened to the conversation with Dr. Lewis. He said he had already gone over the proposal and that he had written to Ottawa advising them that although we had requested support for two years they should give it to us for twenty! We had our grant. The whole story behind this sequence of events came out some years later when Dr. Lewis was Director of Research at the New Jersey Institute of Neurology and Psychiatry. He told me in detail what had happened.

Each request for support was put before a committee called to Ottawa for that purpose. The committee that year consisted of the three most eminent psychiatrists in Canada and three scientists from other disciplines. The psychiatrists were Dr. A Stokes, a professor at the University of Toronto, Dr. E. Cameron, then professor at McGill

University in Montreal, and Dr. E. Hobbs, professor of psychiatry at Western University in London, Ontario. The scientists included Dr. Young and Dr. Devries. Luckily, as already mentioned, these men had been in Regina earlier in 1951 and I had had a chance to talk to them both and gain their enthusiasm for our proposed research. I believe this meeting in Regina in Dr. McKerracher's office was in the end very helpful towards our getting the grant.

In the committee's final vote, explained Dr. Lewis, the three psychiatrists had vetoed my proposal and the three scientists had approved it. The chairman, Dr. Roberts, wanted us to get the grant simply because Saskatchewan had not yet applied for any of the funds for which it was eligible. He felt that each province should get its fair share of research funds. But he did not want to vote against the three top psychiatrists. The three psychiatrists voted against our proposal because they felt it was foolish, much as had the psychiatrists in England to whom Dr. Osmond had first outlined the same ideas before he came to Saskatchewan. Dr. Roberts resolved the impasse by suggesting that the grant request be sent to Dr. Lewis. The committee agreed that they would accept Dr. Lewis's recommendations.

I have never discussed this meeting with Dr. Roberts, but I have reconstructed what probably influenced the thinking of that committee. The three psychiatrists had three major objections to the research. The first was that we were proposing a biochemical model for schizophrenia causation, rather than a psychoanalytical one. The second was that they did not want to see any funds going to Saskatchewan, with the exception of Dr. Stokes, who had in fact advised Dr. McKerracher to initiate a research program in Saskatchewan. The third reason was that neither Dr. Osmond nor I had yet been accepted as fully qualified psychiatrists. The "big three" were not involved in any plot against us. Dr. Cameron and Dr. Stokes had no use for each other. In fact, I doubt whether any of them were friendly with each other. They had come to their decisions independently and believed that any other psychiatrist, especially one as distinguished as Dr. Lewis, would back them up. His support for us must have been very surprising indeed to the Canadian professors of psychiatry.

The stalemate continued for the next four years and almost every one of our grant requests was sent to Dr. Lewis, who always supported them, in which acts he greatly advanced the scientific understanding of schizophrenia.

After our money came through, Humphry and I were suddenly confronted with cold reality. While preparing our application and impatiently waiting for the response from Ottawa, we had been rather like an opposition party, full of confidence that given a chance we would know what to do. Now we suddenly wondered how to get started. We decided to enlist the help of some of the scientists at the University of Saskatchewan. I had close links with several of the professors there and hoped that they might become interested in helping us.

VI

THE SASKATCHEWAN COMMITTEE ON SCHIZOPHRENIA RESEARCH

Accordingly, early in 1952 Humphry and I discussed the creation of a committee that would help guide our research. I wanted to involve several scientists then at the University of Saskatchewan, including Professor Charles McArthur, at that time chairman of the Department of Biochemistry, and Duncan Hutcheon, professor of pharmacology in the department of physiology, then operating under the chairmanship of Professor Louis Jaques. I approached Charles, and he agreed he would join us. He suggested we also invite Vernon Woodford from his department. Professor Hutcheon, with his chief's approval, also agreed to join us. I appointed myself chairman since I would have to do the major work in directing the committee's progress and in obtaining research funds. Of course Humphry was a member, as well as Dr. D.G. McKerracher.

The newly constituted committee met in Saskatoon on April 25 and 26, 1952, in a room behind the library of the medical building. Humphry and I had planned this first meeting very carefully. The three professors knew nothing about schizophrenia. Humphry and I had decided that the first thing we had to do was to arouse their interest. They would be less inclined to help us if they found the subject boring. Humphry opened the meeting by outlining what we knew about schizophrenia, its epidemiology, its clinical characteristics, the lack of available treatment, the number of Canadian hospital beds occupied by schizophrenic patients (50 percent), and so on. I followed with an outline of how little we knew about the causes and treatment of schizophrenia and described our hypothesis. This was followed by a general discussion on procedures for the committee's work. We looked at matters such as communication, coordination of our efforts, and the like.

During my presentation I drew the structures of adrenaline, mescaline, LSD, ibogaine, and harmine on the blackboard. Every one of the hallucinogens was an indole and mescaline theoretically could be converted into one. One could tell at a glance that this two-ring indole structure was the common link amongst all these chemicals. I also discussed Dr. Osmond's observation that when asthmatics inhaled adrenaline that had lost its chemical stability and become discoloured, turning a pink shade (stable adrenaline is colourless), they sometimes had experiences similar to those produced by the hallucinogens or by schizophrenia. The pink compound was one of the oxidized derivatives of adrenaline. We therefore included it in our discussion even though we did not know what it was. At this point Dr. Hutcheon, who had been listening attentively throughout the whole morning and into the early part of the afternoon, spoke up. He asked, "Would you like to know what that pink compound is?" We were all surprised and urged him to tell us. He replied that it is *adrenochrome* and proceeded to draw its formula on the board. There it was, the missing link, an indole that could be made in the body from adrenaline!

Before receiving this information, Humphry and I had believed that the only indoles present in the body were derived from l-tryptophan, an amino acid. We did not yet know that tyrosine (another amino acid) and adrenaline would be found to be other major sources of indoles, including others besides adrenochrome, in the body.

The effect upon us was electrifying. We had suddenly and unexpectedly been presented with a major refinement to the basic hypothesis by which we were hoping to find the elusive schizophrenic toxin. Dr. Hutcheon told us he had studied under Professor

Burns at Oxford and his dissertation had been on adrenochrome. He knew how to make it and he had studied its properties. I am certain that he was the only scientist in Canada at that time who knew anything substantial about adrenochrome. The only other scientist I knew who had worked with adrenochrome was Professor Roger Manning, my first biochemistry professor. To have Hutcheon on our committee represented a major stroke of luck. His expertise undoubtedly saved us a lot of money and many months, perhaps even years, of research effort.

I now sensed a marked change in the feeling tone of the meeting. Before Hutcheon made his comments, the scientists had not really known how they might help. But now they saw possibilities open up and they became enthusiastic. They began to talk about what "we," i.e. the committee as a group, would do. We now had a sense of unity, and a common objective—and every member felt they could make a useful contribution.

In the test tube, adrenochrome is the first oxidation product of adrenaline. In 1952, we could not know whether it was really made in the body, but there is no doubt about this today. It is a very reactive indole and is the precursor of many other indoles in the body, including some of the dark pigments that can be found in the brain and the skin. In the body the oxidation process that leads from adrenaline to adrenochrome occurs in two steps. The new compound formed by the loss of one electron from the adrenaline molecule is very unstable and can rapidly change back to adrenaline if that electron is replaced. Significantly, *if the electron is not recaptured, or if this cannot occur because of a deficiency in the nicotinamide adenine dinucleotide (NAD$\Leftrightarrow$NADH) system, oxidized adrenaline will lose another electron and become adrenochrome. Adrenochrome cannot be changed back into adrenaline.* Adrenochrome too is very reactive and promptly forms adrenolutin and a large variety of other oxidized indoles. Pink adrenaline, or discoloured old adrenaline, contains a mixture of these various oxidized derivatives. The same sequence occurs with other catecholamine hormones, such as dopamine, noradrenaline, and so on. These compounds too are indoles.

We had begun by presenting to the committee our hypothesis that we needed to search for a compound related to adrenaline that shared various properties of mescaline. In light of Hutcheon's information our next step would be to look for the presence of adrenochrome in the body, and if we found it, to establish whether it was related to schizophrenia or not. Thus, we had further narrowed our search. We no longer needed to consider dozens of indoles, including those derived from tryptophan and catecholamines, but only those compounds derived from catecholamines.

A most interesting discussion filled the rest of the afternoon. Osmond and Smythies had conjectured that adrenaline is converted to a hallucinogenic molecule through the addition of a methyl group. Hutcheon thought it more likely that an oxidative product like adrenochrome is formed, and moreover, this would account for the clinical reports of psychotic reactions following the injection of old adrenaline preparations. Woodford then suggested that the intracellular co-enzyme nicotinamide adenine dinucleotide (NAD) could be essential for the adrenaline oxidation. If this proved to be true, supplemental nicotinamide (vitamin B-3) might competitively inhibit this action of NAD and limit adrenochrome formation. (Later, it would be revealed that NAD plays interesting roles in brain chemistry. It is needed to reconvert partially oxidized adrenaline that has lost one electron back to adrenaline; it is also needed in the oxidation reaction that converts oxidized adrenaline to adrenochrome.)

Woodford went on to explain that adrenochrome had been shown by other researchers to slow the Krebs cycle in the body. The Krebs cycle consists of a series of enzymatic reactions that strip energy from glucose in small increments, rather than by burning the sugar up as in a flame. We wondered if inhibition of the Krebs cycle in the brain by adrenochrome could lead to symptoms of mental illness. Woodford proposed a plan of action:

1. He would carry out an intensive study of how the Krebs cycle is affected by the hallucinogenic agents—including adrenochrome, if it proved to be a hallucinogen—as well as their antidotes. By

this study, he might determine at which link in the cycle the inhibition occurred.

2. He would develop a test to detect adrenochrome in urine and blood. One could then attempt to correlate its concentration with the manifestations of schizophrenia. Woodford felt that, for the moment at least, this task would be secondary to the first objective, since much more had to be learned about the chemistry of adrenochrome before it would be easily identifiable in the body. For that reason he did not feel he would need clinical material such as blood or urine at this stage.

McArthur said he would look into the possibility of synthesizing adrenochrome. If it could be synthesized, or if it was available commercially, it could be pharmacologically tested by Hutcheon and then released for clinical trials. On the basis of Woodford's and Hutcheon's suggestions, we also agreed we should try a clinical trial of schizophrenia treatment using massive doses of thiamin, riboflavin, pyridoxine, nicotinic acid, ascorbic acid (vitamin C) and perhaps magnesium injections. The rationale for thiamin, riboflavin, nicotinic acid, and pyridoxine derived from their known effect on the Krebs cycle. Massive doses of these vitamins, we knew, increased the rate of reaction of the enzymes in the cells and might restore energy production in the brain to normal leading to a resolution of schizophrenia symptoms. These considerations also explain the planned use of magnesium in small doses.

The rationale for using ascorbic acid arose from its strong anti-oxidant properties, which could theoretically prevent adrenaline from changing to adrenochrome. Significantly, the richest source of vitamin C in the body is the adrenal gland. The reason for these high concentrations has not been explained to this day. Perhaps the quantity of ascorbic acid in the adrenal cortex is essential to prevent a deterioration of adrenaline from occurring. It is also well known that the ascorbic acid content of the adrenal cortex drops precipitously under stress. The second richest source of vitamin C is brain tissue.

As we continued our discussion, nicotinic acid emerged as the preferred nutrient to consider since its deficiency caused the disease pellagra, which even then could often not be distinguished from schizophrenia and which I today consider a form of schizophrenia. Nicotinic acid is a component of one of the most ubiquitous co-enzymes in the body and is involved in hundreds of reactions. And it is a major antioxidant.

Hutcheon then went on to outline what he knew about adrenochrome's properties. It is a powerful enzyme inhibitor and in laboratory studies it interferes with the metabolism of brain cells. He also told us he knew how to make the compound. At that time he had working for him a Master's student, Mr. Norman Eade. We decided to allocate some of our grant money to Hutcheon, which would allow Eade to synthesize adrenochrome under supervision and to test its properties on animals. As far as we knew, it had not yet been tested this way. After we knew with certainty what its toxic properties might be, we would be in a better position to take the compound ourselves in order to test it for hallucinogenic properties. Because we sought knowledge of its mental and perceptual effects, it had to be tested on people and we did not want to give it to any volunteers until we ourselves had experienced its effect. We were confident that it would not kill us since we were fairly certain it was already being made in the body; we did want to know its lethal dose (LD) 50, i.e. the amount in milligrams which would kill half the animals in a short term study. Hutcheon would also turn over some of the adrenochrome to Vernon Woodford, who would study its effect on brain tissue respiration. Finally, Hutcheon told us about adrenolutin, which was produced in the lab by adding hydrogen to adrenochrome.

Woodford suggested that since adrenochrome interfered with the operation of the respiratory enzymes, we ought to study this interaction more. The respiratory enzymes were derived from three vitamins: cocarboxylase from thiamin, flavin adenine dinucleotide from riboflavin and adenine nicotinamide dinucleotide from niacinamide. Again it struck us as logical to use these vitamins with our patients, as theoretically speaking, they could suppress the toxic effect of adrenochrome. Such therapy would involve giving large doses, which would be feasible, since we knew these vitamins were safe. I was the resident expert on the vitamins since I had taken my PhD on the study of thiamin in cereal products. The committee agreed that Osmond and I should prepare to make clinical trials of these nutrients.

By the end of the meeting we were a coherent, friendly group of psychiatrists and scientists all ready to work toward the same objective, to develop a successful treatment for schizophrenia. Humphry and I had achieved our major objective in calling such a committee together. I have never ceased to be impressed by the number of amazing coincidences that brought this committee together. Had there been even one member missing, the adrenochrome hypothesis could not have been developed and the use of vitamin therapy for mental illness would have been set back many years. I would like to summarize again the skills and expertise of our committee members:

1. Myself, with a background in science and medicine, a strong enthusiasm for psychiatric research and specialized knowledge of nutrition, especially of vitamins.
2. Duncan Hutcheon, perhaps the only scientist in Canada who had studied adrenochrome in depth and who knew how to make it and study its pharmacological properties.
3. Humphry Osmond, the only psychiatrist in Canada who had experienced the effects of mescaline and knew something about other hallucinogens. His work with the "toxin M hypothesis" catalyzed our entire research effort and heralded the adreno-chrome hypothesis.
4. Charles McArthur, willing to participate with his department of biochemistry in our research.
5. Griffiths G. McKerracher, backed by a progressive government willing to support what may have seemed to them to be a hare-brained scheme cooked up by a group of research psychiatrists.
6. Vernon Woodford, deeply familiar with the processes of inter-mediary metabolism in various tissues and his willingness to use his time to help us with our studies.

It is impossible to calculate the odds that these six people with their individual interests and talents could ever have met, and in one of the most remote parts of Canada, Saskatchewan.

Another factor unique to Saskatchewan favoured us. The province offered no complete training for medical doctors. Therefore, no group of physicians motivated by the conservatism inherent in medical schools (who could have attempted to prevent us from starting the research) were present. In a related stroke of luck, both Humphry and I had not been psychiatrists long enough to have become permanently habituated to the old theories then current. I have often wondered whether it would be possible to start a project such as ours today. I have concluded that to do so would be very difficult because there are so many restraints on research today. In my experience, the time and effort required to clear the various committees controlling research nowadays, in ethics, methodology, etc., and the likelihood that the conservatism usually displayed by these committees will squash any truly new ideas, means that many innovative individuals no longer pursue research. Those who persevere often find themselves ploughing the same fields over and over again.

The suggestions that arose during this first meeting of our research committee determined the nature of the coming project and the path that we, the committee, would follow for the next sixteen years. I have used the hypothesis we developed there as a guide ever since. It is an elegant and simple idea which I must have presented some hundred times in my talks all over North America. I have found that lay audiences, unlike many of my psychiatric colleagues, have had no difficulty following the argument. The basic hypothesis can be explained in three steps:

1. Noradrenaline combines with a methyl group and becomes adrenaline.
2. Adrenaline loses two electrons to form adrenochrome.
3. Adrenochrome is one of the main factors in causing schizophrenia.

To prove that the adrenochrome hypothesis is true, the following sub-hypotheses would also have to be shown to be true:

(i) That adrenochrome can be made in the body and that it is made in greater quantities in the schizophrenic person. (I would add now that it is also possible that in the schizophrenic the blood-brain barrier is more leaky and allows more hallucinogenic indoles to cross.) To examine this proposition we needed a biochemical research division that could search for the presence of adrenochrome in body fluids, could study the precursors of adrenochrome creating reactions in the body, for example the enzymes and other catalysts which played a role, and study the ways by which we could inhibit the reactions that lead to adrenochrome production. Our biochemical division became one of the most productive units in our research program. Our chemical studies paved the way for the final development of the method for analyzing body fluids for adrenolutin, and we established that adrenolutin, the second derivative of adrenaline, is made in the body in fairly substantial quantities. The only source of adrenolutin is adrenochrome. Therefore, analyzing adrenolutin gives one an indirect method of measuring adrenochrome. But so far no one has investigated whether elevated adrenolutin levels are related to schizophrenia.

(ii) That adrenochrome or some of its derivatives have hallucinogenic properties comparable to those of mescaline or LSD. We were already gearing up for our LSD studies. Thus, it would not require any major revision of our program to include adrenochrome. If these oxidation products had no hallucinogenic properties, it would be difficult to continue to sustain the adrenochrome hypothesis. Since then it has been clearly established that adrenochrome does have hallucinogenic properties in human subjects and significantly changes behaviour in every animal studied—from spiders to cats to human subjects.

(iii) That preventing or inhibiting the formation of adrenochrome would be therapeutic in treating schizophrenia. To study this sub-hypothesis, we had to create a team of psychiatrists and nurses. This phase of our research eventually became one of the major roots nourishing the development of orthomolecular psychiatry, a term invented by Linus Pauling in the report he published in *Science* in 1968.

After that meeting I began a careful literature search, looking for reports that described the use of vitamins in treating any type of psychiatric disease. I was familiar with pellagra, the vitamin B-3 deficiency disease. This dreadful pre-terminal disease is described as causing the four Ds: dermatitis, diarrhea, dementia, and death. Pellagra, like schizophrenia, is further characterized by the presence of two main sets of symptoms, and a number of secondary symptoms which arise from the first two sets. The main symptoms in both cases are disordered perceptions such as hallucinations of voices and visions, and disordered thought, such as delusions. The greatest number of papers on pellagra were written by pellagrologists between 1930 and 1945. They described how nicotinic acid and niacinamide could be used to treat early and late stages of the disease. Pellagra at one time swept through the southern United States, striking mainly the very poor, who filled the southern mental hospitals. The disease was often indistinguishable from schizophrenia. A history of nutritional problems, typical skin lesions, and a peaking of symptoms in the spring, when sufferers were more exposed to the sun, would help make the diagnosis. When it was discovered that nicotinic acid cured pellagra, it became used as the basis for a diagnostic test. If patients responded to the vitamin they were called pellagra patients. If they did not, they were labeled schizophrenic. This approach unfortunately perpetuated the dogma that only vitamin deficiency states required vitamins for treatment and, conversely, that when a patient did respond to vitamins, he or she must have had purely a vitamin deficiency disease. This dogma unfortunately prevented a serious examination of the use of *larger* doses of vitamins than were given to treat pellagra and the notion of therapeutic amounts was delayed. The pellagrologists had observed that chronic pellagrins required 600 milligrams of nicotinic acid per day to keep them well. This was then considered a huge dose, as it was 50 times as great as the dose required to protect people against developing pellagra. As I read this literature, I was not yet ready to entertain the notion that pellagra psychosis was a form of schizophrenia. That this was so became clear to me much later.

I also discovered a handful of papers that described the results of treating *non*-schizophrenic patients with small quantities of nicotinic acid. These patients suffered primarily from depression and anxiety. By then I was familiar enough with psychiatry to know that diagnosis in this field is very imprecise and that many schizophrenic patients are not assessed correctly the first time they are admitted. Often many admissions occur before the correct diagnosis is finally made. I concluded that the patients in these studies who had responded to the use of vitamin B-3 should likely be re-diagnosed as schizophrenic. I was also familiar with the research by Lewis and Pietrowski, described earlier, which showed that a correct diagnosis of schizophrenia could be made sooner if the diagnostician pays attention to the perceptual symptoms. My speculations turned out to be supported by information that emerged later. It is clear now that patients with manic-depression and depression who have no perceptual symptoms do not respond as well to vitamin B-3, in sharp contrast to those who do have these symptoms. Perceptual symptoms can be measured with the HOD test, which I describe in Chapter Eight. The largest dose of vitamin B-3 used in these studies to treat the depressed and anxious patients was 1.5 grams per day.

I also became familiar with vitamin B-3 as a methyl group acceptor in the body. The resulting compound of this methylation process is N-methyl nicotinamide, which is excreted. In 1950, it was fashionable to diagnose "methyl deficiency disease" which caused liver failure with fatty degeneration due to depletion of methyl groups. Because this vitamin was one of the few methyl acceptors, it was looked upon as a likely candidate for causing methyl deficiency disease. One of the earlier studies on rats asserted that after receiving large doses of the vitamin their livers became fatty. However, this work was shown not to be valid by Dr. R. Altschul, professor of anatomy, University of Saskatchewan in Saskatoon, some years later. He repeated the study and found no increase in liver fat and no histological changes in the rats' liver slices when examined under an electron microscope. Professor Altschul concluded that the earlier rat colonies had been infected with disease, probably a virus, something that was very common then. But the idea that niacin causes liver problems became well entrenched in medicine, on flimsy evidence, and still creates problems for physicians who use the vitamin to lower cholesterol levels. However, even in 1952 it was pretty clear that vitamin B-3 was safer than the condition we were going to treat. Schizophrenia is a very dangerous disease that leads to a host of serious side effects, including chronic invalidism and suicide. Giving nicotinic acid would be the lesser of two evils, if indeed it was an evil at all. It was not until 1957 that I became aware that between 1945 and 1950 Dr. W. Kaufman of Bridgeport, Connecticut, had used nicotinamide in doses of up to 4 grams per day for treating his arthritic patients, with great success. We knew that the LD 50 for animals was about 5 grams per kilogram of body weight. In human terms, one would have to take over half a pound daily to approach danger. This is impossible since the vitamin is bulky and would first cause severe nausea and vomiting, thereby discouraging a person from continuing to swallow more. In the years since our research began, about three deaths have been caused through the use of an unstudied slow release preparation that caused liver damage. But according to the world's top experts in niacin, the vitamin is not toxic to the liver even though its use sometimes elevates liver function tests. The increases in the liver enzymes which may occur when niacin is used do not mean that there is liver damage, unless the test results are very high. Such increases usually mean that the liver is functioning more rapidly. This also very commonly occurs with the use of many drugs that are relatively non-toxic. The liver function tests usually become normal over time even when the same dose of niacin is maintained. Unfortunately the delusion that niacin is toxic to the liver is so widespread that most doctors are afraid to use it even though they have no fear of giving very toxic drugs such as the modern anti-psychotics.

After doing this literature search and taking Woodford's ideas into account, we developed a clear rationale for investigating vitamin B-3 as a schizophrenia treatment in our studies: (1) It was a methyl acceptor and so could decrease the formation of adrenaline from noradrenaline, as it is the methylation of noradrenaline that forms adrenaline. Lowering adrenaline production would eventually mean less adrenochrome would come to be present in the patient's body. (2) It was a major component of NAD, an important enzyme. Giving large doses of the vitamin would help regenerate this enzyme. We hypothesized that this enzymatic activity would counter any possible poisoning effect from adrenochrome and its derivatives. (3) Pellagra was a vitamin B-3 deficiency disease, and it was cured by giving low and high doses of the vitamin, especially to chronic pellagrins. It was also used for conditions linked to pellagra but without the classic symptoms and signs, such as senile confusional states and conditions in adults and children then called sub-clinical pellagra.

In our first major publication in 1957, when we presented the first account of the therapeutic properties of vitamin B-3 for schizophrenics, we listed a large number of possible ways in which it could be helpful. Recently, I have become aware of another way in which it may be therapeutic for schizophrenics. Niacin dilates capillaries and thus improves blood flow and the delivery of oxygen. It also prevents adhesion of red blood cells to each other, i.e. prevents sludging. This also improves delivery of oxygen. It has been shown that schizophrenics have deficient blood distribution to the frontal lobes of the brain and these actions of niacin would counter that problem.

We decided to use vitamin C because it was a powerful antioxidant and we hoped would decrease the oxidation of adrenaline to adrenochrome. This vitamin had been used to stabilize adrenaline solutions. (Subsequent research performed by Dr. Heacock in our laboratory found that it is not very efficient at doing so. Rather, it prevents the pink color from appearing because it catalyzes the conversion of adrenochrome to yellow and colorless substances and so gives the illusion that the adrenaline solution has been stabilized.) We decided to use at least 3 grams each of vitamin B-3 and vitamin C per day in three divided doses. Our reasoning was simple. These vitamins had been given at lower doses with only partial success. We therefore felt that the original trials and pilot experiments had used inadequately low doses and that, given the strong theoretical support for their use, as well as their safety, we should double the largest dose previously given to psychiatric patients. It turned out that the dose we chose is still a good and safe starting amount for both vitamins.

VII

Pilot Trials of Vitamins for the Mentally Ill

Our first practical problem was to obtain vitamins in the quantity required to test our theories. Vitamins were available commercially at the time, but only in tablets containing very small doses, in keeping with the idea prevalent at the time that only small quantities would be required by anyone. These commercially available tablets contained so little active vitamin in fact, that most of their bulk was filler which the makers hoped was inert, but in many cases was not. If we were going to study vitamins as a schizophrenia treatment, we would need almost pure vitamin tablets or capsules. We decided to have 500 milligram tablets made up for the two forms of vitamin B-3 then known (nicotinic acid and niacinamide) and for vitamin C.

I wrote to Merck, one of the largest vitamin manufacturing companies at that time and today. The company had been a leader in determining the structure of vitamins and had at one time distributed excellent information booklets describing each one of the vitamins. I told them what we had in mind and requested that they send us ample quantities of these vitamins. Almost by return mail I received 50-pound barrels of nicotinamide, nicotinic acid, ascorbic acid (vitamin C), and riboflavin. This may have been one of the better investments this company ever made, for by sending us a few dollars worth of vitamins they helped initiate the discovery that niacin lowers cholesterol and elevates high density cholesterol. Today, niacin must be sold by the ton for this one indication alone.

The nicotinic acid, nicotinamide, and ascorbic acid were subsequently made up into 500 milligram capsules by the pharmacists of the General Hospital in Regina and the Saskatchewan Hospital in Weyburn. After I moved to University Hospital in Saskatoon in 1955, their hospital dispensary made up the capsules and later dispensed the tablets made for us by other drug companies. These vitamins were released on my prescription in Regina and in Saskatoon for research use. I think a similar procedure was used at Weyburn. Fifteen years later an experiment conducted at a California mental hospital, Metropolitan, near Los Angeles, proved that we were correct in making up our own capsules. I had given a series of lectures there outlining our work and results. The research group there decided to repeat our work but their pharmacist would not allow them to have any tablets containing more than 100 milligrams of niacin. As a result, they had to give each patient 30 tablets per day. Many patients became nauseated by the tablets due to the fillers, and the researchers had to discontinue the study. This turn of events did not prevent them, however, from claiming that they had tried to repeat our work and had not been able to get the same results we had achieved.

We had planned to examine all the main B vitamins, one at a time, later in combination. As vitamin B-3 appeared to be the most promising, we started with that one. As it turned out, we never did get around to testing large doses of riboflavin because vitamin B-3 proved so effective.

Another practical consideration involved explaining the effects of niacin to my patients. I was by now familiar with the flush it causes since I often took the vitamin myself and had persuaded many of my colleagues to take it as well. I did not like the flush. It came on soon after tablets were swallowed, showing they were readily absorbed. It started in the forehead and gradually worked its way down. In some people the flush engulfs the whole body. In most cases it stops either in the chest, abdomen, or thighs. It lasts several hours and then slowly recedes. Occasionally, it is followed by a general chill which does not last very long. As our research went on, we were able to prepare patients much more thoroughly for the flush experience. We found that very rarely, patients feel faint during or just after the flush. In fewer than ten cases, as recorded over the past forty years, patients have fainted. Interestingly, those patients who need the vitamin the most tend to flush the least. This group includes schizophrenics, alcoholics, arthritics, and elderly patients with coronary disease or high blood cholesterol.

In patients who did flush, the flush would decrease in intensity and duration with each subsequent dose until in most cases it became a minor nuisance or disappeared entirely. The flush becomes very minor in time because the steady use of niacin keeps the body's histamine levels low. I thought the flush was caused by histamine which has been released by the niacin, and when the histamine levels are low, there can no longer be any flushing. Flushing does however, return if a patient does not take the vitamin for a few days. A few patients enjoyed the sensations of warmth associated with the flush, and would often stop for a few days so that they could once more experience it.

In my clinical experience, I have noted that many schizophrenics do not flush at all until after a year or two after treatment begins, by which time they are very much better generally. When ill, their biochemistry prevents the flush, but as they improve, this ability to respond is regained. In some, however, the flush proved so troublesome that the nicotinic acid form of vitamin B-3 had to be discontinued and replaced with nicotinamide which does not cause any flushing in 99 percent of patients. However, very rarely, patients will flush on nicotinamide. They obviously have the ability to convert nicotinamide to nicotinic acid so quickly that they will flush. The best non-flush product, more recently available, is inositol niacinate. It has all the positive features of nicotinic acid and none of its side effects. But it is not as effective as pure niacin in lowering cholesterol levels. The only drawback with this preparation is its cost.

In the 1990s, David Horrobin followed up on my observation about niacin's affects and developed a diagnostic skin test for schizophrenia. In this test, one places a plastic strip containing four pockets on the skin. Each pocket is filled with a different concentration of niacin. The strip is taken off after five minutes and the skin examined. Schizophrenic patients, as compared to healthy controls, flush very little—the areas which have been exposed to the niacin seldom turn pink or red while the skin of the non-schizophrenic control much more often does. Horrobin's research has been confirmed by several universities but his test has not yet been approved by the United States Food and Drug Administration (FDA). Given that about 50 years ago it approved the use of large doses of niacin for lowering cholesterol levels, this refusal to approve Horrobin's test surely represents one of the strangest decisions of this agency.

A few days after I had received the first shipment of bulk vitamins, I drove to Weyburn to meet with Humphry and give him his first supplies of the nicotinic acid and ascorbic acid. Later, in the afternoon, a senior psychiatrist came in. He told Humphry that a patient, Ken, about 21 years old, was in a catatonic stupor and was dying. He suggested that Ken's relatives should be notified immediately so they could come in to see him. Ken had been in the hospital for several months and had not responded to insulin coma therapy nor to a series of ECT sessions. That day he lay on his bed unresponsive, not able to eat or drink. Catatonic deaths were not uncommon many years ago. Usually at autopsy there would be no pathological findings to account for the death. We decided to make him the first patient to receive massive doses of the two vitamins I had just delivered. We were certain we could not do Ken any harm since he was so close to death. We all went to the ward and inserted a tube into his stomach since he could not swallow. Then we poured in a mixture of 5 grams of nicotinic acid and 2.5 grams of ascorbic acid. We waited anxiously by his bedside after this treatment and felt relieved that he seemed to grow no worse. This fact also reassured us that the dose we had used was non-toxic, at least for this patient. He was given the same dose later that day, twice on the next, and this regimen was continued. On the second day he was able to sit up and drink his solution of vitamins. One month later he was completely normal! His family came to see him again and after their visit demanded that Ken be discharged. The psychiatrist suggested that this would be premature since he had been well for only such a short period of time, but they insisted, saying that he was well as far as they were concerned. He remained well, even though he was not given any follow-up vitamins. I interviewed him in Saskatoon many years later. He told me he had no recollection of ever having been a patient at the hospital. He was now a successful businessman and chairman of the local board of trade. As far as I could tell he was normal. Ken was the first schizophrenic patient ever given large amounts of nicotinic and ascorbic acids.

Ken's initial recovery alone was very surprising and encouraging. It showed that we could safely give large doses of niacin and vitamin C. Compared to the dangers of insulin coma treatments and ECT we could classify the vitamins as safe. In this case, they also seemed clearly effective. We ruled out the possibility of a placebo response since the whole setting had absolutely no similarity to a situation in which placebo responses are apt to occur. I do not think that putting a tube into a comatose patient is conducive to a placebo response. The fact that Ken recovered showed that at least one member of the population of schizophrenics had responded to a therapy that until then had existed only as a hypothesis. We now had to search for others who might be helped and to find a way to determine for which patients this approach would work.

The second was Miss G., a patient of mine at the Munroe Wing. She had just been admitted for the third time, and this time was placed under my care. She had been a stenographer for a large Saskatchewan corporation. Several years before this admission she had attended a Christmas party for employees and others. Following this party, she became paranoid, delusional, and fearful. She began to think that she was involved in a love affair with her boss when in fact there was no relationship. She was certain that this affair would destroy his marriage and she became very depressed. During her first admission she was given a series of ECT sessions and was well for a while afterwards. She was back at work by spring. The following

Christmas she went to such a party again, and after that the same delusions recurred. Again, she responded to a second series of ECT treatments and once again she was back at work by spring. The whole sequence was repeated for the third time the following year, when she was placed under my care. In our first interview, before I had a chance to talk to her, she hid in a closet and tried to strangle herself. I did not think there was any point in giving her more ECT and it appeared likely to me that if no improvement could be created, she would have to be committed to the Saskatchewan Hospital at Weyburn. I thought she would make a good first subject for me since the best mainstream psychiatry had to offer then did not show promise in her situation. I started her on nicotinic acid, one gram three times daily. For the first few weeks I saw no improvement. Then, slowly, she began to respond. I discharged her a few months later, advising her that she must remain on the vitamin. I arranged to see her on a follow-up basis.

A few months later her sister came with her to tell me that Miss G. was paranoid again, that she had stopped taking the nicotinic acid and would not go back on it. I was very stern with the patient and told her that if she did not keep taking this vitamin, she would end up in hospital again. She resumed her medication and was well in a few months. She eventually went off the vitamin three times. Each time the paranoid delusions recurred and each time they cleared when she resumed the vitamin. Several years later, when she had been well for a long time and working at her old job, she approached me and discussed with me whether she could try to go off once more. This time I agreed she could. She has remained well since then.

I also began to give nicotinic acid to other patients in order to gain experience with it. We had to know the optimum doses, the side effects—if any—and how best to deal with them. On May 8, 1952, I wrote to Humphry about a patient I had started on nicotinic acid one month before. I had seen her first at a one-day clinic in Swift Current, Saskatchewan. We serviced this clinic from Regina, going there by plane for the day. This is what I wrote:

One month ago, when I was in Swift Current, I saw a Mrs. R. who was recently discharged from the hospital at Weyburn where she had received ECT, diagnosis: depression. When I saw her she was quite retarded, her thinking processes were slow, she was unable to sleep or eat, and unable to perform her household activities. She appeared confused and her memory was bad. Following our nicotinic acid hunch, I placed her on one gram of nicotinic acid per day. I saw her again yesterday and there was a remarkable change in this woman. She walked in alert, relaxed, claimed that her memory had come back and she had lost all of her post-shock headaches of which she had previously complained. I was rather impressed by this and wondered if we should not try a run of nicotinic acid after shock or concurrent with shock, to prevent the memory loss, disorientation and confusion that sometimes occurs.

After these initial successes, the Saskatchewan Committee on Schizophrenia Research met for the second time at the medical school in Saskatoon on June 30, 1952. Dr. J. Lucy, a psychiatrist working with Humphry at Weyburn, was helping him with his research. He reported to us that the study of histamine as a schizophrenia treatment I had requested had gotten under way. The treatment trials at the Munroe Wing had already been started and the results were published in 1955 by Parsons and myself. Dr. Lucy found that chronic schizophrenic patients could tolerate enormous amounts of histamine by injection before their diastolic pressure went down to zero. When measuring blood pressure two readings are taken, systolic and diastolic. It was amazing to see patients lying comfortably on their bed with a zero diastolic reading after receiving their histamine injections. Humphry and I would spend many hours discussing the implications of this abnormal tolerance to huge amounts of histamine.

Dr. Osmond reported the results of giving nicotinic acid to six schizophrenic patients in the hospital at Weyburn.

1. Mr. P.B. was referred to the Saskatchewan Hospital from the Munroe Wing because he appeared to have either a chronic Alzheimer's disease or catatonic schizophrenia. After arrival at Weyburn, he was very quiet for a few days but then became

acutely psychotic. He had delusions about his clothing, and expressed fears that he would be killed, poisoned and executed. He was started on nicotinamide, one gram daily, and in four days his behaviour returned to normal. He remained in hospital for six months and was discharged well.

2. Mr. K.C. was the first patient who had been given vitamin treatment, as described earlier in this chapter, and had recovered from a coma to become normal.

3. Mrs. L., age 50, had had several previous admissions. She showed both manic and schizophrenic symptoms. She had responded temporarily to ECT. She believed that everyone was listening in on her, that radio broadcasts were being made about her, so she began to try to tear up the air registers and plug the pipes. She was started on five grams per day of vitamins C and B-3, and within two weeks was much better and no longer presented a nursing problem. However she relapsed a few weeks later, but not back to her original psychotic state.

4. Mrs. L., age 25, was a post-partum schizophrenic. She was given ECT at the hospital, which provided temporary relief. Later she received 60 insulin coma treatments, which brought no improvement. She was started on niacin and vitamin C. One week later she was better and two weeks later she was well enough to be discharged.

5. Mr. M., age 32, was severely disturbed. He was noisy, tiresome, frightened the staff, and exhibited severe anger. He was started on nicotinic acid, given three ECT treatments and was well within three days.

6. Mr. M., age 39, was very ill when admitted. He repeatedly said, "It is too late." He masturbated openly, paced aimlessly, was dirty and unkempt. This was his second attack in 18 months. He was started on 10 grams of each vitamin daily and within three days was well.

I reported on two patients who had recovered with vitamin B-3. The first was Miss G. I have already described her response above, and I summarized her case for the meeting. The second was a Mr. F., age 39, who had been ill for three months. He was very depressed on admission and had an interesting, very firm delusional system. He was a veteran of World War II and had served well and honorably. On discharge, he went back to his farm in rural Saskatchewan and ran it successfully. Before admission he began to suspect that everyone in the community was opposed to him, that even the Canadian army had plotted against him. During the war, he and two friends had moved too far from the Canadian lines and, as they had raced back, his two friends had been killed and he, wounded. In his paranoid state he had concluded that the whole exercise had been set up by the army in order to test him; he could not believe his two friends were really dead. He then received a copy of his regimental history and there he saw his friends listed as killed in action. He concluded that the army had printed a special issue just for him so as to maintain the conspiracy. He was given one gram of nicotinic acid per day. Ten days later he left the hospital without notice. When his father brought him back he told me that Mr. F. had been so convinced the whole community was talking about him he had had to go home to check the situation out. I increased his vitamin dose to one gram twice daily, and after a few weeks he began to become doubtful about the validity of his delusions. He was discharged and recovered at home on maintenance nicotinic acid.

These brief descriptions are an account of what occurred in the first eight attempts at high-dose vitamin therapy with diagnosed schizophrenic patients. Today I know we were actually giving small doses.

All of us were tremendously excited, but, so strong was the belief by psychiatrists that there was no effective treatment for schizophrenia, we remained very cautious about publishing any information. We considered these results to be part of a preliminary pilot that would help us determine optimum doses and potential toxicity levels. We discussed starting well-controlled studies. Humphry and I believed that the reason ECT and insulin coma were in the long run not effective was because no chronic disease can be expected to respond to occasional treatment. The schizophrenia treatment protocols of the time could be compared to treating a diabetic for a few weeks and then taking the patient off insulin. Dr. Osmond now discussed the need for continuous long-term treatment with the committee. It was possible to give it with nicotinic acid. We also considered some of the mechanisms by which the vitamin might act.

We discussed how changing what is called the pyridine ring in LSD (one of the two rings of atoms that create the indole nucleus of the molecule) by adding something to it removed LSD's hallucinogenic action. We theorized that this occurred because the changed pyridine ring could not be absorbed in certain critical brain centres. We wondered if flooding the body with nicotinic acid might act as an antidote against LSD, by supplying a substance that was added to the pyridine ring. Woodford discussed the role that l-tryptophan might play in the genesis of schizophrenia since it is an indole and its derivatives are indoles. Closure of this protein's side chain would produce a substance very similar in structure to harmaline, also a hallucinogen. After a few routine business matters were taken care of, we agreed to meet again at the Saskatchewan Hospital in Weyburn. By regularly changing meeting locations, we felt we would be able to involve people from all the research units as they developed.

After that second meeting, I continued to plan and carry on our research program. We had selected vitamin C as a research topic because of its antioxidant properties. But I had not yet used it alone, only in combination with vitamin B-3. At this time, an opportunity arose for testing out the effect of vitamin C alone. A middle-aged psychotic woman was brought into the hospital. She had had a mastectomy many weeks before, and following this had developed a massive infection that had lasted for weeks. The wound would not heal. Then, her psychiatrist diagnosed her schizophrenic and decided to give her ECT, the only effective treatment available to us. I approached him and asked whether he would consider delaying the use of ECT so that I could test her response to vitamin C alone. He agreed he would withhold the ECT for four days and start her the next Monday, rather than on Friday, as he had planned. My initial plan had been to give her three grams per day, but when I realized I had only a few days, I saw that this approach would be futile. I therefore decided on a really massive dose. I ordered she be given one gram of vitamin C each hour, day and night. If she slept for five hours, for example, when she awakened she was to be given the five grams that she had missed. We started on Saturday morning. By Monday morning she had taken 45 grams of vitamin C. When her psychiatrist came to give her the ECT treatment on Monday morning, he found that she was no longer psychotic. In addition, her infection had begun to heal. She was discharged as mentally normal, but was not given any follow-up vitamin prescription. She died six months later from her cancer, still mentally normal. I had no interest in cancer but was impressed with her response to the vitamin C, which had cleared her psychosis and saved her from ECT. This experiment proved that even massive doses of the vitamin were safe and that some psychotic patients would respond to it even when used alone. I did not pursue this line of inquiry any further at that time, but later tried a few more therapeutic trials of isolated vitamin C using 10 grams per day over a long period of time. Based on my clinical observations, it became my policy to always use vitamin C in combination with vitamin B-3, except in our double-blind experiments (described in the next chapter) where the design in order to facilitate statistical analysis, called for only one vitamin as the main therapeutic variable.

In the summer following this second meeting, I also continued to study the psychiatric literature by reading as much as I could, and by participating in the training program all we residents were doing to prepare ourselves for the specialist examinations in psychiatry. There was then no formal set of requirements for a fellowship, but a training program had been instituted at all Canadian mental illness care facilities which allowed residents in psychiatry to write a set of written exams after four years, and if these were passed, to undergo oral exams at one of the psychiatric centres. Our specialty training included regular seminars at the Munroe Wing. These were attended by the nurses and social workers as well. There were also two types of conferences. The most important were case conferences where patients' histories were presented, the patient was interviewed, and vigorous discussion about the diagnosis ensued. Treatment suggestions were made. These conferences could last several hours.

After the second year of training, the resident staff fell into two points of view with respect to causes and treatment. Psychoanalysis had grown very quickly and had become the branch of psychiatry to which most residents aspired. We, therefore, had a group of physicians who became strong believers in Freud and interpreted all their patients' problems in Freudian terms. I had also started out as a Freudian, I think simply because there was no other paradigm available which promised so much. However, I became more and more skeptical the more experience I gained in psychoanalysis. During my first two years in residency, I gave every one of my patients three hours per week of psychotherapy. Since I had twelve to thirteen patients on my list it was not possible to give them each that much individual therapy. Group psychotherapy was becoming very popular at that time and we had had several seminars on groups. I decided that I would see each one of my patients once per week individually and twice each week in group therapy. I divided my patients into two groups, each with six or seven members. I was the group leader. I thought I could research group therapy as well. My first secretary, paid for through the first research grant we received in 1952, sat in with each group and recorded its conversations in short-hand. At first I thought her presence would inhibit free and open discussions, but it did not. In fact, once the groups were established, she became an integral part of the meetings. On several occasions, when she could not be there, the group could not get going. We had more fruitful discussions when she was there.

All in all I conducted four group sessions each week for several years, spending about 17 hours in psychotherapy per week, or about one-half the required working hours. (The rest of the time I did research, met in conferences, dictated the clinical notes, and participated in the teaching program for the nurses.) After each group session, I would dictate my notes using one of the first dictating machines then available and the secretary would then transcribe the notes. I finally completely lost interest in the practicality of analysis after I began to prepare a series of articles describing the psychodynamics of the seven "psychosomatic diseases." These were the same diseases that had been studied by Franz Alexander at the Chicago School of Psychoanalysis. The result of all this activity was that I concluded that although group therapy was interesting and patients found it helpful, I did not see any major improvement in their symptoms.

I had proposed to the psychiatric staff of the Munroe Wing, the Weyburn hospital, and the hospital in North Battleford, that we publish a departmental journal which could be used in our training efforts and for presenting our research findings to one another. (The Saskatchewan Hospital at North Battleford was the second large mental hospital in the province, located about 100 miles northwest of Saskatoon. It had a small research unit.) The journal would be available to every psychiatrist in Saskatchewan's Psychiatric Services Branch. I volunteered to be the editor, provided the resident psychiatrists would also do some of the writing. I called it the *Saskatchewan Psychiatric Journal*. The venture did not last very long because very few psychiatrists contributed what they had promised and I got tired of writing most of it myself. I had arranged that we would do a series on psychodynamics for the seven psychodynamic diseases, assigning each disease to a different psychiatrist. But no manuscripts came in. I prepared the first one. Then, when I needed more material, I prepared the second one, and I believe I finally wrote a third. By that time, it was clear to me that every psychodynamic interpretation was exactly the same for all the diseases. They all had to do with sex, with the relation between a concavity, the vagina, and a convexity, the penis. It simply did not make any sense to me to call on the same dynamics to explain diseases as diverse as hyperthyroidism and ulcerative colitis. I finally concluded there was nothing to psychoanalysis.

To return to the training program, we also held a conference every morning concerning admissions and general problems; it began every morning at 8.00 am. The chief nurse, Marg Callbeck, would tell us about patients admitted the previous day and the reasons for their admission as well as the problems presented by other patients. Often these morning conferences ran more than an hour.

Each patient conference ended in vigorous discussions of the patient's psychodynamics, the correct diagnosis, and the best treatment. Of course, the only treatments then available were ECT and psychotherapy, so this last part of our discussion remained rather limited. Since we could not spend much time talking about treatment, we spent most of it talking and arguing about dynamics and diagnosis. Diagnosis was very imprecise and was heavily influenced by psychodynamics. I recall one conference very vividly; the psychiatrist presenting the case of a paranoid schizophrenic stated that underlying it was his homosexuality. This surprised me since no evidence had been presented that the patient had ever engaged in homosexual activity, nor that he was even what we then called a latent homosexual. (The word "gay" had not yet become a noun.) I asked the psychiatrist to provide evidence for his conclusion and he replied hotly that since the patient was paranoid, therefore he had to be a homosexual, according to Freud. Freud had described only one case in which he had come to this conclusion, but already this case was becoming the basis for a universal statement of fact in the psychiatry of 1952! These conferences did force us to examine the principles of psychiatry very carefully. I believe we learned more this way then had we simply been given a series of lectures outlining the same material. Most of the candidates for their specialty who I trained with would pass their exams.

In addition to these internal lectures and conferences, Dr. McKerracher regularly arranged to bring in from elsewhere well-known psychiatrists who would give us seminars from their own field. The most prominent of these was Dr. Karl Menninger, who by then was world famous. Dr. Menninger came with his young wife and son and spent two weeks with us. He gave us a series of lectures on psychoanalysis at the Munroe Wing. Psychiatrists came from Weyburn to participate in this program. Dr. Menninger did not try to proselytize. He was matter-of-fact about psychoanalysis. He considered it a research tool, not a modality which was particularly beneficial as a treatment. He did not advise that all psychiatrists be analyzed. He was a very good speaker. Many years after I met him, when he was in his eighties, he wrote to me. He said that he was concerned about his memory and wanted to know what kind of a vitamin program he ought to follow to reverse the changes he was experiencing. He had been advised to write to me by a former resident of the Menninger Clinic with whom he had maintained a close relationship, an enthusiastic orthomolecular psychiatrist. I immediately sent Dr. Menninger a long letter outlining what I thought he ought to be taking. Whether he followed my program I have no way of telling. He did live many years after that, into his nineties, and remained productive to the end of his life.

The training program Dr. McKerracher organized for us was very good, in spite of the fact that we did not have a medical school and very few formal lectures. I must give a great deal of credit to Dr. McKerracher for his wisdom in constructing such a thorough program. We wrote our final exams in 1954 and I passed. Later, Dr. McKerracher told me that I had come in with the second highest mark in Canada for that year. Then we went to Edmonton by train for the oral psychiatric finals. I passed these as well and in due course received my certificate qualifying me as a psychiatrist. A few years later the Royal College of Physicians and Surgeons set up the psychiatric fellowship degree which is current today. All who then had certificates were automatically awarded the fellowship. I was pleased at the time that I did not have to write another set of examinations.

VIII

DOUBLE-BLIND THERAPEUTIC TRIALS OF NIACIN

I was familiar with biostatistical methods for evaluating the results of drug trials since I had studied these methods as applied to agriculture. If one wanted to study the effect of fertilizer on crop yield, one would divide the land into plots, and according to a random scheme, apply the fertilizer to some plots and not to others. By measuring the growth of the plants in fertilized and non-fertilized plots, one could arrive at a true comparison between the effects of fertilizer as compared to no fertilizer. The technique worked well because one dealt with large numbers of individual plants. Using this approach in human studies immediately raised the issue of how could one randomly select subjects. With plants and animals one did not need to be concerned about the effect of faith or attitudes. With human subjects, these are so essential to the therapeutic process that it is virtually impossible to assign patients to random groups. Indeed, in the 1950s, awareness of the placebo effect (a positive response to fake treatments) was emerging in the literature to the point that, for a time, a new professional group called placebodologists plied their trade. They seem not to be around anymore. I wondered even then why anyone found the discovery that patients' expectations and hopes played a role in determining how they responded to treatment surprising. This should not have been surprising. It is patently obvious that if a patient has no hope, he or she will not even follow through with any treatment regimen. In my opinion, the power of placebo was grossly exaggerated. But it was in response to the placebo's distorting influence as well as to the problem of researcher bias, that the "double dummy" experiment was introduced in England and soon was taken over by American scientists and dubbed the double-blind technique.

In a single blind experiment, patients do not know whether they are getting an active drug or a dummy or placebo pill. Only the evaluating physician knows what the patients are getting. It is therefore possible that the physician's own biases and faith may determine how that drug will be assessed. If the physician is very pleased with the drug or if he has received a large grant of money to persuade him to do the study, he may be tempted to overvalue the remedy's efficacy. In a double-blind test, the evaluating therapist also does not know what the patients have been getting. As the word spread, the medical establishment assumed that the double-blind experiment design represented a superb way of eliminating both the patients' placebo effect and the evaluating therapists' bias.

In 1952, I and my research team had not yet even heard about the double-blind method. We had begun our pilot studies and planned on doing large scale open clinical experiments of the type that had been the mainstay of experimental medicine for centuries. This method depended upon the clinical acumen of the treating doctor, who would evaluate results by comparing them against what would have been expected from other treatment or from no treatment at all, i.e. against the known natural history of the illness. As previously described, we had applied to Ottawa for grant money with which to do such open clinical studies. Soon after submitting our proposal, in the early months of 1952, we heard from Dr. C. Roberts, with the Department of Health and Welfare in Ottawa, about a study that had recently been completed in Montreal by a chemist named Seguin. Seguin had discovered a protein compound (a particular type of nucleotide) that he said produced a fifty percent response in schizophrenia patients. He had managed to interest a drug company in making the material and selling it as a treatment for schizophrenia.

However, the Department of Health and Welfare wanted further studies to be completed before the new compound became freely available. None of the eastern research groups were interested, so Dr. Roberts contacted us. Intrigued by a potentially valuable new treatment, we agreed to add Seguin's compound to our research program.

Humphry and I went to Ottawa to meet and make arrangements with the Department as well as the drug company. In Ottawa, we also met Dr. Roberts' employee, Dr. Bud Fisher. Dr. Fisher was a virologist who had unfortunately been infected and severely damaged by a virus with which he had been working. He was ordered never to go into the laboratory again and was given the job of evaluating grant requests. He was also a biostatistical consultant. He had just completed a new application form that would be used by grant applicants in future. The application form contained questions having to do with how the project results would be evaluated, what mathematical techniques would be used and so on. He introduced us to the double-blind technique. With Dr. Fisher's help, we prepared a study protocol that would test Seguin's preparation via the double-blind method. These studies were begun before our vitamin B-3 trials got underway. On completion, the results would indicate that the compound Seguin was using was useless in schizophrenia treatment. In this work with Roberts and Fisher, we quickly realized that our chance of getting the grant would be much better if we indicated that we were willing to shift from open to double-blinded studies. We were desperate for the money and having no understanding of the limitations of the method, we immediately decided to take up this new technique. Fisher advised us that in the double-blind study, only one treatment could be examined at a time. We decided to drop ascorbic acid from our planned research, but refused to discontinue ECT. In the short run, it was the only effective treatment and if we had not been able to use it we would have given up the main therapy capable of controlling very aggressive, hostile behaviour on the ward and would also have lost a way of helping patients with severe suicidal depression. We therefore worked ECT into the design of our first double-blind experiments.

We did not know that in following Ottawa's lead on this issue, we would become the first psychiatric group anywhere in the world to do double-blind experiments. (Perhaps if we had known this, and if we had looked upon the method as a significant improvement, we would have published our study design and results immediately, and with great fanfare, in 1952.) We finally published the method we had used in the *Menninger Bulletin*, in 1954.

The design we used for the first vitamin B-3 double-blind therapeutic trials is also described in my book ***Vitamin B-3 & Schizophrenia: Discovery, Recovery, Controversy***, CCNM Press, Toronto, 1998, pages 38 to 54. We used three treatments: placebo, niacinamide, or niacin, giving patients one gram three times per day for thirty days. We could not use only niacin and placebo, because the niacin flush would immediately betray to staff who was taking it; with niacinamide there was no flushing. However, we informed clinical staff that only niacin and placebo were being used. They therefore thought all patients who flushed were on niacin, and that the remainder were on placebo. In fact, half of those patients who did not flush were on niacinamide, and the other half were on placebo.

The three treatments were assigned randomly. After discharge the patients were visited by a trained social worker, Mr. I. Kahan, who administered a standardized questionnaire. They were seen by Mr. Kahan every three months until one year had passed. His evaluations were also conducted blind. After two years the code was opened up.

I was not surprised by the results since I had already seen so many patients respond well to vitamin B-3. Nine of the 30 patients received placebo and three were well one year later. Ten received niacin and eight were well one year later; eleven had received niacinamide and nine were well. Niacin had improved the two-year recovery rate from 33 percent to 80 percent as compared to placebo.

We reported these results to the province's psychiatric workers at a clinical meeting attended by physicians, nurses, and social workers. The reaction was mixed; there was no sudden burst of enthusiasm. I believe it was difficult for these professional workers to believe that a vitamin could help a disease as stubborn, terrifying, and mysterious as schizophrenia. Dr. McKerracher, our chief, remarked that if these results held we would get the Nobel Prize. I became very uneasy on hearing this, for it was an ambivalent statement It could as well have meant that since it was highly unlikely that we would ever get that prize he thought it was also highly unlikely our results would hold. He urged us not to publish as it would be premature to do so and to conduct further controlled studies. This we were happy to do. All the controlled studies that followed yielded the same results in favour of niacin therapy. Altogether, we completed six double-blind controlled, randomized trials between 1953 and 1960 with adults, and two additional such studies with children. These studies all showed a major improvement in the two year recovery rate, from 35 to 75 percent.

We did finally announce our results in 1957, in the ***Journal of Clinical Experimental Psychopathology*** published by Arthur Sackler, one of the Sackler brothers whose histamine work our group had corroborated. By then, we had published our adrenochrome hypothesis, eliciting intense controversy, as few scientists believed adrenochrome was produced in the body or that it had hallucinogenic properties. To this day, I wonder if our first paper on schizophrenia treatment with niacin would even have been published, had Arthur Sackler not been both my professional colleague and friend.

Few psychiatrists were aware that we were the first to do psychiatric double-blind experiments and the first to publish the method in the psychiatric literature, and as a result, we have been criticized for not having done controlled experiments with vitamin B-3. Today, I find this criticism ironic. For the truth is, the more Humphry and I did double-blind studies, the less we came to respect them.

A primary problem with blinded studies, single or double, is that they are unethical—they involve lying to patients. In this context, the giving of informed consent is impossible. If patients are told of the experiment, they are advised that they may or may not be getting the active compound. Usually patients are not even told of the experiment since they do not like the idea of being fooled, of taking something which is inert. Those who agree to take part in a blind study usually end up feeling foolish and they lose trust in their doctor, who has played this trick on them. Many years ago, I tried to run a blinded experiment with my patients when I was in private practice, in which I planned to compare an older, well-known antidepressant against a new one which was supposed to be even better. I explained all this to my patients, assuring them that by participating in the study they could never be any worse off and were taking a fifty percent chance that they would respond much better than to the old drug. A small group agreed to take part. But after I started my study, I found that within this group, the number of patients who failed to keep their appointments became so great I could not complete the study. Normally, about five to ten percent of patients do not keep their appointments. In this study the percentage climbed much higher than that. I concluded that when I offered these patients the chance to participate in the study, they lost their confidence in me and showed it by not coming back to see me any more. They did not like feeling that I knew something about their treatment that they did not. I have never tried to run this kind of therapeutic trial since.

Another issue to consider is the blind faith research physicians have that this type of study eliminates placebo and bias effects. Not a single experiment designed to test this basic proposition has ever been done, yet it has become one of the strongest articles of faith in the research community. I call this attitude faith because it is not scientific to use a technique which has not passed the test of hard experiment. My observation over the years has been that these studies do not eliminate bias as it's usually possible, even easy, for patients to figure out what they're getting and break the code. Drug companies also routinely manipulate the results of double-blind studies by testing compounds on those populations least likely to experience side effects.

Following our original use of the double-blind experiment in psychiatry, Dr. Osmond and I published a series of papers questioning the method and describing why, in our opinion, it was defective.

Today, many research scientists are opposed to it on principle. I have not, however, seen anyone claim it produced defective results in our original trials. In any case, those results have been confirmed in my clinical practice, and the practices of numerous other psychiatrists, over and over again.

In the double-blind study, we have our new naked emperor, clothed by the imagination and misconceptions of research establishments. I consider it an expensive, inappropriate, unethical way of testing treatment in people, useful only for obtaining research grants and for making it easier to publish in standard medical journals. I cannot recall a single successful new medical treatment that has emerged over the course of my career that depended upon the double-blind method for its introduction.

The HOD Test

Research is always an unpredictable enterprise. We never intended to get involved in opposing the double-blind experiment. Neither did we expect that our trials would indirectly help us develop two new diagnostic tests for schizophrenia. This turn of events could just as easily have happened had we done open trials; but since we did not, the origin of these tests is linked to our double-blind studies.

As we moved into our research, I asked Dr. Neil Agnew, our first psychologist and later the Munroe Wing's chief research psychologist, to examine the world literature for a diagnostic test for schizophrenia which we could use in our studies, as back-up to our clinical assessments. We also sent him to the United States to work for several months with a famous psychologist, Dr. James Cattell, who had developed a comprehensive set of tests for mentally ill patients. After Agnew came back, he selected those tests from all the ones he knew about that he thought would be most helpful. We incorporated his selections into the protocols that we used in testing vitamin B-3 as a schizophrenia treatment. The tests were included in our first two double-blind studies, during both pre- and post-treatment assessment. I met with Dr. Agnew after these studies were completed to ask him what he thought of the tests we had used. His conclusions were highly unsatisfactory to me.

He said that not one of the tests had yielded results that correlated with our clinical findings. Dr. Agnew went on to maintain that no accurate test for schizophrenia would ever be developed because the diagnosis was subjective; psychiatrists could not agree amongst themselves as to who had the illness and who did not. His ideas were certainly correct insofar as at the time, schizophrenia diagnosis was largely subjective and major disagreement did exist among psychiatrists as to the proper criteria for a diagnosis. At times our discussion became heated. At one of these moments I remarked that since psychology had failed to come up with something helpful in diagnosis, I would have to develop an objective test myself. I added that the test would be so objective, its accuracy at detecting schizophrenia would be comparable to a weigh scale's ability to measure an object's weight.

That evening, I pondered this conversation and the problem of creating a good objective diagnostic test. For the first time since becoming a physician, I asked myself how I established a diagnosis. The first step I took, I realized, was to ask questions that helped me establish the history of the disease. By wording my questions carefully, I guided my patients to and through the relevant material. Patients generally responded with either a yes or a no; sometimes they could not be certain. But the majority of the questions I asked could be answered "yes" or "no." I determined the diagnosis according to the number and nature of the questions answered with a "yes." For example, I as a physician may ask, (1) "Do you have pain in your chest?" (2) Does it hurt more when you breathe?" and (3) "Do you have a cough?" If the patient's answer to these three simple questions is yes, then I begin to suspect that the pneumonia syndrome is present. But that syndrome may involve a bacteria, virus, fungus, or cancer, and so on. The second stage of diagnosis, therefore, consists in running specific tests that will rule out an incorrect diagnosis, rule in the correct one, and reveal the underlying factors at work in the illness. I realized that I saw the difference between a good and less skilled diagnostician as lying in the ability to ask the correct questions.

I had by this time accepted Dr. John Conolly's definition of schizophrenia, made in the nineteenth century, as a disease of perception combined with an inability to tell if the perceptual changes experienced were real or not. Schizophrenia therefore presents a combination of perceptual disturbances (visual and auditory hallucinations) and thought disorder (thinking based on the false perceptual material). Mood and behavioural changes are usually secondary, and arise as reactions to the basic changes in perception and thinking. As I thought about the way in which the illness manifests, it struck me that what was needed was a simple psychological test that would work with the experiential world of the patients. Both Humphry and I had a pretty good idea of what that experiential world was like, both from the hundreds of patient interviews we had conducted, and from our own experiences with the hallucinogenic effects of mescaline, adrenochrome, and LSD.

It further occurred to me that we often asked questions of the patient intended to elicit a description of the perceptual world being experienced, for example, "Do you hear voices?", "Do you see visions?", and "Do you think that people are talking about you?" I suddenly saw that the same questions could be asked by writing them down on cards, one question per card, and asking the patient to answer by placing each card in one of two boxes—one marked true, the other false. The cards placed in the true box would describe the world as perceived by the patient at the time the test was given. The schizophrenic patient would choose as true those cards that described the perceptual world of an individual with schizophrenia. As a patient became well and perceptual changes disappeared, many cards first chosen as true would be placed in the false box.

This test would be more objective than those currently available because patients would take it on their own. The test would provide a quick, easy way of asking patients a large number of questions, a larger number than would be possible otherwise, as asking and answering all those questions verbally would be tiring to patient and examiner both. If we assigned each card a point value, we could generate a number that could be correlated to the intensity of a person's perceptual changes. The higher the number, the more certain we could be that the patient was suffering from schizophrenia.

I discussed these ideas with Humphry; he thought they had great promise. Our next step would be to develop an appropriate set of questions. Both Humphry and I worked on this, drawing on our assessments of what the average schizophrenic patient experienced. Our second step would be to administer the test to a large population of patients of all types and to compare the results against their clinical diagnoses as well as against those obtained with normal subjects. After this exercise, we would be able to narrow down the questions to those most likely true for schizophrenic patients.

We prepared 145 cards, each with one question on one side and a number on the other. I began to test my patients. I also left two sets of cards at the University Hospital psychiatric ward and instructed the nursing staff to give the test to every patient admitted to the psychiatric ward. Each day I picked up the test results and examined them. I did not want to leave this data at the ward where these patients' therapists might be influenced by it. After I had accumulated about 30 test results, I compared the outcomes against the diagnosis established at the hospital. This first assessment of the new test indicated that it was viable. It sorted the schizophrenics from the other patients with a high degree of certainty. Such was the beginning of the Hoffer Osmond Diagnostic test (HOD).

We eventually used a final version of the HOD test with thousands of patients and normal subjects. With time, I found that when a disagreement existed between the test results and the initial clinical diagnosis, if I waited long enough, the clinician, even without knowing what the HOD test had shown, would very often change the diagnosis to agree with the test. Our positive results with the HOD test are recorded in the medical literature. In my opinion, it remains one of the most valuable diagnostic tests for schizophrenia available.

In 1962, Professor Harold Kelm, Professor of Psychology at the University of Saskatchewan, joined us and made major and valuable contributions to the refinement of the test and to the publication of our book which described it.

In 1960, I met Dr. L.J. Meduna in Chicago. He was Editor in Chief, *Journal of Neuropsychiatry*, and Professor of Psychiatry, University of Illinois College of Medicine. Dr. Meduna had discovered ECT as a schizophrenia treatment while working in Budapest under Karl Schaffer at the Interacademic Brain Research Institute. In the United States, Dr. Meduna remained dedicated to taking a biologically-based approach to this disease, in sharp contrast with American psychiatry's ongoing desertion of medicine in favour of psychoanalysis. I told Dr. Meduna about our work with the HOD test as well as a chemical test we had developed for some forms of schizophrenia, based on the mauve factor, described in Chapter Ten. He agreed to publish our papers on these topics, and in an unusual display of generosity, gave us almost the entire journal, Volume 2, No. 6, August 1961, which was published with a dedication to our research group.

In 1962, Dr. Osmond, by that time director of psychiatric research at the Bureau of Neurology and Psychiatry at Princeton University in New Jersey (where he had taken a post formerly held by Joe Tobin after leaving our unit in 1961), used the same basic strategy as had informed the creation of the HOD test to develop the Experiential World Inventory test in collaboration with his chief research psychologist, Moneim El-Melegi. The EWI is a more sophisticated test than the HOD, utilizing a much larger number of questions and a different scoring system. It is probably the most accurate diagnostic test for schizophrenia available. I have given both the HOD and the EWI to hundreds of patients and the EWI will often indicate the presence of schizophrenia when it has been missed by the HOD test. Unfortunately, only a few psychiatrists practising today actually use these tests. The vast majority remain unaware of them, as is also true for almost all psychologists. Both tests are available in convenient computerized versions, so the scores can be tabulated very quickly— and immense sums of money can be saved when an early accurate diagnosis of schizophrenia is made. (See *Healing Schizophrenia*)

IX

Pure Adrenochrome: Its Synthesis and Hallucinogenic Properties

When we first announced it, the adrenochrome hypothesis of schizophrenia elicited huge controversy. Many psychiatrists and researchers maintained that adrenochrome could not be made in the body, and as a result, our niacin treatment for schizophrenia must be worthless, since it was based on a faulty hypothesis.

I will start this chapter on adrenochrome and its properties by leaping into the compound's future.

In 1989, Professor Robert E. Beamish and his group of researchers at the Division of Cardiovascular Science, St. Boniface General Hospital Research Centre and the Department of Physiology, University of Manitoba, in Winnipeg, published on adrenaline derivatives in the body and their effects on the heart. They showed that it is primarily in the heart muscle that adrenaline is converted into adrenochrome. They settled the question of whether adrenochrome is made in the body once and for all.

Now, back to the 1950s. We held our third meeting of the Saskatchewan Committee on Schizophrenia Research in Weyburn on September 4, 1952. We discussed a number of business items. The first was a trip to New York that I planned to take with Humphry Osmond. We had contacted the Dementia Praecox Committee of the Scottish Rites Masons and had been invited to meet with them and present our research program. This presentation and the results it obtained will be discussed in detail later.

Secondly, Professor Woodford reviewed his work with brain tissue metabolism. He had found that whole cells were not inhibited by mescaline and LSD, that the cell membrane had to be broken for this to happen. This meant that these two substances could not enter the intact cell.

During the months in which we had undertaken our first double-blind trials of niacin therapy, we had also given small sums of money to the University of Saskatchewan so that Professor D.E. Hutcheon could synthesize and study the properties of adrenochrome and adrenolutin. Norman Eade, Hutcheon's student, had made adreno-chrome and had tested it on rats to determine how lethal it was. At this meeting, Professor Hutcheon reported he had made pure adrenochrome and that its toxicity was 3 milligrams per mouse for a 20 gram animal. This result indicated that it would be safe to give adrenochrome to human subjects, at least from a physical point of view. He also found it lowered the body temperature of the animals. He stored the adrenochrome under nitrogen in glass-sealed contain-ers and we kept it in a deep freeze. At room temperature it was very unstable, quickly becoming black and developing black specks. He also mentioned he had given some to Professor Woodford for use in tests on cell metabolism.

Fourthly, our research psychologist, Ben Stefaniuk who was working with Humphry at Weyburn reported on experiments with LSD given to volunteers and the method he and his group had devised for studying LSD-related phenomena. The next morning he took 200 micrograms of LSD to demonstrate the compound's effects to those members of the research committee who were interested.

Finally, we had a distinguished visiting psychiatrist at this meeting, Dr. D. Blaine, then president of the American Psychiatric Associ-ation. He told us about work that Professor Robert Heath was doing at Tulane University. Heath was placing electrodes deep into the brains of schizophrenic patients and finding irregularities in their electroencephalogram readings. He also told us that at Cleveland

Accepting Hospital they were giving chronic schizophrenia patients 300 milligrams per day of cortisone and that they became well and stayed well as long as they remained on the medication. (In the long run, this latter study could not be confirmed. Since then, cortisone has been found capable of inducing psychosis.) We then planned our next few meetings, to be held in Saskatoon.

Our first experiments in 1952, intended to test adrenochrome's hallucinogenic properties, were performed with the unstable product Hutcheon had described at the meeting. We took precautions to use it as soon as possible after we opened the vials in which it had been sealed. We agreed that before we asked any volunteers to take adrenochrome we would take it ourselves. This would give us a good deal of information about what it might do and would later give us confidence that we would not harm our volunteer subjects when they took it. We did not know what the effective dose would be. We guessed it would be somewhere between the effective dose of LSD, about 100 micrograms, to the effective dose of mescaline, about 300 milligrams. We decided to start with a very small dose given intramuscularly and then to increase the dose each time until we found what we thought to be the most effective dose. One of us would start, then we would switch to the other with the new dose, then back to the first one, each time increasing the amount. This is how we described these early experiments in 1954: "The first subject (Abram Hoffer) received what we supposed was 0.1 mg in 1 cc of water subcutaneously. This makes a fine port-wine coloured liquid. The injection was accompanied by a sharp and persistent pain at the site of the injection. There were no recognizable psychological changes. Blood pressure and pulse readings taken every five minutes for half an hour showed no change. The second subject (Humphry Osmond) was given what we believed was 0.5 mg. Again there were no pressor effects but there were marked psychological changes. Later Abram Hoffer and his wife both took 10 mg doses intravenously and had marked changes, particularly in affect and behaviour. Abram Hoffer became overactive, showed poor judgment and lack of insight. Rose Hoffer became deeply depressed for four days and endured a condition which was indistinguishable from an endogenous depression.

Here are a few excerpts from Humphry Osmond's account: "After the purple red liquid was injected into my right forearm (October 10, 1952) I had a good deal of pain. I did not expect that we would get any results from a preliminary trial and so was not, as far as I can judge, in a state of heightened expectancy. After about 10 minutes, while I was lying on the couch looking up at the ceiling, I found that it had changed colour. It seemed that the lighting had become brighter. I asked Abe and Neil if they had noticed anything but they had not. I looked across the room and it seemed to have changed in some not easily definable way. I wondered if I could have suggested these things to myself. I closed my eyes and a brightly coloured pattern of dots appeared. The colours were not as brilliant as those which I have seen under mescal, but they were of the same type. The pattern of dots gradually resolved themselves into fish-like shapes. I felt that I was at the bottom of the sea or in an aquarium among a shoal of fishes.

My experiences in the laboratory were, on the whole pleasant but when I left I found the corridors outside sinister and unfriendly. I wondered what the cracks in the floor meant and why there were so many of them. Once we got out of doors the hospital buildings, which I know well, seemed sharp and unfamiliar. As we drove through the streets the houses appeared to have some special meaning, but I couldn't tell what it was. We reached Abe's home where I felt cut off from people but not unhappy.

Later Dr. Osmond took adrenochrome again, five milligrams of it. This time the changes were more clear to Humphry and to the observers. We noted that he withdrew from people and his behaviour became very uncharacteristic. He became preoccupied with inanimate objects, became negativistic, showed loosening of the associative process, anxiety, and distractibility. After I took my fourth or fifth dose of adrenochrome, I became depressed for two weeks with paranoid ideas which suddenly lifted as if a weight had been removed from my back. I will never forget those two weeks.

Based on these early experiments and others, we reported in a large number of papers published in the psychiatric literature that there was little doubt that adrenochrome and also adrenolutin, its first derivative, were hallucinogens. However psychiatrists were not convinced, dredging up a variety of reasons why they could not accept this data. We created a major controversy and to our surprise Dr. J. Smythies, who had worked so closely with Humphry in England and later in Weyburn, joined the side of the disbelievers. By then he was located at the University of British Columbia and he joined the attack on us by claiming that none of these experiments meant anything since they had not been done double-blind. However none of the critics tried to repeat our work, with the exception of Dr. Max Rinkel. But he used a product he thought was adrenochrome and in fact was not. In 1995, Dr. John Smythies reassessed his position and joined us in furthering our views. He published an excellent series of reports in the psychiatric literature describing some of our earlier work and bringing it up to date.

It was many years before we discovered that our adrenochrome was unstable because it was contaminated with the silver ions used to oxidize adrenaline to adrenochrome. Until then it had been believed by students of adrenochrome that the compound was inherently unstable. The solution to the conundrum came about as follows. In 1957 I was invited by Dr. Max Rinkel, from Boston, to come to a meeting of the Northeast neuropsychiatric group. They had also invited Dr. Robert Heath, Chairman, Department of Psychiatry, from Tulane University to present his findings regarding taraxein. This was a substance he claimed to have isolated from the blood of schizophrenic patients, and he said it made his test monkeys psychotic. I was to be one of three discussants of his paper. I concluded that I would have to visit Professor Heath in his laboratory if I was to give an intelligent discussion of his research.

From March 10 to 23 I went to Boston via Vancouver and New Orleans. In Vancouver, I met with members of the local neuropsychiatric group and also had lunch with an English organic chemist. I spoke to him about the inherent instability of adrenochrome preparations and the difficulty that that fact generated for our research. He remarked that in general, organic preparations tended to be unstable if they were contaminated, and that very pure organic preparations were stable. Our product therefore must be "dirty." We had been making adrenochrome using the standard procedure of oxidizing an adrenaline solution with silver salts. It immediately occurred to me that the powder undoubtedly was too rich in silver and that we could make our product stable by removing these impurities. During my flight to New Orleans via Los Angeles I wrote to Dr. N. Payza, my research chemist, telling him to dissolve his adrenochrome and run it through a charcoal filter to remove the silver ions.

I returned home with high expectations of seeing stable adrenochrome for the first time. As soon as I could I asked Dr. Payza whether he had prepared the pure adrenochrome. He had not. I became very angry and ordered him to do it immediately. About 4 o'clock that afternoon, he called me in to show me the first pure adrenochrome crystals ever made. He had followed my advice, allowing the solution which had passed through the charcoal to stay in a glass dish and slowly, the adrenochrome coalesced into beautiful, dark-coloured crystals. These were so stable that they did not decompose even when placed into solution for several hours at room temperature. After that it became much easier to do adrenochrome research. This work was taken up by Dr. Ronald Heacock, who completed the most thorough chemical investigation of adrenochrome and adrenolutin and their derivatives that had been done to date. Later, we synthesized stable adrenolutin but we did not ever succeed in making stable noradrenochrome. Dr. Osmond had some fun with the stable adrenochrome, which he carried about with him in a small vial. On one occasion he was told by the chief chemist of one of the major drug companies that adrenochrome would never be made stable. After Humphry had been repeatedly assured of this fact, he pulled out the vial and showed it to the chemists. This little joke was symbolic of the larger scope of our work. When we started our research, no one believed that adreno-chrome was a hallucinogen, or that niacin would help schizophrenic patients. We enjoyed proving to ourselves how wrong the authorities so often were.

Once we had stable adrenochrome, we also began to investigate the effect of both adrenochrome and nicotinic acid on the brain wave pattern of epileptic patients at the Munroe Wing. In this research, Szatmari and I found that adrenochrome given intra-venously to epileptic patients intensified their electroencephalo-gram (brain wave) abnormalities when these were present and revealed them when they did not show at first. The changes came within ten minutes after the injection. We theorized that, as Vernon Woodford's research was increasingly suggesting, adrenochrome inhibited energy production in the brain via the Krebs cycle reac-tions, intensifying abnormalities already present or revealing latent ones. We also found that if we gave the patient 100 milligrams of intravenous nicotinic acid at the height of the abnormal brain wave patterns, the EEG abnormality would resolve itself within a matter of minutes. This, we felt, occurred because the vitamin helped restore normal Krebs cycle activity. Nicotinic acid, we further found, has anticonvulsant properties when used as an adjunct to anticonvulsant treatment, but by itself cannot stop seizures. Since these early experiments, I have found it very helpful for my epileptic patients. Its use makes it possible to decrease the dose of their anti-convulsant drugs by up to fifty percent and thus greatly diminish their side effects. The results of our research with adrenochrome and epileptic patients were published in the following article: Szatmari, A., Hoffer, A. and Schneider, R: The Effect of Adrenochrome and Niacin on the Electroencephalogram of Epileptics. *Am J Psychiat,* 3:603-616, 1955.

X

LSD, Niacin, and Alcoholism

LSD, one of the hallucinogenic indoles, was discovered in 1938. Humphry and I felt that like mescaline, it induced an experience similar to schizophrenia. Thus we were keen to explore its effects more deeply. We began to study the compound's effects on normal volunteers in Regina in 1952; the compound was still legally available then. Giving LSD to normals was called inducing a model psychosis.

We decided to conduct most of our LSD experiments under Humphry's direction, as he was the only one of our group who had had direct experience with any hallucinogen. Mr. Ben Stefaniuk, a psychologist, joined us and worked at Weyburn with Humphry. We did not give LSD to any volunteers who showed any psychopathology, nor to patients, except for the alcoholics whom we later treated with psychedelic therapy. By then, it was also clear from other studies, especially some that had been done in Greece, that when first order relatives of schizophrenics are given LSD, they are prone to undesirable and prolonged reactions. Our volunteers had to sign special consent forms after the experience was described to them. They were given the LSD in hospital, and Mr. Stefaniuk, a doctor, or a nurse stayed with them at all times. After the experience was over, they were allowed to go home if someone would be with them, otherwise they were kept in hospital overnight and released the next morning. Our use of LSD is described in detail in *The Hallucinogens*.

Our studies with LSD led to valuable new information. Many of our doctors and nurses volunteered to take the compound and gained a far better understanding of what it is like to be psychotic. These professionals became much more empathic therapists after the LSD experience. We also gained a deeper conceptual understanding of the importance of perceptual changes as a factor in our patients' experience. This understanding helped catalyze the development of the HOD and EWI tests.

Another important finding was that niacin moderated the LSD experience. By the time we started working with LSD, we already knew that the vitamin was helpful for schizophrenia. We reasoned that it might therefore also be helpful as an LSD antidote, that the psychological similarity of the schizophrenia and LSD states meant that an underlying biochemical similarity existed in the body during these two states. This line of reasoning proved correct in practical terms. Giving intravenous niacin to normal subjects or alcoholic patients who were having a distressing or overly lengthy experience helped the individual come out of the experience quickly in every case. A few reports have since emerged in the medical literature telling of emergency room physicians who have used the vitamin with the same results. I am convinced that niacin is the safest and quickest compound for bringing an LSD subject very quickly out of an undesirable or prolonged reaction. It does not leave patients groggy and disoriented, as tranquilizers do. Niacin also reverses the hallucinogenic effects of adrenochrome, given intravenously, and reverses the electroencephalogram abnormalities that show up in human subjects injected with adrenochrome. I know of no reports of the use of niacin to reverse the effects of other hallucinogens.

Shortly after we had begun our LSD studies, Mr. Sid Katz, a reporter for *Macleans* magazine, visited Humphry at Weyburn and heard about this work. He volunteered to be a subject. Humphry and I discussed his request carefully and decided that it would be valuable to us for information about our research to be made public. In any case, we did none of our experiments in secrecy. Mr. Katz described his experience in an issue of the magazine which sported a lurid front cover. The story was accurate and well done but generated much criticism of us from some psychiatrists in eastern Canada. For instance, many years later I was told by one of his former students that Dr. Robert Jones, then professor of psychiatry at Dalhousie University, decided that none of our research thereafter could be taken seriously; he could not trust anyone who had worked with LSD. It is possible that some of the hostility our adrenochrome hypothesis and niacin treatments for schizophrenia would generate had their beginnings in our willingness to be open about our LSD research. Perhaps other psychiatrists felt, as Jones did, that we could not be taken seriously if we were willing to experiment with an hallucinogen.

Further, at this time, in the early 1950s, psychoanalysis was striking boldly into North American psychiatry; many psychoanalysts proclaimed that schizophrenia was not a disease. They saw it as a reaction, a way of life, induced by intrapsychic conflicts or by conflicts with authority figures (usually the mother), and so on. Although the psychoanalysts claimed to be devout followers of Freud, they seemed willing to disregard their master's caution. He himself had advised his followers to be wary of treating schizophrenics and did not hold out much promise for psychoanalysis as a schizophrenia treatment. In any case, our exploration of LSD, which was based on the assumption that a biochemically-active compound could produce symptoms similar to those of schizophrenia, was a direct challenge to the growing psychoanalytic view. Our work with adrenochrome and niacin fell into the same category.

The Psychedelic Experience

Early in 1952, Humphry and I were invited to Ottawa by Dr. C. Roberts to discuss nucleoproteins as a possible schizophrenia treatment, as already described. We flew to eastern Canada on a slow, noisy, and very uncomfortable airplane. On the way, I developed a cold. We arrived in Ottawa very late and by the time I got to bed I was too exhausted to sleep properly. As a result, I spent part of the night thinking about our research, especially the LSD experiments that had started running. I also found myself thinking about how in some cases alcoholics were able to turn their lives around after having a devastating physical or emotional experience. Alcoholics Anonymous (AA) believed that many alcoholics would not do well until they became deeply motivated by "hitting bottom." "Hitting bottom" often meant going through a bout of *delirium tremens*, a dangerous physical condition that carried a 20 percent risk of death. Obviously we could not force our alcoholic patients into such experiences in order to motivate them. It struck me that the LSD experience in some ways resembled the *delirium tremens* experience but that it was safe and easily controlled. I wondered if we could use LSD to give our alcoholic patients an experience something like "hitting bottom." In contrast to going through real *delirium tremens*, the patient would be able to remember everything that happened and thus their chance of benefit from the experience would be increased; as a result, perhaps these patients would be motivated to stop drinking, whether members of AA or not.

I discussed the idea with Humphry the next morning; he thought it a hypothesis worth pursuing. I decided we would begin running trial LSD treatments for the alcoholics in our wards as soon as possible after returning home.

On our return, Ben Stefaniuk and Humphry began this work with some of the alcoholics in the hospital. We started by inviting those who had failed to respond to any previous treatment to try LSD. As with our healthy volunteers, we explained the procedure in detail, required the signing of a special consent form (beyond that required on hospital admission), and made sure that no patient was left alone while under the influence of the compound. We used one gram of niacin if the individual did not come out of the experience quickly enough; occasionally we gave 100 milligrams intravenously. We did not give any LSD to schizophrenic patients even if they were also alcoholic, and we did not give it to patients who were in the hospital involuntarily.

By the time we had worked with a number of patients, we knew that we could not reliably induce an experience that in any way resembled *delirium tremens*. A very few patients did have quite a rough time. But the majority of the patients had exciting, interesting experiences in which they felt at ease, developed some insights, and enjoyed most of what happened. In fact, Weyburn alcoholics given LSD so often had a pleasurable, beneficial experience, that Humphry realized we were dealing with a different phenomenon than that of the induced psychosis (psychotomimesis) we were anticipating. Since it was different, it would have to be given a different name, for no phenomenon can be studied if it is not dignified by a name. Humphry thought about this matter for some time and also discussed the question with Aldous Huxley. He eventually decided on the word "psychedelic," by which he meant "mind manifesting." The Greek word "psyche" means "mind," the word "delos" means "to make visible." He announced this new term at a meeting of the New York Academy of Sciences in New York City in 1957. Here is his statement from page 132 of our book, *The Hallucinogens:* "A psychedelic compound is one like LSD or mescaline which enriches the mind and enlarges the vision. It is the kind of experience which provides the greatest possibility for examining those areas most interesting to psychiatry and which has provided men down the ages with experiences they have considered valuable above all others."

We did not expect that "psychedelic" would become a household term around the world.

I recently looked up the word in the *American Heritage Dictionary* and found it defined as: "Of, characterized by, or generating hallucinations, distortions of perception, altered states of awareness, and occasional states resembling psychosis." This definition misses entirely the spirit and meaning of the word psychedelic, and probably reflects the anti-hallucinogen hysteria that later developed in governments and conventional society, partly due to the abuses of some of LSD's advocates, and partly due to the discomfort some people feel at the frontiers of their own awareness.

After we had recognized the phenomenon Humphry would name the psychedelic experience, we looked for those factors that favoured this type of response to LSD. It had become clear that the psychedelic reaction was much more powerful in changing our alcoholic patients' attitudes than the harsh imitation of a crisis we had originally hoped to elicit. We found that in the wake of the psychedelic experience, patients had more insight and more understanding of the self. To achieve it as consistently as possible, we increased the support we gave our patients, worked to make them more comfortable, and included music, pictures, and photographs in the session. We found, for example, that pictures of Van Gogh paintings catalyzed very interesting and beneficial responses in our LSD subjects. Duncan Blewett, PhD, and psychiatrist Nick Chwelos made important contributions to our knowledge of how to bring about the psychedelic experience rather than its opposite. They wrote a report describing their findings. A mimeographed copy apparently fell into the hands of Timothy Leary at Harvard. He later used this information as a basis for his work with the hallucinogens, but never gave our Saskatchewan group credit. The methods we finally came to use are described in detail in our book *The Hallucinogens*.

We would eventually treat roughly 2,000 alcoholics in five Saskatchewan hospitals using the LSD psychedelic experience. Our follow-up surveys showed that about half of them were helped. We published reports on this work in a number of journals.

A very eccentric person, Al Hubbard, made a major contribution to our psychedelic research. Mr. Hubbard was a millionaire who lived on Canada's west coast. Through his own experimentation, Al had become very excited about the psychedelic experience and decided that it was so valuable and beneficial to humanity that it would be desirable to induce it in every member of the top management of the Fortune 100 companies. I met him through Ben Webster, a businessman who had agreed to try LSD under Al's supervision and been deeply positively impressed. Al informed Ben that he must look me up as one of the experts in this arena, which Ben did. Ben and I would become good friends and he later played an important role in the Huxley Institute for Biosocial Research (described in Chapters Seventeen and Eighteen).

Meanwhile, Al had begun working with Dr. Ross McLean, a Vancouver psychiatrist who owned a private hospital in that city. Dr. McLean began working with alcoholics in that hospital, drawing on Al's expertise. They utilized some of the techniques we had developed, but took them even further. When I eventually met Al, I was impressed with his enthusiasm and invited him to demonstrate his approach at University Hospital, with some of the alcoholic patients we were then treating with LSD. Our final method became a mix of his ideas and ours, and probably the ideas of many others as well— Al was in contact with groups in California interested in psychedelic research, as well as with Aldous Huxley.

Al became discouraged when LSD was later placed in the same category as narcotics by North American governments and removed from official and medical use. The heavy arm of the law came down on LSD largely because of the irresponsibility of Timothy Leary.

I was very unhappy about Mr. Leary's move into psychedelic therapy. I did not have any direct contact with him, but read reports on his work in the press, and received updates from Humphry and Aldous Huxley. During the time that Leary was flying high with his Harvard professorship and his psychedelic unit, Aldous Huxley, after talking it over with Humphry, warned Leary that he was playing with fire and that he underestimated LSD's potential for harm. Dr. Leary totally ignored this advice, dismissing it with the statement, "What do doctors know about LSD?" I believe his own heavy use led him to make errors of judgement; he took both LSD and psilocybin (an hallucinogenic mushroom) several times weekly.

Thanks to Leary, after LSD escaped from the clinics into the streets, it spread very quickly. I too was aware of its potential danger when used in uncontrolled settings and had already seen a few students who had abused it and were suffering serious, prolonged, almost schizophrenia-like side effects, in some cases long after they had stopped taking the drug. Most of them had been very curious because of the publicity given to Leary and other advocates of unlimited use.

I heard Leary speak only once, when in 1966 I was in San Francisco at a meeting on the Berkeley campus that was also addressed by him and Allen Ginsberg. I presented my work on the treatment of alcoholism with LSD and received a reasonably enthusiastic reception. (Leary's presentation, on the other hand, was received with wild abandon by a crowd that seemed not to care that he was merely quoting himself in sound bites of which I could make no sense. I realized his audience did not care what he said, they simply wanted to hear and adore him. They had already accepted his message.) After my presentation, Berkeley students crowded around me, wanting to talk about LSD. I advised them that the compound must be used with great caution. I added that I did not expect they were likely to follow my advice, but that if they did use LSD, they should at the very least take certain precautions. These were: (1) to select a physician whom they could trust and let that doctor know what they were going to do in case they ran into any difficulty from which they could not extricate themselves; (2) to have ample supplies of niacin on hand to help themselves come down from the experience. At least one or two of these students took my advice about niacin seriously and later that year it appeared in the *Village Voice*, the weekly New York City paper.

Later, Dr. Russell Smith from Detroit would tell me of an occasion on which he had been called to help the police identify vitamin B-3. They had seized white tablets from some student and they did not know what they were. Dr. Smith recognized them as niacin tablets. In Detroit, apparently, so-called responsible dealers were advising their clients to have niacin on their person in case they needed it to come down from an LSD experience. They would not sell the drug unless the buyer also took the niacin. So-called irresponsible dealers did not bother to advise the use of niacin.

One evening during that trip to San Francisco, I received a call at my hotel from Allen Ginsberg, the poet. He wanted to meet with me but did not tell me why. I was busy all day, so I suggested he come to my hotel and join me for breakfast. He groaned and said he never got up before noon or later. I pointed out that unfortunately I was already committed. He said he would come. I had heard him also on the platform. He was short, wore a beard to his navel, and wore his hair like a sunburst halo around his head. His face was barely visible.

The next morning I went down for breakfast early and waited for Mr. Ginsberg. He arrived a few minutes later. I saw him come to the door of the dining room and wait there for someone to direct him to me. But the waiters very studiously avoided him. I then called my waiter and told him very sternly that Ginsberg was my guest and to please bring him to me. Over breakfast he told me a remarkable story.

I already knew that Ginsberg had been in a mental hospital, as had his mother, both diagnosed with schizophrenia. Ginsberg and his lover had started a campaign to take all those other of their relatives residing in New York State mental hospitals out of these institutions one by one and to rehabilitate them. They did this by moving these individuals into their apartment and providing them with support, kindness, and help of all kinds. The relatives all gradually got better. I saw no contradiction in this method with what I was recommending, i.e. the use of vitamin therapy and nutrition. Dr. John Conolly had shown in 1850 that with support, humane treatment, and good nutrition, he could get half of his patients well. And the New York State hospitals were so awful that almost any other environment would have been much better.

Ginsberg and his lover had assisted a large number of their relatives in this way and were finally trying to help one of the last. This man proved to be a very difficult patient. He was so deteriorated that he smeared feces all over the apartment. Ginsberg told me that he and his partner could no longer stomach the horrible stench. He then came to the reason he wanted to see me. He had heard my presentation at the meeting and now wondered how much niacin he should be giving his relative. I discussed the matter with him. I have not met him since, nor do I know what happened to the last of his "patients".

I was interested in Ginsberg's own mental state. He had not kept secret the symptoms from which he suffered. I experienced him as normal in spite of the fact that he had been treated for schizophrenia and had taken hallucinogenic drugs so frequently. I concluded that he had cured himself by taking these drugs. One of the biggest problems many schizophrenic patients face is the fear generated by the perceptual disorder. I guessed that by taking hallucinogens so frequently, Ginsberg had trained himself to be comfortable in the experiential world of the schizophrenic as well as in a world free of the perceptual distortions brought on by the disease. Over the years since, I have found that people who have taken these drugs and then later become schizophrenic are not nearly as disturbed by and fearful of the perceptual disorders produced by the natural disease. They also find it easier to accept the explanation that their body is producing something like LSD.

Our work with the psychedelic experience also led directly to the development of a diagnostic test for certain types of schizophrenia. Dr. Neil Payza played a significant role in this development. He was a biochemist who worked with us for a time before being let go because of personality problems. He had already managed to produce pure, stable adrenochrome, as described earlier. I had gotten the idea that there might be a new compound present in the body after LSD was taken. Since the LSD and schizophrenia experiences were so similar, I reasoned, perhaps this compound would also appear in the bodies of schizophrenic patients.

We had already been examining the urine of patients using a particular test (paper chromatograms). One day in the late 1950s I gave Payza two samples of urine from an alcoholic patient, one taken just before he was given LSD, and the second sample taken two hours later, at the height of the experience. I asked him to examine both urines and to look for something which appeared only after the LSD had been given. A few days later he was able to show me a mauve spot on the paper strip—this substance was not present in the pre-LSD urine sample. Further work confirmed that the presence of this compound in a patient's urine frequently meant that they suffered from a form of schizophrenia we initially called malvaria, later pyroluria. The mauve factor can also appear when an individual is experiencing severe oxidative stress.

Niacin and Alcoholism

As we began to treat large numbers of schizophrenic patients in the early 1950s with high doses of vitamin B-3, we inevitably found ourselves working with a few who were both alcoholic and schizo-phrenic. We learned from these patients that niacin is a particularly good treatment for alcohol addiction.

For example, one of my patients told me that she had joined AA in order to stop drinking, but whenever she succeeded, she would begin to hear voices. She found these voices worse to live with than the consequences of drinking. She would return to the bottle to get rid of them. Her dilemma was a terrible one: should she be a sober member of AA and suffer auditory hallucinations, or should she free herself of them by living the life of an alcoholic? I offered her a way out—high dose niacin. Within a few months, she was able to stay sober without any recurrence of her voices. She later became a member of the first Schizophrenics Anonymous group I helped organize in Saskatoon in 1960 (described in Chapter Fourteen).

Something about her case twigged in me the idea that alcoholics would likely respond to elevated niacin consumption whether or not they were schizophrenic. I began using it with the alcoholic patients on my wards and did indeed see good results. I shared this discovery with Bill W., co-founder of AA, in the early 1960s. Bill was intensely interested and started taking one gram of niacin three times daily. As a result, he was relieved of severe exhaustion, tension, anxiety, and insomnia within two weeks. Bill W. went on to become a major advocate of the use of niacin in the treatment of alcoholism. This work is described in greater detail in Chapter Eighteen.

In the late 1960s, Dr. Russell Smith, the medical director of a hospital in Detroit which specialized in the treatment of alcoholics, began using niacin. He found that the response rate of his patients was very high, ranging from 63 to 100 percent, depending on the year in question.

Most of the patients he initially treated with niacin wanted to stop drinking, but he also persuaded a number of individuals who had no interest in giving up the habit to begin taking the vitamin. After a few years, more and more of this group were drinking less. This was not surprising to me. A well, relaxed, and healthy individual will very rarely become alcoholic. The person must first have a problem that seems to be helped by alcohol consumption.

Since these original discoveries, our knowledge of how to treat alcoholism with nutrients has expanded significantly. Inspired by my and others' research, nutritionist Joan Mathews Larson PhD, began a clinic for alcoholics in Minneapolis. Her recovery rate is around 75 percent. Her books and those by Dr. Joe Beasley provide important information about the treatment of alcoholism.

Niacin has since been investigated for its possible helpfulness in drug and nicotine addictions and shows promise for these conditions as well.

Mescaline and Peyote

Our work with LSD sparked my interest in mescaline, the compound Humphry Osmond had first worked with. Mescaline is present in the peyote plant, a cactus that grows in the southwest United States and Mexico. I studied that plant as well and in this way, became acquainted with the church that had adopted the peyote plant as its sacrament, the Native American Church of North America. My knowledge of this plant landed me in opposition to the government of the day.

In 1953 or 1954, the Canadian newspapers suddenly carried in banner headlines announcements that the national government was starting a major effort to suppress the use of peyote by the Canadian native peoples who were members of this church. This action had been catalyzed by a question asked in the House of Commons in Ottawa by a member of the Cooperative Commonwealth Federation (CCF) party, Max Campbell, from North Battleford, Saskatchewan. I was astonished. I had considered the CCF to be a left wing party and tolerant of all religions. The local Regina newspaper, the *Leader Post*, asked what I thought about the government's actions and I replied that in my opinion they were totally unwarranted and a lot of nonsense. I was then widely quoted across Canada. I also wrote to Mr. M.J. Coldwell, the CCF's national leader, demanding to know why Max Campbell had asked that question. I would later discover the question had been planted by the government—it had wanted an opportunity to announce its new campaign to suppress the use of peyote. Max Campbell represented a region where lived the Red Pheasant tribe, some of whom belonged to the Church. He was properly concerned about the plight of the tribespeople and had been persuaded by the Department of Indian Affairs that one of the reasons for their poverty and high alcoholism rates among the Red Pheasant tribe was the use of peyote.

Several years later, Mr. Campbell wrote to me, wanting to meet, which we did in my office at University Hospital. He was angry and hostile at first and I was very careful with him. I explained that members of the Native American Church upheld several important articles of faith, including honesty and abstinence from alcohol. They were probably the most responsible members of the tribe. I also pointed out that the peyote was safe, as they used it within a carefully controlled religious ceremony. After he understood the real issues, Campbell and I became close friends.

During this period of political controversy, I decided that Dr. Osmond and I should really find out firsthand what happened during the all-night rituals that the First Nations people claimed as an essential part of their religion. I wrote to one of the Church leaders, Mr. Frank Takes Gun, and asked him whether he would allow myself and a number of my colleagues to participate in an upcoming ceremony. I waited many weeks to receive his reply. He had taken the time needed to ascertain that we were not another arm of the government trying to sabotage the Church.

A few months later, I drove to the reservation with Dr. Osmond, psychology professor Duncan Blewett, research psychiatrist Dr. T. Weckowicz, and Dr. Neil Agnew, our Chief Research Psychologist. We also had a tape recorder with us.

The Church members had set up a teepee in which the ceremony would be held. Dr. Osmond took peyote and later wrote about his experience in detail. I fell asleep for a major portion of the ceremony. I do remember with amusement one of the chief celebrant's comments. At midnight he said this was the best time to pray because all the white men were asleep.

The mescaline and peyote experiences are not the same, I think there are several reasons for this. Mescaline, when used alone, is taken in high concentrations, up to 750 milligrams in one dose. It would not be possible to get that much mescaline from the number of peyote buttons taken in a typical ceremony. Secondly, peyote contains other similar compounds, including mescaline precursors and derivatives, and I expect these would markedly modify a person's response. Finally, the context of an all-night ceremony around a ritual fire in a smoke filled teepee is so far removed from the experience of the usual mescaline user that this in itself would make for a marked difference.

So far as I know, the Government of Canada did not pursue any further its attempts to suppress the use of peyote after this imbroglio I was involved in. I do not know the present status of the Church in Canada.

The professional use of LSD was, however, effectively wiped out in the wake of the public reaction to people like Timothy Leary and Montreal's Dr. Ewen Cameron, who abused the compound. It became illegal to use LSD in Canada in the early 1960s, and the requirements for doing LSD-based research became so rigid that all work in this area essentially came to a halt. For many years it was essentially impossible to do research with LSD, but very easy to obtain it in any number of schoolyards. Within the last decade there has been a resurgence of interest in psychedelic therapy and the US FDA has started to approve therapeutic studies with hallucinogens, including LSD. This I see as a very positive development that in the long run must benefit our understanding of mental illness, addiction, and the potential of the human mind.

XI

Niacin and Cholesterol

An unexpected offshoot of our work with niacin and schizophrenia was the discovery that niacin (but not niacinamide) is an excellent total cholesterol-lowering agent. Further, if cholesterol levels are very low to begin with, niacin will increase them to more normal levels. Only in the past few years have I found out why. Niacin elevates high density lipoprotein (HDL) cholesterol levels, sometimes called "good" cholesterol. This is a more important therapeutic effect than in lowering total cholesterol.

The first study indicating niacin's cholesterol-lowering properties was published in 1955 by myself, Professor R. Altschul, and Dr. J. Stephen. Our report has been credited with starting a new paradigm in the use of vitamins, the vitamin-as-treatment paradigm. This paradigm later expanded into the orthomolecular medicine paradigm that I mention throughout this book. "Ortho" is Greek for "correct". This term "orthomolecular" literally refers to using the "correct molecule" to treat disease. Linus Pauling proposed the term in his famous 1968 *Science* article, "Orthomolecular Psychiatry." He presented the view that any biochemical imbalance could be restored by providing the person who suffered from it with the right substances in optimum amounts. Thus the treatment of schizophrenia with niacin is an orthomolecular therapy.

The cholesterol-lowering effect of niacin was unexpected. We made this discovery because Professor R. Altschul, Chairman, Department of Anatomy at the University of Saskatchewan, was studying athero-sclerosis in rabbits. He had found that he could elevate cholesterol levels in these animals by feeding them cooked egg yolk. Raw eggs did not have this effect. Then he discovered that he could decrease the elevated cholesterol levels by exposing the rabbits to ultraviolet radiation. He wanted to find out if people would respond the same way, but was not able to secure the permission of any Saskatoon physicians to work with their patients. He approached me in 1954.

He and I then discussed the idea of working with some of the enormous number of chronic patients in the Saskatchewan mental hospitals. Dr. Osmond and I decided to cooperate with him. We were convinced that the amount of ultraviolet radiation our patients would receive in Dr. Altschul's studies would be minimal and safe. We even thought this exposure might be beneficial, as these patients were indoors almost the whole year, and seldom received natural sunlight. We predicted that Dr. Altschul's treatment would increase their vitamin D levels. We also hoped that we could use his research as a resource in further training our clinical staff in research methodology. Finally, we felt that the attention these patients would be getting would be helpful to them. Psychosomatic medicine was very prominent at the time and it was generally believed within this school of thought that attention was a powerful factor in helping patients get well. In other words, we were convinced we would not harm our patients, that we might help them, that the clinical staff would benefit, and that we might help Dr. Altschul discover something valuable.

Before starting the research, we agreed that Dr. Altschul should come to Weyburn to visit Dr. H. Osmond and address the medical and nursing staff.

Dr. Altschul took the overnight train from Saskatoon to Regina, where I met him and drove him to the hospital at Weyburn, about 72 miles southeast of Regina. The trip took about one and a half hours. There and back, we discussed his findings. He described to me his hypothesis that the main factor in the genesis of hardening of the arteries was pathology in the intima, the innermost lining of the blood vessels. He maintained that at sites of increased blood turbulence, for instance at arterial junctions, or places where arteries curved sharply, excessive wear and tear on the intima took place. As long as the intimal tissue could repair itself as fast as it was being damaged, there would be no deposition of plaque, which he understood as a type of stopgap measure introduced by the body, similar to a scab on the skin.

These ideas seemed sensible to me and reminded me of a recent experience. Roughly a year and a half earlier I had been increasingly bothered by severe bleeding of my gums, despite the fact that my teeth were in relatively good shape and I consumed three grams of vitamin C daily. My dentist had been unable to help. During this period I was also giving some thought to the niacin flush. Many of my patients did not like it and I would often have to explain carefully that it was not harmful and would likely stop happening in time. I had begun to wonder what would happen if a patient of mine taking niacin were to sue me because of the flush. I did not have the usual defence, namely that I was doing the same thing as other doctors. At the time, Dr. Osmond and I, as far as I knew, were the only two physicians in the world that I knew of giving niacin in large doses. I decided that I should take the niacin long enough that I could be my own witness. Then, if I were sued, I could tell the judge that in my opinion niacin was safe not only because of the many animal studies indicating so, but because I myself had been taking it for months. Accordingly, I began taking three grams daily. No one has ever sued me—and my experiment with the vitamin had a surprising result. One morning after I had been taking the niacin for two weeks, I began brushing my teeth and suddenly came to with a start. My toothbrush was clean; my gums were not bleeding. I saw my dentist a few days later and he confirmed that my gums were in much better condition than previously. I could only conclude that the niacin had increased the ability of my gum tissues to repair themselves, an ability which slows down with aging. I did not know then that niacin is a healing vitamin for all body tissues. It does, indeed, increase the rate of repair everywhere in the body.

I asked my dentist whether he would be willing to try the treatment on some of his other patients with similar gum problems. He did and found they all experienced improvement when they took niacin.

As Dr. Altschul told me his theories about the intimal lining of the artery and how it must repair itself quickly so that plaque build-up can be avoided, I immediately thought about my experience with niacin and my gums. I told Professor Altschul about the research we had done on niacin as a schizophrenia treatment and also described the flush it causes. I suggested that the vitamin might increase the rate of healing of the intima, and if this were the case, could be beneficial in preventing the development of arteriosclerosis. He asked me where he could obtain some. I promised to send him a pound from my stock. This I did a few days later.

Three months had passed when I received a call from Dr. Altschul one evening. He was very excited and repeatedly exclaimed, "It works, it works!"

What works?" I queried. I had completely forgotten about having given him any niacin.

He replied that he had given niacin to rabbits in whom he had induced high cholesterol and that it had lowered their cholesterol levels to normal. He had done enough tests to be sure of his conclusion. Then he added that it was now important to run some human trials. I agreed and replied that I would discuss the matter with Dr. J. Stephen, pathologist for the General Hospital in Regina. I acted as biochemical consultant to him and knew him well.

The next day, I spoke to Jim Stephen, outlining Altschul's findings as well as my own experience with niacin, which by then I had been taking for about two years. Dr. Stephen agreed that we should give niacin a trial in human patients with high cholesterol. I expressed my concern that we would have to talk to each hospital patient's admitting doctor for permission. To my surprise, he replied that there was no need to do so, and added that the doctors did not know what was going on in hospital anyway. He said he would select a large number of patients, order cholesterol level tests, then place them on niacin and after two days again order cholesterol level tests. These events occurred in 1954. Today, such a simple procedure would be totally impossible. One would have to run a gauntlet of various therapeutic and ethical committees first.

I received a report from Dr. Stephen a few weeks later. As I scanned the data, it became clear within a few minutes that two grams of niacin daily, the average dose used by Dr. Stephen, lowered cholesterol in people.

I called Dr. Altschul that evening and gave him the happy news. I said I would send him all the data for him to write up and we could publish this finding as a report by Altschul, Hoffer, and Stephen. He surprised me by asking whether it was necessary to include Dr. Stephen. I replied that in my opinion it was, and that unless we included him in the paper I would not agree to publication. Professor Altschul was much more familiar than I with the tendency of scientists to steal one another's ideas. He was very careful to observe the ethical rule of science that one gives credit to any prior publication—and he zealously guarded his own contributions to the march of research.

Altschul and I then began a series of additional studies on the relationship between niacin and cholesterol levels. We found that the vitamin elevated cholesterol if the initial values were very low.

The next year, I was invited by the Mayo Research Foundation to come to Rochester, Minnesota, and talk about the use of vitamin B-3 as a schizophrenia treatment. I accepted this invitation and gave a series of lectures and seminars at the Foundation. The Foundation generously arranged a banquet for the last night of my stay. I sat next to the Chairman of the Division of Psychiatry, Dr. Howard Rome. By this time I was tired of the subject of niacin and schizophrenia. I began to tell Dr. Rome about the effect niacin had on cholesterol levels in rabbits and people. The next day I returned home.

A few days later, I would find out, Dr. Rome went to an evening meeting that the Chairman of the Division of Medicine, Dr. Allen, was having with his residents. Dr. Rome was a duck-hunting buddy to Dr. Allen. Apparently he said something like, "I have just been told by some crazy Canadian that you can lower cholesterol levels with niacin.

This statement sparked the interest of the senior resident, Dr. Willim B. Parsons, since his ward included several patients with high blood cholesterol levels. He asked Dr. Allen for permission to make a trial of niacin with these patients. He received it and Dr. Parsons was soon in possession of data that confirmed ours. He published as well, and his report was very important, as it alerted the medical profession. Our paper had been published in a rather obscure journal as far as physicians were concerned, and this was before the days of computer-driven search engines and indexes. When the Mayo Clinic first report appeared, Dr. Altschul became concerned. He said to me, "One day they will try to steal our idea." Surprised, I asked how that could possibly happen, since we had already published. He pointed out that in their first paper they had referred to our prior work and that they would do the same in the second paper. But after that they could choose to refer only to their own papers and we would be left out. I did not really think this would happen, but to allay Dr. Altschul's fears, I suggested that since we had already done significantly more research since publishing our first paper, that we publish as quickly as possible in a variety of journals, so that it would be impossible for anyone to steal the idea or claim credit for our work. We followed through with this strategy. Dr. Altschul also eventually wrote a book on niacin and cholesterol, which was published posthumously due to his untimely death. Dr. William B. Parsons Jr. and the Mayo Clinic were scrupulously honest and always acknowledged the original idea. Dr. Parsons and I have remained good friends. He is the world's expert on the use of niacin for normalizing abnormal cholesterol levels. If, in the field of psychiatry, one psychiatrist outside of Saskatchewan had acted the same way Dr. Parsons did, orthomolecular psychiatry would have been advanced at least 30 years.

A few months after our niacin paper appeared, I spoke to the Deputy Minister of Health for Saskatchewan, Dr. Burns Roth, and advised him that the government would do well to take out a use patent on niacin as a cholesterol-lowering agent. I informed him that we had one year after the date of our publication in which to apply for such a patent and that we could make substantial sums of money for our research from it. He agreed to discuss the possibility with the Minister of Health. When I next saw him, he said the Minister did not want to apply for such a patent since he felt niacin should remain in the public domain and not be subject to royalties and control. I was not experienced enough at the time to take the action I would in the same situation today, namely to apply for the patent on behalf of myself and my two co-authors, and after receiving it, inform the government. My concern was that once the treatment entered the public domain, it would no longer be patentable by anyone, and therefore no drug companies would become interested in developing and marketing it. And as it happened, about a year later a British pharmaceutical concern patented clofibrate, the first major cholesterol-lowering drug. They must have made millions from it, as it became the standard treatment, while niacin, by comparison, languished. Yet it has been firmly established that niacin, unlike the cholesterol-lowering drugs, has the power to extend life-span. It is not only amongst the most effective and safe substances for decreasing cholesterol, but also very economical. But drug companies will never promote it in its current form. This situation may change if someone discovers a way to deliver niacin that duplicates its cardiovascular protective effects while removing its ability to cause a flush. In 2003, one drug company did launch sales of a patentable preparation of non-flush niacin and this compound sells for significantly more than ordinary vitamin B-3.

The Mayo Clinic went on to publish a number of excellent reports on niacin, including a study of its effect on the liver. For the previous decade it had been feared that niacin taken in high doses would produce a methyl deficiency syndrome, since it binds with methyl groups in the body to form compounds that are then excreted. Methyl deficiency, in turn, produces deposition of fat in the liver. Between 1945 and 1955, a number of papers had been published dealing with this topic. One group of researchers had reported that giving niacin to rats caused these animals to develop fatty livers. But the Mayo Clinic examined the livers of rats who had been on niacin for one year and found no pathology. Dr. Altschul also repeated this earlier study in his laboratory and found no evidence of liver damage in his specimens. He told me he thought the original study was probably invalid because in the period in which it had been done, it had been very difficult to obtain animals free of viral infection. He suspected that the animals used in the earlier study had been infected and this had caused their liver problems.

The next major development in this area was a study by Dr. E. Boyle, who worked with the National Institutes of Health (NIH) in Bethesda, Maryland. He became interested in niacin after reading the Mayo reports. He started a large number of his patients on niacin, and followed them all very carefully for ten years. He summarized his findings in a publication prepared by Bill W. and distributed to AA physicians in 1968. (See Chapter Eighteen for more information on Bill W. and his efforts to promote niacin use amongst recovering alcoholics and others.) Dr. Boyle said that in this group of patients, all of whom had suffered one heart attack, six deaths occurred over the ten years. Normally he would have expected 60 deaths. With niacin, he had decreased the death rate by 90 percent. After publishing these results, Dr. Boyle became one of the consultants to the Coronary Drug Study, a massive collaborative study financed by the NIH that ran between 1966 and 1974 in forty hospitals. The results of this study, published in 1986 by Canner et al in the *Journal of the American College of Cardiology*, established niacin as being one of the safest and most effective substances known for lowering cholesterol levels.

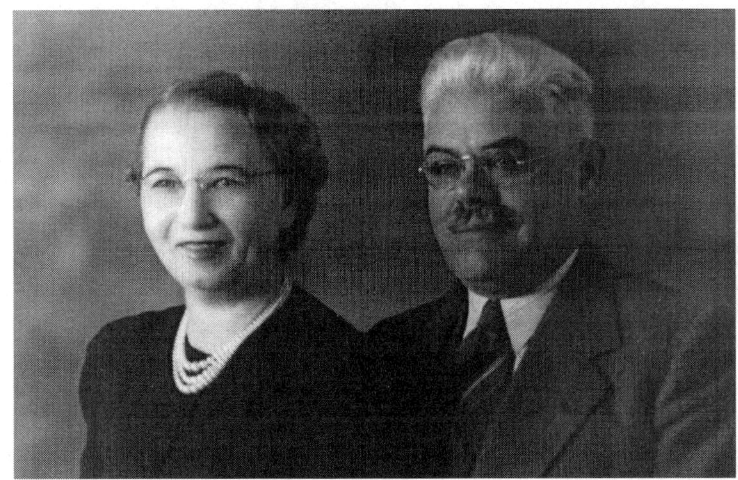

My parents, Clara and Israel Hoffer sometime between 1920 and 1930.

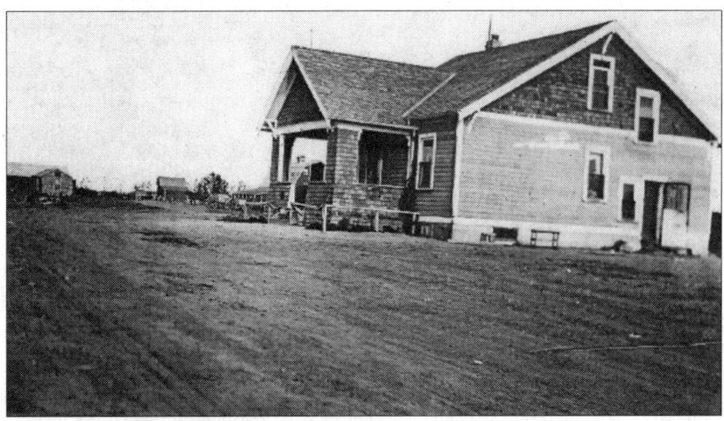

The Hoffer homestead in Saskatchewan around 1917.

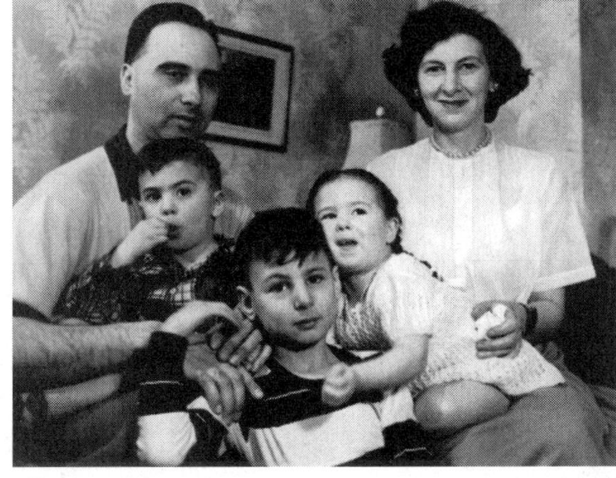

Young family: me, Rose, John, Miriam, Bill.

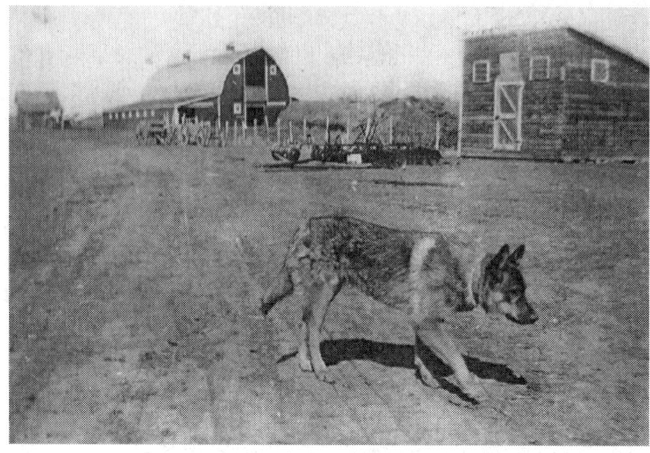

Laddie, my favorite dog; around 1930 on our farm in Saskatchewan.

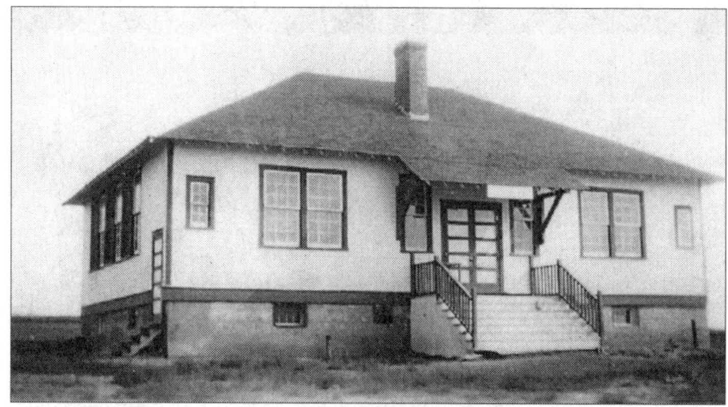

The school I attended from 6 to 12 in Hoffer, Saskatchewan. The village Hoffer no longer exists. This picture stems from around 1930.

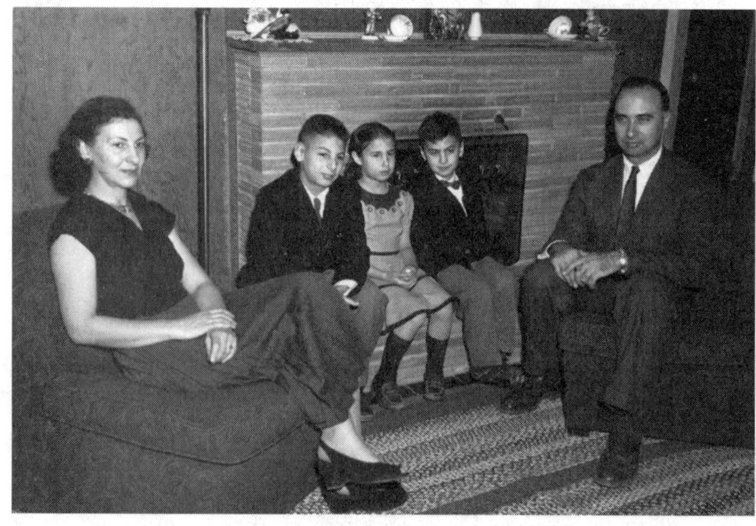

My wife and I with our children in the 1950s.

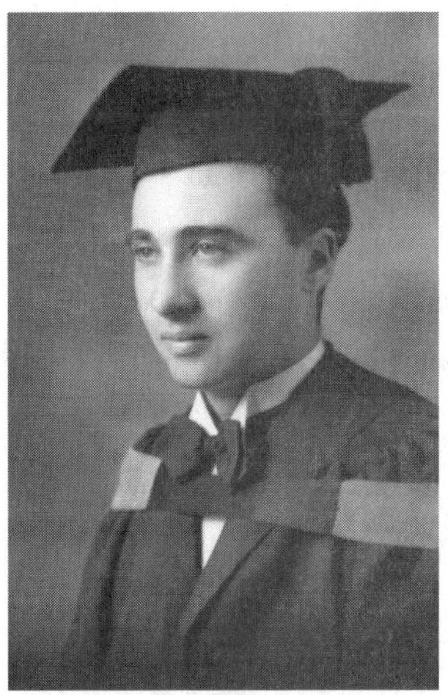

I received my Bachelor of Science in Agriculture (BSA) degree in 1938 at the age of 21.

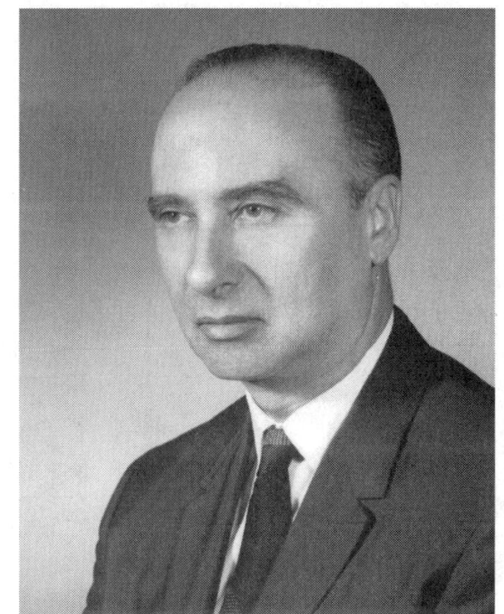

At the University of Minnesota in 1944.

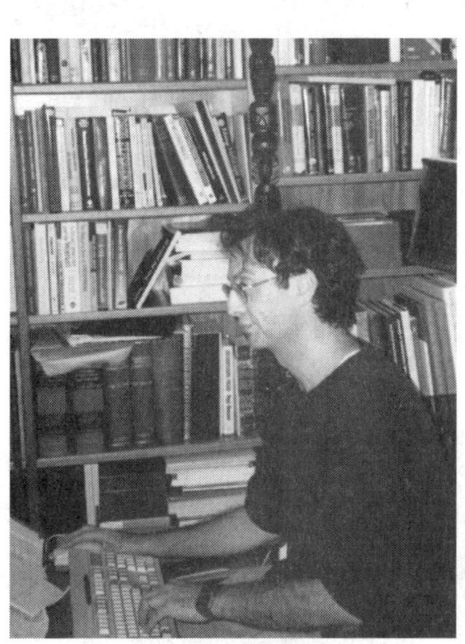

My son John Hoffer in the late 1990s in my library. John is professor of medicine at McGill University in Montreal, Quebec.

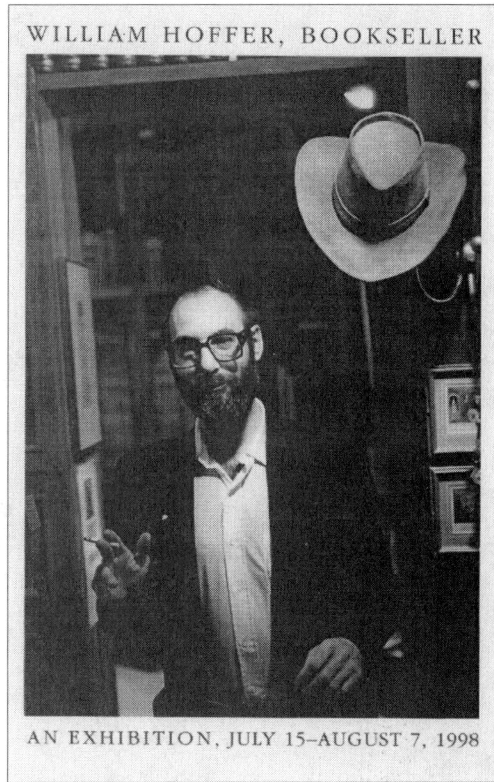

My son William who died in 1997.

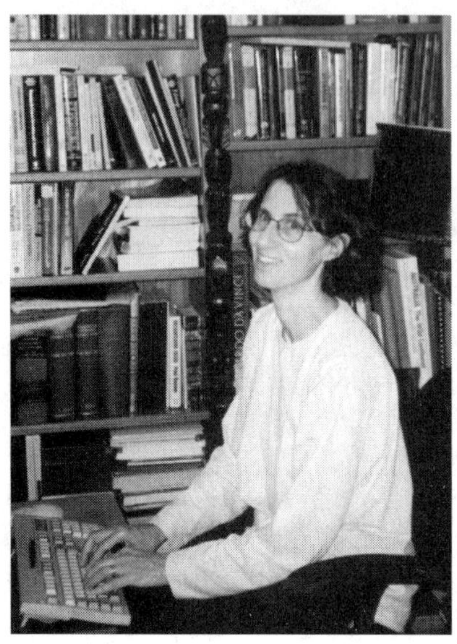

My daughter Miriam who is a dietician
at Women's College Hospital in Toronto.

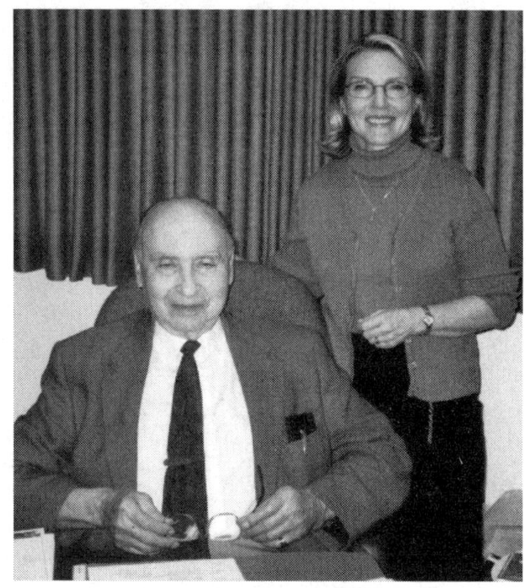

In my office in Victoria, B.C., with
my secretary Fran Fuller in the late
1990s.

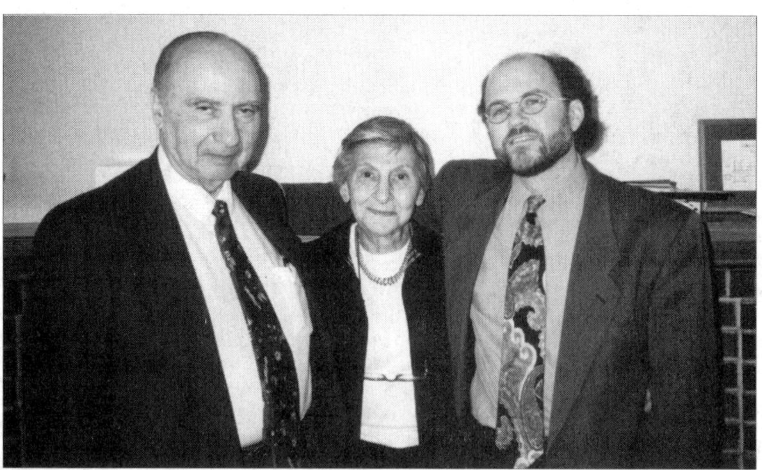

With my wife Rose and Steven Carter, the Executive
Director of the International Schizophrenia Foundation
in the late 1990s.

XII

THE ROCKEFELLER FOUNDATION

Our relationship with the Rockefeller Foundation began in 1952. Dr. McKerracher was advised by Dr. William Malamud, Professor of Psychiatry at Boston University and Dr. Hudson Hoagland, Director, Worcester Foundation, near Boston that the Rockefeller Foundation might be interested in our research. Dr. Malamud had at one point been one of the distinguished United States psychiatrists invited to spend a few days with us in Saskatchewan to give a series of lectures and seminars. I had met Dr. Hoagland on my first tour of American research centers, in 1951. These men told Dr. McKerracher about the Dementia Praecox Committee, a research group organized and chaired by Dr. Nolan D.C. Lewis. They were both members. Dr. Lewis had created this group right after the war, in order to keep the flame of biological psychiatric research burning. He knew that psychoanalysis was going to sweep the nation. Although he was also an analyst, having been anointed by Dr. Freud himself, he did not want to see biological research die. The committee was funded by the Scottish Rites Masons. They gave annual small grants, usually of around $5,000, to various investigators. These investigators then reported the results of their research at the next appropriate annual meeting of the Committee.

We were invited to attend the 1952 meeting as observers. Our expenses were not paid, as we were not grantees. The meeting itself was held in the Waldorf Astoria hotel, in the Canada room. I thought this very appropriate. Before the meeting, Dr. Osmond, myself, and Dr. McKerracher held a conference in the latter's room to decide how best to present our data. We had our adrenochrome hypothesis by then and had started our vitamin B-3 clinical trials. I recall how careful Dr. McKerracher was as he cautioned us not to use the word cure when talking about our vitamin data. We would, after all, be surrounded by some of the greatest American psychiatrists and research scientists. Humphry and I decided not to tell the group we were working with adrenochrome but merely to outline the basic indole hypothesis that we were going to examine. We did not want them to know about adrenochrome because we did not quite trust them not to steal the idea from us. I know now that we need not have worried, since the idea had really been too novel for anyone to even want to steal. When my turn came, I outlined our hypothesis very carefully, in about the same way I had done at the first meeting of the Saskatchewan Committee on Schizophrenia Research. After I had finished my presentation, Humphry and I were astounded when Dr. H. Waelsch, the well-known biochemist working with Dr. Lewis at the Psychiatric Institute, asked whether we had considered adren-ochrome. We immediately had to discard our secrecy plan and told the group that we had synthesized it and were going to make studies of it. Dr. Osmond then reported on our vitamin research. I cannot recall the reports that were made by the other scientists. I do recall that the Dean of Johns Hopkins University Medical School spoke to Humphry and me privately during a break and told us very seriously not to be deterred from our work, as he warned us of the negative reaction he was certain it would generate. He turned out to be absolutely correct—and nothing could have deterred us.

We had come to this meeting with no expectation that we would receive support from the Dementia Praecox Committee. We had been invited as a courtesy to Dr. McKerracher, under the firm condition that we would not apply for a research grant. But the con-tacts we made there paved the way to the Rockefeller Foundation. We would apply for a grant from them in 1954.

In the meantime, as 1953 unfolded, Dr. McKerracher was busy with plans for the new Department of Psychiatry for the College of Medicine at the University of Saskatchewan. The college was being upgraded from one which gave only preclinical lectures in anatomy, physiology, and histology over two years into a complete medical school. The University Hospital was under construction and would be completed in 1955. Dr. McKerracher was pretty certain he would be appointed the first Chairman of the Department.

We decided to move our research headquarters from Regina to Saskatoon in order to be close to the new college of medicine with its resources and because we would have ample space in the new hospital then under construction. In Regina, in the Munroe Wing, we had only a few small offices in the basement of the building. It was a dark, dingy area with the usual pipes and other services overhead. Given the space available, it had been impossible to set up a research laboratory. I had to plan the move from Regina to Saskatoon.

This situation was the backdrop when in 1954 I applied to the Rockefeller Foundation for a grant requesting over $300,000 to support our research over three years. In this application I outlined our adrenochrome hypothesis, describing what we had observed by then, i.e. the hallucinogenic properties of adrenochrome and the therapeutic properties of vitamin B-3 for early schizophrenia. Later that year, Dr. John Weir, Medical Director, Rockefeller Foundation, came to visit us for a few days, since the foundation did not award grants until the potential recipients were visited. I was still based in Regina. These on-site visits were the main means by which the foundation assessed the quality of the grant proposal and of the investigators who would do the research. Dr. Weir spent a couple of days with me and Dr. McKerracher, observing our work and the hospital, and going over the ideas we had developed. I drove him to Weyburn one morning so he could meet Dr. Humphry Osmond and his research staff. Humphry showed us through his hospital and then we had a meeting with his medical staff. On the way back to Regina, Dr. Weir was unusually quiet. Eventually I asked him what he had thought of the hospital. Humphry and I had planned to let him see the worst part of the hospital as well as some of the better wards. We had shown him wards which housed up to 70 chronic patients. These are indescribable. They had bare concrete floors, gouged with holes. The patients in the female ward did not like to keep their clothes on, and for this reason the temperature of the ward was kept around 80 degrees Fahrenheit so that they would not get pneumonia. When someone came onto the ward, some of the patients would crowd around the visitor, but most were apathetic and submerged in their psychosis. Dr. Weir replied that he considered the hospital at Weyburn one of the three worst he had ever seen. I asked with interest where the other two were. He replied, "One in Egypt and the other in Jamaica".

The following day we drove to Saskatoon. I had asked Mr. Fred Mendel, a good friend, whether he would be willing to organize a social event in the evening for Dr. Weir and some of the faculty members of the new medical college at Saskatoon. It was our intention that after our group moved to Saskatoon to the University Hospital in 1955 that the research grant would be administered by the University of Saskatchewan. Fred very graciously invited a number of the faculty and a few others. We met at his private art gallery, near his meat packing plant.

From Saskatoon, John Weir flew back to New York. Before he left he told me that he was going to recommend to the board that they give us the grant, and that the odds were very good that the board would accept his recommendation. I asked him whether he would want an annual report from me. With all the other grants I had received I had to submit annual reports before we could obtain the following year's money. He replied, "Hell no. We do not want to hear from you again. You will be given the grant in order to spend it on research, not in writing useless reports." I found this very refreshing, then asked if he would mind if I sent him copies of all the research reports which we published with the aid of Rockefeller money. To this he agreed. This foundation had a good reputation for supporting what would be valuable research. Their desire at that time not to burden their investigators with useless work was I believe, one of the reasons they were successful.

The Rockefeller Foundation three-year grant began in 1954. It was administered by the University of Saskatchewan. All expenditures had to be approved by me and I had to follow a detailed budget which I worked out with the help of Dr. Osmond, Dr. McKerracher, and Stan Rands, his administrative assistant. We continued in this manner for the duration of the grant, which eventually ran for six years. The first three-year grant gave us just under $180,000 and the three-year renewal gave us less. I applied for the renewal after receiving a pledge from the Saskatchewan government that as the amount of money allocated through the Rockefeller Foundation each year went down, it would take up the slack. The foundation liked the fact that their grant would be used as seed money that would establish our research group. I consider the amounts we received to be substantial. To put them into perspective, consider that in 1954 a top chemist with a PhD would be lucky to obtain a salary of around $6,000 per year. Today that same position would pay up to ten times as much, or more. The rest of the money we needed came from the provincial government, from federal health grants, and in the form of small sums from other foundations.

While the foundation was very generous in refusing to ask for reports, the first grant did come with one condition attached. Dr. Weir explained that the foundation wanted me to visit psychiatric research centers in Europe and would make me a Rockefeller Travel Fellow. They proposed a three-month tour. I replied that I could not leave Rose and our son Bill alone in Regina for that amount of time and would want to take them with me. He said that on the daily allowance they would be giving me I would be able to pay for all three of us including hotel and food charges. I then agreed to go. We left in March of 1954, flying to New York and then sailing on the Ile de France for England. We left our two younger children, John and Miriam, with Pearl and Jack Wilner—Jack was then a scientist working for an experimental farm. He later became known for his work in assessing winter hardiness in plants using electrical measurements.

I had with me a list from John Weir of the research centers in Europe that the foundation suggested I visit. I had written to these establishments and arranged an itinerary.

In London we stayed at Ciba House, owned by the Ciba Foundation, a creation of the drug company Ciba. It served as a combined hotel and conference centre for physicians and scientists. While in London I had a useful meeting with Dr. Jonathan Gould, a psychiatrist. He had developed a vitamin B complex injectable preparation which he had found useful for bringing patients more quickly out of any type of delirium. He told me about a study he and his group had just completed. They had treated about 70 children with poliomyelitis. Half were given vitamin C in large doses and half were given placebo. The ones given the vitamin all recovered. In the placebo group about 20 percent of the children were left with residual impairment. I asked him whether he planned on publishing these results. He replied that there was no point, since the Salk vaccine had just been announced. I wish they had reported their vitamin C results as it would have supported the work done by Dr. Frederick Klenner of Reidsville, North Carolina, in the United States. He had announced to the American Medical Association in 1949 that intravenous vitamin C injections could cure polio, but the information had been rejected, due to the fact that earlier studies on vitamin C and polio had had conflicting results. The lack of success in some studies may have been because not enough vitamin C was used.

In London we rented a Morris Minor car, probably the smallest car I have ever gotten into, but very cheap. By the time we and our luggage were stowed away there was no room for anything else. We drove to Wales to visit Dr. Derek Richter. Dr. Richter had done some work with adrenochrome but had never drawn the same conclusion from his studies that we had. This was during a period when indoles were being examined as a possible cause of schizophrenia. The indoles were thought to be products of bowel metabolism. Most scientists, Dr. Richter among them, thought that high levels of any indole would be necessary to produce schizophrenia and these quantities were not found in the blood nor the urine. We also met with Dr. Hemphill, who had studied schizophrenics carefully for many years in a search for biochemical markers. One of his findings was that about ten percent of schizophrenics have either over-or underactive thyroid glands. From Wales we drove north to Birmingham where we met Dr. Joel Elkes. None of these meetings were eventful, nor had any effect on the nature of our research.

From London we flew to Paris. We knew no French and had difficulty getting along. We visited Professor Henri Baruch. He was working with bile extracts which he had given to animals to induce changes in behaviour. This work was part of the search for hallucinogenic indoles made in the bowel. He told me about his pigeon experiments, in which he produced a kind of catatonia in these birds. Professor Baruch was one of the few investigators studying the production of model psychosis in an attempt to reproduce some of the manifestations of schizophrenia. Several years later, at University Hospital, I repeated his experiment, using adrenochrome which I injected into homing pigeons. After the injection of adrenochrome, the pigeons also remained passive (catatonic), even while perched on a person's head or shoulder.

From Paris we flew to Switzerland. There I met with the research group at Sandoz (we had been obtaining LSD from Sandoz Canada for our research) and learned all about the interesting work they were doing with LSD. I also met Dr. Peter Witt, the spider scientist. He had found that spiders given hallucinogenic drugs wove distorted webs and he used this fact as a marker for detecting hallucinogenic activity in a compound. Adrenochrome also distorted the pattern. We rented another small car in Switzerland and drove across the Alps to Italy. In Rome we met with the discoverer of ECT, Dr. Cerletti. I was very pleased to meet him. He was still doing research, and had developed the hypothesis that ECT released a naturally occurring antidepressant chemical in the brain. He was trying to extract such a chemical from the brains of animals given ECT. He was not eventually successful. Perhaps with modern techniques such a substance might be found.

From Rome we flew to Frankfurt, West Germany, where I planned to visit the university. Huge piles of rubble still sat in the centre of the city from the bombing it had received ten years earlier. I learned nothing useful from the researchers there. After only a few days, we went on to Copenhagen, where I visited the Institute at Herstedvester for men. Here men found guilty of violent crimes, most of them criminal sexual psychopaths, were incarcerated forever. They had a real life sentence unless they could prove to the psychiatrists running the place that they would never repeat their violent acts. They were treated humanely. I learned that about half of the inmates were eventually released, most of them after volunteering to be castrated. As a result, the Institute boasted a very low recidivism rate. Then we came back to London for a few more weeks and returned by ship to New York. We were met at the immigration dock by a representative of the Rockefeller Foundation who whisked us through and escorted us to the hotel. We were very happy to be back in North America, where we could finally warm up.

I found this European tour very helpful because it demonstrated to me that nowhere in Europe was any work on schizophrenia being done that I could count of real value. Given the weakness of our competition, I returned home more confident that we could firmly establish our research program.

Early in July 1954, I and my family moved to Saskatoon so I could begin work in the new University Hospital. Psychiatry was given two wings in the new building, 5D and 5E, on the top floor. The new research area contained two large chemical laboratories across the hall from each other, equipped with fume cupboards, benches, and all other services considered essential in a modern laboratory. The labs also included offices for a psychologist, a chief research nurse, myself, and two secretaries whose work was needed to administer the research. The wing housing the labs, 5E, did not contain any patient beds, but did include therapy areas.

Here I and my staff continued our work according to policies I had established from the beginning. Each of my chief investigators were expected to give half of their time to the overall research program. They could give the other half to their own projects on condition that they could show these were related to the whole investigative program. I also established that only workers who had made a direct contribution to the research involved would have their names on papers. At that time it was the custom in many research units for the director to attach his name to every paper that appeared and thereby soon rack up an enormous number of publications. While this strategy advanced many an academic career, I did not consider it fair or appropriate. Every paper bearing my name contained a substantial contribution from me and any paper that I co-authored also contained the names of all workers who had made a significant contribution to it. A large number of papers which I did not co-author were also published by our research unit members. As part of the preparatory process for publication, and to facilitate strong, ongoing research, I also read all the manuscripts generated by our work, discussed them with the authors, and then submitted them to members of the Saskatchewan Committee on Schizophrenia Research for review.

Three members of the research staff who had worked with me in Regina moved to Saskatoon. Neil Agnew, M.A. (he later received his PhD) was our chief research psychologist. He and I published one paper together on our finding that nicotinic acid and nicotinamide greatly reduced the intensity of the LSD reaction in normal volunteers. Biochemist Dr. Roland Fisher was with us for several years, but was not productive and was eventually asked to leave. Miss M.J. Callbeck, RN, was our chief research psychiatric nurse. She had been head nurse in the Munroe Wing when I arrived there in 1950. Before that, she had received postgraduate training at the Allan Memorial Institute, part of McGill University in Montreal, and as a result had been in charge of psychiatric training for nurses at the Saskatchewan Hospital in Weyburn for about two years. When I began my research program at the Munroe Wing I needed the full cooperation of the psychiatric and nursing staff. Marg Callbeck was a very good nurse who became extremely helpful to the research program. Her enthusiasm ensured that the rest of the nursing staff would be supportive. As time went on, the nursing staff in general had become much more interested and cooperative than the Wing's medical staff. They had to work more closely with the patients and were soon aware that a new dimension had been added to the treatment of schizophrenia when they began to see recoveries unlike any they had witnessed before.

After I learned that the first Rockefeller Foundation grant had been approved, I informed the staff of the Wing. A few months later, Marg asked me whether she could join our research group. She wanted to give up her position as chief nurse. We did not have much of a budget and she agreed to work for substantially less than she was making. This showed me she was highly motivated and I was glad to add her to our staff, as I needed a research nurse to look after the patients in our division. A research nurse looks after records, makes sure all the orders are properly carried out, interprets the research studies to the regular nursing staff, and meets with the rest of the research staff to advocate on the patients' behalf from the nursing point of view.

After we moved to Saskatoon in 1954, we decided we wanted to create an entire research nursing division. The Rockefeller Foundation was intrigued by this idea and offered us a grant that would allow Marg to visit psychiatric research centers in the United States. We arranged for her to spend several weeks with Professor Robert Heath at Tulane Medical School in New Orleans. I was by then familiar with his work with taraxein. This was a protein fraction rich in copper that he had extracted from the blood of schizophrenic patients; when injected into monkeys, it made them psychotic. I was extremely interested in this research, and wanted Marg to observe the experiments Health's group was doing. After that she went to New York City and worked for several months at the Psychiatric Institute under Dr. Nolan D.C. Lewis, with their research nursing division. Then she returned to Saskatoon to head up our own newly-formed research nursing division, consisting of herself. She remained in this post until we both left the University Hospital in 1967. Miss Callbeck became co-author of ten reports to the psychiatric literature. She was one of the four authors of our first report on the treatment of schizophrenia with vitamin B-3. She was also co-author of four reports on cholesterol and nicotinic acid, two on the autonomic nervous system, one on the HOD test, and one on a personal experience in an experiment she had volunteered for. On the basis of my theoretical reasoning about the effects of LSD (that it catalyzed adrenochrome production) and my observations that penicillamine was therapeutic for schizophrenia when combined with vitamin B-3, I got the idea that if a volunteer took penicillamine and then was given LSD, the LSD reaction would be prevented. Marg agreed to be a volunteer. She had already taken LSD twice and was familiar with its effects. But in combination with the penicillamine, something went wrong. She did not, indeed, develop the usual LSD reaction—and lost her affect. For two weeks she was not able to feel any emotion. I was very concerned and watched her very carefully but also felt certain that this effect would be washed out in two weeks. She recovered almost to the day I had predicted. However I decided never to run that experiment again. We published an account of it in the following paper: Hoffer, A. and Callbeck, MJ: Drug-Induced Schizophrenia. *J Mental Science*, 106: 138-159, 1960.

In their support of our group's research and professional development over six years, I believe the Rockefeller Foundation got their money's worth. Our work became one of the main roots of a new type of medicine that would be given the name "orthomolecular" by Linus Pauling. We opened up a number of new areas to research, some of which are just now being investigated, although they should have been followed up several decades ago. The adrenochrome hypothesis and its offshoots alone, including niacin therapy for schizophrenia, represents a splendid return on the Foundation's investment. We received altogether about 400,000 1954 to 1960 dollars or about 2,000,000 of today's dollars. One schizophrenic patient treated by tranquilizers or one not treated at all will cost the state about $2,000,000 over their lifetime. Every schizophrenic patient treated successfully with orthomolecular methods saves their community that same $2,000,000 and to date, there have been thousands so treated. Over 90 percent of early and relapsing patients will recover if given orthomolecular treatment for up to 2 years.

After the Rockefeller Foundation in 1959, I approached the Rockefeller Brothers' Fund in New York. Each of the brothers provided a portion of the monies this fund paid out, and they retained personal control over how the fund was disbursed. During my second meeting with him, the director, who was interested and sympathetic to our work, told me that I would be invited to New York within the next few months to present my grant request before the Rockefeller brothers. I was indeed invited, but a few days before I was to leave I received another call. Nelson Rockefeller had just announced that he was going to run for the governorship of New York. As a result, he would no longer have time to meet me. Nor would the other brothers, since they would be involved in the campaign. That was my last contact with the Rockefellers.

XIII

The Book:
How To Live With
Schizophrenia

I first discovered Dr. Donald Johnson, British Member of Parliament (MP) in 1951. He was a doctor who later became a lawyer and then an innkeeper before his election to parliament. I had been searching the literature for information on substances like mescaline or LSD, compounds we defined as chemicals which caused changes in perception and in thought without mental confusion or disorientation. I ran across a citation for a pamphlet called "The Hallucinogens" by one Dr. Johnson. I located him and he sent me a copy, and, as already described, we adopted his term for the compounds we were studying. In this pamphlet he described the effects of hashish. He had obtained much of his information from several commissions which had examined the problem of hashish addiction, especially in India. We began to correspond and later Dr. Osmond and I met with him in London. Several times we had tea with him at the Parliament Buildings, in a room overlooking the river Thames. He told us that he had written the report after he had recovered from a transient psychotic reaction.

He had been running an inn at the time. One day a wine salesman brought with him an opened bottle of wine. Normally the bottles were sealed and would be opened only in the buyer's presence. This time, without thinking much of it, he began to drink from the previously-opened bottle. While he was doing so, his wife came in. He offered her some from the same glass. She drank about one half of what he had. The following day both Dr. and Mrs. Johnson became psychotic, he more so. His wife called for help and Dr. Johnson was committed to a mental hospital under an old mental health act. His wife remained at home and was well within about three days. During his admission interview with the psychiatrist at the mental hospital he was told that he would never get well and would have to spend the rest of his life there. He was denied visiting privileges. However, after a few days he began to recover and soon was able to smuggle notes out via other visitors to his lawyer, who arranged for his discharge. The double psychotic reaction he and his wife had experienced puzzled him very much and he began to search for an answer. He could not accept that they had simultaneously developed schizophrenia and concluded that he and his wife had been poisoned by the wine they had consumed. He had no enemies he knew of and could not guess how this could have come about. But the event initiated his search for natural compounds which might have been placed in the wine. He also informed the police, but they would not take him seriously and no investigation was carried out. He had never been ill before this experience and he remained well afterward. For many years he had run for the Conservative party with no success. After his psychotic experience he ran once more and this time he was elected. It is a pity his claims were not investigated as his explanation appeared logical to us. He described his experience in a book later on. By the time he met us he had already become a publisher. He was one of the main MPs who introduced new mental health legislation into England. It might be a good idea for every legislator to have a similar experience with our mental hospitals and psychiatric wards.

Early in the 1960s, I was in London and called upon Dr. Johnson. As we enjoyed our afternoon tea on a balcony overlooking the Thames, he suddenly asked me if I had any books I would like to have published. My immediate reaction was negative, but after awhile it occurred to me that there was a book that was very badly needed, a book for schizophrenic patients and their relatives. I asked Dr. Johnson what kind of book he had in mind and he replied that it would be up to me, he would publish anything I wanted. Dr. Osmond and I were then organizing the American Schizophrenia Association. I thought it would be most helpful to families if they could be given correctly hopeful information about schizophrenia. The only other potential sources of information were their relatives' doctors, who generally refused to talk about schizophrenia, or psychiatric textbooks which invariably gave the most depressing views about the condition and its prognosis. One of my patients had once made a serious suicide attempt after reading this type of material. He had been treated in University Hospital in Saskatoon over several admissions but had not been told his diagnosis. A few months after discharge he was in his doctor's office near his home. The doctor had to leave the office for a moment. This young man immediately looked into the file and found that he had been diagnosed with schizophrenia.

That evening he looked into an old dictionary at home and found *dementia praecox* defined as a hopelessly incurable disease. He took a 22 rifle into the garage and shot himself in his chest, missing his heart by 1 centimetre. He was readmitted, repaired, and came under my care. Then I discovered what had happened. After I discussed schizophrenia with him as a biochemical disease that could be treated and controlled, he accepted the diagnosis.

I thought Humphry Osmond would be interested in writing such a book with me. I suggested to Dr. Johnson that we would prepare the first draft and then ask my sister Fannie to rewrite it into the type of language that would be comprehensible to the layperson. When I saw her after returning home I asked her whether she would be willing to translate our text into plain English. Fannie agreed, Humphry thought the project a good idea as well, and we decided to split the royalties three ways. The book was published by Johnson Publications Ltd., 11-14 Stanhope Mews West, London S.W. 7, in 1966. The foreword was written by the Right Honorable Christopher Mayhew, MP, and its last sentence read, "This book has an interest and importance far beyond its immediate subject matter, and deserves the widest circulation." It was published at about the same time in the United States by a small house, University Books. The foreword for the American edition was written by Dr. Nolan D.C. Lewis. The book was revised and published again in 1974 by Citadel Press and updated again in 1993, again by Citadel Press, New York, NY. Since then, the book has been revised once more by myself and is available as *Healing Schizophrenia*, published by CCNM Press, Toronto, 2004. I believe the foreword Dr. Lewis wrote for the first American edition remains an excellent description of the book's aims and contents, and I offer it here:

This is a unique book in two ways. It is the first book written for the schizophrenic and schizoid patients, instructing them in what attitude they should take to live with the disorder. Secondly, the authors have accomplished the difficult task of presenting a longitudinal picture of the whole problem in perspective, utilizing only those terms that can be readily understood by the general reader.

The authors' description of the nature of the disorder including its universality, inheritance aspects, physical and physiological changes and psychological phenomena, such as changes in thought processes, mood changes, behavior oddities and numerous examples of depersonalization phenomena, afford the necessary orientation desirable to approach the more complicated items and theories concerning causes described in subsequent sections of the text. Biochemical, psychological and sociological factors are discussed and particular attention is devoted to the description of the action of several psychoactive drugs used currently, including the personal experiences of the authors with adrenochrome, a substance of great importance discovered by the authors.

The excellent biological survey emphasizes quite clearly that man is a multi-determined being existing in a complex of interrelations and that biology is one comprehensive basic science in which all aspects of living things blend. The person must be considered as a biological unity, the product of numerous and complex factors, including the historical, the genetic, and pre-birth influences, the family life and formal education, social circumstances, and cultural traditions. These are blended into a true integration, that is, into something reactively different from any of the ingredients that compose it.

This being true, in order to get at the pathology of behavior we must not only study the individual in action, but also the brain and the other organs of the body, particularly those that support the brain directly, and finally the whole individual. We should not yield to the modern trend to explain everything in psychodynamic terms, which may seem fairly satisfactory to us, or even help the patient adjust to the world, to some extent, but we should continue to seek correlations in the physiological and structural parts as well as in the psychological. Although we can as yet approach a human being only objectively, our attitude should remain holistically oriented at all times. It may help to remember that we are always in an "organic" state from conception to final complete disintegration.

In the section on therapy, one finds detailed instructions for a total attack on the disorder, directed throughout to the patient and his relatives, with a comprehensive discussion of the pharmacological approaches, including an informative presentation of the nicotinic acid therapy as originated and applied by the authors in their research and practice. Concerning pharmacological studies, there are results that are worth mentioning, in support of the interest in this field. To enumerate just a few of the important achievements of psychoneuropharmacology that have appeared during the past 15 years, one may mention (1) contributions to the knowledge of the structure-function of brain cells as well as of other body cells; (2) demonstration of a biochemical individuality of the brain and the providing of methods for the study of a chemical basis of learning; (3) emphasis on the dependence of some of the pharmacological responses on the situational and social settings; (4) renewal of interest in the placebo response for careful scrutiny, testing and evaluation; (5) indications that the so-called drug-produced experimental "model-psychoses" are in some way linked to enzyme systems in the brain; (6) certain impressions running through the results of published biochemical research showing similarities sufficient to suggest that a chemical factor or factors are involved in schizophrenia. It would seem to be established that there is something different circulating in the blood of schizophrenics than in that of other people. The contributions of the authors of this book have been extensive and outstanding in several of the areas included in the term 'psychoneuropharmacology'.

How To Live With Schizophrenia was the first "how to" book published in the medical literature. It appeared during a time when it was considered almost unprofessional conduct for any psychiatrist to tell their patients that they had the disease schizophrenia. Karl Menninger had published a paper just a few years earlier strongly condemning such a practice. About 100,000 copies have been sold since it first appeared. The title, *How To Live With Schizophrenia*, reflected our intent to make the book's contents clear, as well as my son John's observation that "how to" books sell very well. The book has been translated into French and Portuguese. A good companion book is my volume, *Common Questions on Schizophrenia and Their Answers*, published by Keats Publishers, New Canaan, Connecticut, 1988.

The book has had an impact. Over the years I have received numerous letters from grateful individuals telling me how they had used the information to recover or to help a family member recover. It has not been reviewed in medical journals, probably because the idea that one can treat schizophrenic patients with large doses of a vitamin was—and remains—anathema to many psychiatrists. It has also been universally acclaimed by patients and their families who felt relieved of their guilt when they read that schizophrenia is a biochemical disease and not caused by so-called schizophrenogenic mothers. Psychoanalysts had promulgated the view that certain cold or "refrigerator" mothers were responsible for causing the illness in their children.

This idea persisted far too long. In August 1991, I was consulted by a young mother whose seven-year-old daughter was clearly schizophrenic, and suffered from visual and auditory hallucinations. She had been seen by a psychiatrist in Vancouver several months earlier. I was astonished to learn that he had told the woman that she was the cause of the problem. She left his office crying. They returned to their family doctor and complained bitterly about this psychiatrist. The doctor then admitted that he had heard similar complaints from other patients. He had referred the child to him because he would be able to see her the soonest. Given this psychiatrist's attitude, I was not surprised he was not very busy. After seeing me, she read our book and was freed of the guilt generated by the psychiatrist. Surely her circumstance must be very rare today—at least I hope so!

I have received surprisingly few critical letters, but one I recall most vividly also had to do with the mother issue. It was written by a woman who complained bitterly that our book was wrong since she had been impressed by her psychiatrist with the fact that her mother had been one of these "refrigerator mothers" and it was she who had made her ill. Her language against me was most vile and intemperate. Only a few physicians have shown interest in the book. One was a Boston psychiatrist who came to Saskatoon to observe me in my work after he read it. He began to practice with vitamins but unfortunately died a few months after I met him.

Bill W., co-founder of Alcoholics Anonymous, read our book and recommended it to Dr. E. Boyle, Director, Miami Heart Institute. When he got hold of it, Dr. Boyle spent the whole night reading the book. Early the next evening he phoned me at my hotel in New York. He thought it was a great book and was especially well written for doctors. He thought we had written it for the average physician. I corrected him by stating it had been written for the average layperson. Because we had done so, I explained, average physicians who generally knew little more than average laypersons about schizophrenia would be more willing to read it and able to grasp its message. They would not think it had been written down to them. Boyle and I became close friends. He later acted as an advisor to the Drug Coronary Study which eventually established nicotinic acid as the most effective compound for accomplishing two tasks that lower the risk of heart attack or stroke, namely lowering cholesterol and increasing high density lipoprotein cholesterol. His work with about 90 patients who had had a coronary attack found that over a ten-year period only six instead of the expected 60 died when nicotinic acid therapy was used.

In his public lectures, Professor Linus Pauling often told how this book had been a major factor in arousing his interest in the use of megavitamin therapy. After he read our book, he decided that he would not retire as planned, but would enter a new phase in his contributions to medicine and science. How our book came into his hands makes for an interesting story. In 1960, a doctor from

California called me in Saskatoon. He told me about his twelve-year-old son, a patient in the psychiatric ward of a University Hospital in California, crying as he spoke of his son's disease. The psychiatrist had told him that his son would never get well and that the best course would be to have him committed to a mental hospital for the rest of his life. The doctor could not accept this advice. Instead, he began to spend as much time as he could in the medical library, hoping to read about a better treatment. There he ran across our first report, published in 1957, in which we described the use of vitamin B-3 for the treatment of acute schizophrenia. In our report we referred to the double-blind controlled studies where we had compared niacin and niacinamide against placebo. The results with the use of this vitamin were twice as good as they had been with nothing (placebo). I recommended that he place his son on niacin, 1000 milligrams three times daily. But in 1960, 500 milligram tablets were not commercially available: the largest tablets were 100 milligrams. These were of little value since they contained a lot of filler in order to make a tablet which would be not too small. Taking thirty each day would load the patient with filler and make him sick. The California doctor found a company in Seattle, Kirkman Laboratories, willing to make up 500 milligram tablets. They were the first United States company to do so. With a bottle of niacin tablets in hand, he went to the hospital and spoke to the psychiatrist in charge. He told him about his conversation with me and about the results we had published in the 1957 article. He asked him to start his son on the vitamin. The psychiatrist surprised him when he vehemently refused to consider this. He told him two lies, first that niacin would fry his son's brain, and second, that they had tried the vitamin treatment already and seen no response. The first lie merely showed how ignorant the psychiatrist was of the effects of niacin. It dilates the blood vessels near the skin, but not those leading into the brain, so it cannot possibly heat up the brain. The second lie was merely a forerunner of a large number of lies that the establishment used successfully from that point on. When there was no toxicity they invented it, and when they claimed vitamin B-3 had been tested and did not work they simply lied outright, because to them the end justified the means. The "end" as explained to patients was the desire to protect them from false optimism. The real end was to protect themselves against the need to do a better job treating their patients.

The psychiatrist finally told this man that if he insisted, the boy would immediately be discharged. This was a major threat, as the boy was too psychotic to be cared for at home. The boy's father went home depressed. After talking it over with his wife he asked her whether she would go to the hospital every day and give their son the niacin. She was too timid to do so. He therefore began to feed it to his son on regular visits, as they walked around the hospital grounds. He did not want to give him the tablets directly as this would be too obvious. He therefore reground the tablets, placed the powder on bread, covered the bread with jam, which his son loved, and fed him these niacin-jam sandwiches. His son did not know he was taking anything, so this was a single blind controlled experiment with one subject. After about three weeks, his son said, "Daddy, whenever I eat the sandwich I turn red." His father became worried that his son would tell his psychiatrist and promptly began to put niacinamide in instead of niacin. Twelve weeks after the vitamin treatment was begun his son said, "Daddy I want to go home." His father got him discharged. His son completed Grade 12, finishing in the top five percent of all US students that year. I suggested that he remain on the vitamin for at least 12 months. To be on the safe side, his father kept him on for 18 months. Then he discontinued. A few months later, the boy began to relapse. His father put him back on the vitamin but this time he did not respond as fast. I have observed this phenomenon in my clinical practice. He called me again and I suggested he give him penicillamine in addition. I had found this copper chelator useful in the treatment of schizophrenics. Within a few weeks of starting this second chemical, his son recovered. He has remained well since. He became a physician, later a psychiatrist. He worked for one summer at the Linus Pauling Institute and later went into research in California. He has published some papers. As far as I know he is still well today. I later described this case in my paper, "Five California Schizophrenics," published in 1967 in *The Journal of Schizophrenia*.

This "miraculous" recovery occurred in a small Southern California community and became known to another family living there. Their daughter had become paranoid and had failed to respond to several years of intense treatment including family therapy, drugs, and group and individual psychotherapy. Her family told me about her and I agreed I would accept her at University Hospital in Saskatoon. She came by car with her parents. On the way she tried to strangle her mother. She arrived at our hospital in a very psychotic condition. I promptly placed her on the vitamin program and gave her a small series of ECT. She made a complete recovery and was discharged within 30 days. She then went home and with the exception of a few minor relapses has remained well since. She was the subject of a special film made a few years later, *Schizophrenia—Shattered Mirror*, made with N.I.M.H. support. Her father looked upon her wellness as a miracle and decided to proselytize the treatment in his community. He purchased copies of *How To Live With Schizophrenia* and began to call upon each doctor in the area to discuss his daughter's case and to leave a copy of the book. Few cared to listen, but he did leave a copy with a psychiatrist who agreed to read it. Later, Dr. Pauling and Ava, his wife, were invited to tea at this psychiatrist's home. She had left the book on her coffee table. On this visit, Dr. Pauling glanced through the book and asked the psychiatrist whether he could borrow it. She was pleased to lend it to him. He began to read it that evening and like Dr. Boyle, read all night. He was amazed by the fact that we were using such high doses of vitamin B-3 and vitamin C when every indication in the liter-ature suggested that only low doses were needed. However our work started him thinking about how these high doses could possibly be helpful. As already mentioned, he decided not to retire from his academic work and took a position as a distinguished professor of chemistry at the University of California at San Diego (UCSD). Without Dr. Pauling's ensuing research and advocacy, it is likely that the present increasing interest in vitamins as therapy would have been delayed many decades. Millions of people today owe their better health to his work. I am unhappy that not a single university offered him an honorary medical degree. He did not need any more PhDs and DScs. The medical profession owes him a major apology for having treated him as shabbily as they have.

XIV

THE CANADIAN MENTAL HEALTH ASSOCIATION AND SCHIZOPHRENICS ANONYMOUS

Both the Canadian Mental Health Association (CMHA) and Schizophrenics Anonymous (SA) were groups that involved lay members. My association with the CMHA lasted about 16 years, from 1951 to 1967. It was warm and friendly at first but did not stay that way. This chapter tells why. My connection with a groundbreaking group called Schizophrenics Anonymous was a much happier one, that led to much benefit for patients. First, an account of my history with the CMHA.

The CMHA

The CMHA, established in 1950, was organized largely by Dr. Claire Hincks, a Toronto psychiatrist. He envisioned it as a national organization that would aim to improve psychiatric care for the mentally ill. Each province was expected to create its own division. Saskatchewan was the first to do so. As previously described, while I was interning in Saskatoon, Dr. D.G. McKerracher came to the city to speak to the first group of CMHA lay volunteer workers. I heard about that meeting, and after Dr. McKerracher's presentation, I spoke to him about the possibility of getting a job with the Saskatchewan Department of Public Health. I began to work in this

Department's employ, in the Psychiatric Services Branch, on July 1, 1950, at the Munroe Wing, as a direct result of this conversation. The following year, Dr. McKerracher asked me whether I would be willing to become Chairman of the Scientific Advisory Committee of the Saskatchewan Division of the CMHA. I agreed to do so and was appointed by the board at Dr. McKerracher's recommendation. I remained in this position until I resigned in 1967.

At the outset, The CMHA, Saskatchewan Division, desired chiefly to improve the treatment provided for mentally ill patients in the community and in the mental hospitals of Saskatchewan. The government, under Premier T.C. (Tommy) Douglas, (he also served as Minister of Health), had already decided to bring the Psychiatric Services Branch into the twentieth century. At the time, Saskatchewan's two mental hospitals and one hospital for the mentally retarded, called a training school, were amongst the worst in the world. Premier Douglas did not need any urging or encouragement, but he did need public support to spend the money which would be needed to rebuild the hospitals, obtain psychiatric staff, train nurses, and provide all the facilities and staff any modern hospital required to treat their patients properly. He thought that the CMHA could play a most useful role in educating the public about the needs of the mentally ill. The CMHA succeeded in doing so. They began to talk openly about mental illness, especially schizophrenia. They arranged for family members and other interested parties to travel to the hospitals to see for themselves what they were like.

Weyburn, where Humphry worked, was about 70 miles southeast of Regina. The roads were still to a large degree dirt or gravel and it could take two hours by car to travel to that hospital from Regina. This made it difficult for family members to visit their relatives in the hospital. The CMHA therefore arranged for buses to bring people there. Dr. Osmond was by then superintendant, and he welcomed these visitors, explained to them what he and his staff were trying to do and showed them the wards of the hospital. These actions represented a major change from previous protocol, when the policy had been to never show relatives the wards. When family members came to visit patients, they waited in a visiting room; their relatives were brought to them. Many years before, my parents and I had had to wait in a visiting room for several hours to see a cousin. Later I discovered that they had taken him from the ward, given him a bath, and changed him into clean clothes, then brought him out. After the visit he was taken back to the same ward and given back the same clothes as before. I found this out only after I had become familiar with the hospital as it was under Dr. Osmond's direction. Even then, the housing conditions were still terrible. But I wonder if the patients were not relatively better off than are similar individuals now living on the streets of our major cities without shelter, medical care, or nursing care. In 1950, society did not know any better, but today we do know how to operate modern humane hospitals—we are simply unwilling to spend the money needed to do so. If we took all the real but hidden costs of chronic, unresolved mental illness into account though, I am certain we would find we are not saving any money at all.

The construction of the Saskatchewan Hospital at Yorkton, a town about 200 miles northeast of Regina, was accelerated because of the public campaign run by the CMHA. The story behind this hospital's design is an interesting one. Kyo (Joe) Izumi, a well-known young architect in Saskatchewan who had already designed and built several notable buildings, had been retained by the government to upgrade our mental hospitals. He became interested in finding out how to design the most therapeutic building. Joe, Humphry, and I had many discussions regarding the needs of the patients. We were especially interested in providing them with privacy, non-existent in the mental hospitals of that day; they were characterized by huge dormitory wards housing up to 80 patients. Dr. Osmond frequently made the point that if patients could be given a choice of living in a modern motel rather than in the hospital, they would undoubtedly choose the motel. But how could we reconcile the patients' needs for privacy and the community's need to provide the best possible housing at the least possible expense? Joe was familiar with our LSD studies, in which we reproduced much of the experience of schizophrenia in normal volunteers. It occurred to us that a volunteer under the influence of the drug could spend time in various types of hospital wards and corridors and would then experience what patients with similar perceptual distortions experience. After recovering from the drug, the person could use the memory of the experience to design a structure that would have a minimal negative impact on the patient.

It was not possible to interview patients and get their views since they were too disturbed and would have had difficulty describing their perceptual worlds. Joe therefore decided he would become a volunteer, take LSD, and spend time on the wards of the hospital at Weyburn under Dr. Osmond's supervision and also on the ward of the University Hospital in Saskatoon, then called 5DE, under my supervision. This he did. After he came out of these experiences he had a good idea of the types of building which would make patients either comfortable or uncomfortable. He designed a small hospital which won a silver medal from the American Psychiatric Association for excellence. He prepared the architectural plans and the government decided to build the first such hospital in Yorkton. It was to be the first of a series of regional hospitals, so located that no one would need to travel more than 50 miles to visit a sick relative. The overall vision for this hospital construction was called the Saskatchewan Plan. But at this time Premier Tommy Douglas left the province to lead the national Canadian Cooperative Federation, a left wing political party, and another man became premier of Saskatchewan.

Mr. Woodrow Lloyd had a different style of governing. Mr. Douglas had known what he wanted and provided massive support for the transformation of the psychiatric services branch into a modern entity. Mr. Lloyd depended more on the advice he was given by his administrators. The new government announced that due to financial problems, they were postponing the construction of the hospital at Yorkton. I then decided that it would be appropriate for the CMHA to become actively involved and to pressure the government not to delay the construction. I was, as mentioned, Chairman of the Scientific Advisory Committee. I had not been notified by any of my superiors within the government that I must not get involved in such a public campaign. I suggested to the CMHA that they initiate a public program that would let the people of Yorkton know what was happening and encourage them to pressure the politicians to go ahead with the building. We had a series of meetings with public speakers. The people of the area responded massively and sent about 700 letters to the premier. Later I heard that he had become extremely angry and put out by this mail—but the government did change its mind and proceed with construction. These events are described in an excellent book written by my sister, Fannie Kahan, *Brains and Bricks: The History of the Yorkton Psychiatric Centre* and published in Regina by the Saskatchewan Division of the CMHA in 1965. As far as I am concerned, this campaign represents the last time the Saskatchewan chapter of the CMHA accomplished anything meaningful or useful, at least as far as treating patients more successfully is concerned.

Unfortunately, while the hospital at Yorkton and others were eventually built, the basic principles of the Saskatchewan Plan were violated. The plan had envisaged a number of regional hospitals. But they were to be hospitals, not first aid stations. The idea was to keep patients in hospital until they were well enough to carry on at home, to work, and to be productive members of the community. If they did not reach this state, they were to be kept in hospital, as they would have been in the older mental hospitals. But the appearance of the tranquilizers in 1955 changed the whole picture. It now became possible to quickly settle down disturbed patients. This gave the treating doctors the illusion that the disease had been brought under control. The older style of keeping patients in for very long periods of time was replaced by a revolving door policy. Patients rapidly circulated from home to hospital and back again, and more recently, from home to hospital to home to various alternate facilities, and finally, to the streets. The Yorkton Hospital administration did not take advantage of the superior new design, did not keep their patients in long enough to establish that they were well and soon prided itself on the fact that they did not need the number of beds which had been planned. Discharging patients became a virtue in and of itself. In 1960, full-blown deinstitutionalization mania took hold and the two large mental hospitals (at Weyburn and North Battleford) were down-graded and their patients scattered all over the province into inadequate nursing homes, hotels, and the streets. Patients in the old style hospitals that could provide no treatment never got well; now, the new style of control with drugs also ensured that patients never got well.

My various attempts to address this situation (which was spreading across Canada) via the deployment of CMHA resources were sadly unsuccessful. I was appointed onto the Scientific Advisory Board of CMHA Toronto by the then Chairman, Dr. McKerracher in the mid-1950s. In that capacity, I attended a meeting in Toronto devoted to the topic of how bad mental health facilities were in Canada. I heard a lot of complaining, moaning, and groaning about the situation. I agreed that the situation was not good, but became impatient with the slow pace of the meeting. I moved that the CMHA appoint a subcommittee to do a survey of facilities in Canada and bring in a report. This proposal was seconded and passed. One of the members of the Toronto CMHA committee was Dr. James Tyhurst. He had carried out some sociological research in Pictou County in Nova Scotia so he was looked upon as the expert in this area. He was named chairman of this subcommittee and I was added to it as well since I had moved the original motion. But later Dr. McKerracher asked me whether I would mind not being on that subcommittee and of course I was pleased not to join. (My guess is that he was beginning to cave in to pressure from the Canadian psychiatric establishment, which did its best to utterly reject my work.) This subcommittee carried out some studies in a desultory sort of way. Eventually Dr. Tyhurst stated he was too busy to write the final report. Another person was appointed to complete it. Nonetheless, this document became known as the Tyhurst report. Its statements helped accelerate the destruction of the mental hospitals, but did nothing to encourage the development of facilities in the community equal to or better than the ones being obliterated. Dr. Tyhurst later became the first

Chairman, Department of Psychiatry, at the University of British Columbia medical school.

While there, he became a persistent critic of the work we were doing in Saskatchewan and attacked me personally. This last I still find surprising, for I never had anything to do with him on a personal level. But Tyhurst told the Food and Drug Directorate (FDD) of Health Canada in Ottawa that I was supplying LSD to the underground. I discovered this when the father of a young girl I was treating came to me. He had asked for an appointment and I arranged to see him in my office at University Hospital. To my surprise he was very embarrassed during our meeting and eventually confessed he had been ordered to talk to me by the FDD. He told me that Tyhurst had reported me to them. I was so surprised I burst out laughing. After a few minutes of conversation he said he was immensely relieved and that he would now inform Ottawa that they could never believe anything Tyhurst ever told them. On another occasion Tyhurst wrote a letter to the University of Saskatchewan Dean of Medicine, Wendell McLeod, advising him to fire me. McLeod, of course, could not do so even if he wanted to because I was working for the provincial government. However, Dean McLeod simply sent Tyhurst back the terse message, "Go To Hell." Since then, Tyhurst has been tried and found guilty of sexually abusing some of his female patients and one of them has become a patient of mine. He is no longer practising psychiatry.

I went to a second CMHA Toronto meeting that occurred several years after the one that set the Tyhurst report into motion. The CMHA, yielding to pressure from families who were demanding that their schizophrenic children be treated with vitamin B-3, announced it would grant $25,000 to Dr. Lehmann and his assistant Dr. Thomas Ban at the Verdun Protestant Hospital in Montreal, later renamed the Douglas Hospital. Dr. Ban had prepared a plan for testing our claims for vitamin B-3's effectiveness and had sent it to me. At this meeting he was to present his plan and I was to approve or disapprove it. I found the three-phase treatment plan he submitted to me acceptable, so long as minor modifications were made.

In the first phase, vitamins would be supplemented with drugs if necessary, such as antidepressants and tranquilizers. Those patients who responded would continue on this treatment. Those who did not would then be given penicillamine. This is a copper chelator; I found it improved the recovery rate. Failures from this phase entered phase three and here they were given a series of ECT. I stated that if Ban and his team followed this outline they would obtain the same excellent results that I was seeing. The second major agreement between Ban and the CMHA Scientific Advisory Committee was that he and his group would not release any results from their study until the entire three phases had been completed. Unfortunately Ban and Lehmann broke every one of the pledges they made to the CMHA at that meeting. They did only the phase one studies. They made no attempt to follow through with the phase two and phase three treatments. This meant that many of their chronic patients were given only vitamin B-3. In their report to the psychiatric literature they described these patients as newly admitted. This was true, but they did not add to their description that these newly admitted patients were chiefly chronic failures from other Montreal psychiatric wards found in general hospitals. A psychiatrist who did not know the Montreal situation would assume that these newly admitted patients were acute schizophrenia sufferers, but they were not. The chronic schizophrenics were the group that had showed the least response in our Saskatchewan trials. For them, phases two and three, as described here, are often necessary treatments. In one of Ban's studies they used eight grams of niacin daily. This dose is too strong for many and many of their patients suffered from severe nausea and vomiting. But they would not reduce the dose. It is difficult to understand how any patient could improve on any treatment if they were continually nauseated during the therapeutic trial. Finally Ban's team refused to publish the results of the HOD tests they had done. The HOD test is more sensitive than clinical evaluation and I suspect that it had revealed significant improvements in many of the patients. Despite these numerous shortcomings in their work, Ban and his team began to release their results almost as soon as they had analyzed them. By this time, the double-blind method had become much more popular, so they also began calling their experiments double-blind when they had actually been designed and run as single blind studies. Dr. Ban also traveled across Canada and the United States to claim that his group had repeated our work and had not been able to confirm the results we said we were getting. The tone of his papers and the enthusiastic reception he received in print and in person made it obvious to me that psychiatrists were immensely relieved to hear that they would no longer have to be concerned about using vitamins to treat their patients. Ban's claims were based on a partial lie, which in scientific circles is probably worse than a complete lie since it can appear to be the truth. He and his team had repeated a few aspects of our original studies, but had used different patients, had used a design that was not double-blind, and had failed to follow the entire procedure we had described. It would appear that these studies were designed to destroy the use of vitamin therapy, not to examine it objectively. The Mayo Clinic did exactly the same to Linus Pauling when they falsely claimed they had repeated his earlier work and could not replicate his results. My suspicions were strengthened when years later, Dr. Ban told me that his salary at the time the studies were done had depended entirely on drug trials financed by major drug companies. I had not earlier been aware of this major conflict of interest. Working for the drug companies he would have had little incentive to properly examine the claims for a product in which the pharmaceutical firms had no interest. Vitamins cannot be patented, protecting the seller's profit.

As a third year medical student at McGill, John Hoffer made the first analysis of Ban's studies, and published it under the title, "The Controversy over Orthomolecular Therapy" in the *Journal of Orthomolecular Psychiatry* 3, 167-185, 1974.

His work had an offshoot. In 1973 the American Psychiatric Association had completed its cursory and fatally incomplete study of our claims and published their task force report, which will be discussed in more detail later, "Megavitamins and Orthomolecular

Therapy in Psychiatry." This report was distributed widely and became the bible on vitamin therapy for the profession. Humphry and I were so fed up by then with our critics' irresponsible behaviour and claims, we simply ignored them and continued our work. But later, encouraged by John's report, we published a rebuttal. Our reply, "In Reply to The American Psychiatric Association Task Force Report on Megavitamin and Orthomolecular Therapy in Psychiatry," published August 1976, can be downloaded at *http://www.iahf.com/orthomolecular/ reply_to_apa_tfr_7.pdf.*

As a direct consequence of our research into effective treatment, in the late 1950s the CMHA in Saskatchewan began to pursue not only more enlightened government policy, but improved treatment results in the mentally ill. I had kept them fully informed of our research by presenting them with written reports and by outlining our data at their annual meetings. Our double-blind controlled studies showed that vitamin B-3 added to any other treatment improved the results substantially. But despite the fact that our results were obtained via the method considered most rigorous, and legitimately published, the psychiatric profession did not like it or believe our assertions. For our findings violated several basic beliefs then common to psychiatry: (1) *That schizophrenia was not a disease, it was a way of life resulting from conscious or subconscious psychosocial problems.* Psychiatry had adopted the Freudian hypothesis with so little critical examination that it considered all studies which had established a genetic basis for schizophrenia as faulty, even totally wrong. The profession's opinion was that since the disease had no biochemical basis, giving any vitamin, no matter the dose, would do no good. (2) *That not even the healthy needed to supplement their diet with vitamins, since the average diet in North America provided everything that was needed.* It followed that giving vitamins was useless, wasteful, and even dangerous because of hypothetical toxicities. If studies found no real toxicities, they were invented. A striking example of this phenomenon was the claim made by Dr Victor Herbert that vitamin C would cause kidney stones. After he gave a series of lectures to medical schools, this idea became accepted dogma even though millions of people have taken this vitamin for several decades and not a single report yet exists of an instance in which a definite relationship between vitamin C and kidney stones has been established. Yet I still find doctors who are afraid of vitamin C because of this myth. (3) *That vitamin B-3 was only needed to prevent the development of pellagra, the classical B-3 deficiency disease.* Schizophrenia was not pellagra and therefore it was idiotic to think that this vitamin could be helpful.

In the face of hard data that this vitamin in fact did help, the opposition concluded that there were other explanations. Perhaps we had made many wrong diagnoses; perhaps we were seeing a placebo response. These accusations were made in spite of the facts that double-blind experiments are supposed to eliminate bias and that our diagnoses were not made by any member of the research team, but by the clinical psychiatrists responsible for treating these patients. I also heard accusations that my patients got well not because I used vitamins but because of my therapeutic personality. Such statements were flattering but totally wrong, since the same therapeutic personality had little effect when I used only the standard treatments every other psychiatrist was using. Because we persisted in providing data to support our conclusions and because the CMHA Saskatchewan Division continued to publicize our findings, we became more and more unpopular with other psychiatrists in Canada.

Dr. Jack Griffin was director general of the Toronto CMHA chapter in the mid-1960s and he was one of the leaders in expressing opposition to our findings. This chapter went on to apply great pressure on Dr. McKerracher and on the CMHA, Saskatchewan Division, to moderate or cease entirely to make any claims about vitamin B-3 and to withdraw support for our work. The pressure gradually accomplished its aims; both Dr. McKerracher and the CMHA, Saskatchewan Division, became less supportive and less enthusiastic as the war of words continued. These events represented my first major experience with attempts to suppress my work and the claims coming from it. By 1967, I saw no alternative but to resign from my involvement with the organization.

As a result, the CMHA must bear a major share of the credit for having delayed a very promising treatment for schizophrenia from widespread use by several decades. Every patient denied this treatment and given only tranquilizers in or outside of hospital will remain ill indefinitely and will cost the country $2,000,000 or more over their lifetime.

Schizophrenics Anonymous

In 1964, I met Gregory Stefan, a recovering schizophrenic patient, in New York City. He had been looking for help, went to an AA meeting and found that one of the people there was a schizophrenic. This person told Gregory he had been able to find a fellowship in AA he had not found anywhere else. Gregory Stefan immediately began to think about forming a similar group for schizophrenics. He spoke to the chaplain of the Veterans Hospital, who thought it was a good idea but would not support it because the hospital psychiatrists were opposed. When he then discussed his desire with me and Humphry, we immediately agreed he had a very fine idea and encouraged him to continue with his effort to start a group. He began with a few interested patients, but their psychiatrists refused to be supportive. In addition, these patients were on drugs only. It is impossible for schizophrenics taking tranquilizers alone to be able to interact effectively in any group. After hearing this news, I decided to try the idea in Saskatoon.

SA was a novel effort. There is an element of will involved in alcoholism. But schizophrenics have nothing to do with becoming sick. The element of will enters into their experience only if they receive appropriate treatment, that allows them to recover to the point where they are aware that they can control the illness by continuing to follow proper treatment procedures. I also knew such a group could only work if its members had recovered to the point where they would be able to interact with one another. Many years before, one of the psychiatrists working with Dr. Osmond at the mental hospital at Weyburn, Dr. Ian Clancy, had met for two years, one hour each week, with chronic patients from the ward in group sessions. But he saw no more interaction at the end of those two years than at the beginning. The patients were too deeply immersed in their own misery, in their own psychotic worlds, to be able to relate to and communicate with others. However, the patients treated with nutrition and large doses of vitamin B-3 were a different group altogether. They were able to interact. It became important for me to determine whether schizophrenics who had reached this stage could be helped by a group modeled at least in part on AA. I discussed the idea with Bill W. and he agreed that it would be worth trying. We decided to use the usual twelve steps except that instead of saying in step number one, "I am an alcoholic", group members would say, "I am a schizophrenic."

By this time I was treating a large of number of schizophrenic patients as outpatients. Some were still quite ill, others nearly well, yet others, somewhere in between. About two or three were also alcoholic and they had had experience with AA groups. I thought that these individuals could instruct the new group and help direct it for the first few months. As it turned out, these patients did play an extremely important role in getting these meetings underway. I then spoke to about 12 of my patients individually and explored the idea with them. I told them that I would be at the early meetings as a resource person but that I would not direct or lead the meetings. I had had enough experience in running group therapy sessions during my earlier years at the Munroe Wing to know what not to do. They all were interested and agreed to come to the meetings. SA held its first closed weekly meeting in October 1964 and its first open meeting in March 1965. In the fall of 1965, a local radio station did a program on SA. In July 1966, the CBC-TV *Cross Canada Show* did a fifteen-minute documentary on SA.

For my part, I was amazed at how quickly the group developed and became cohesive. Before long the members were ready to take over entirely for themselves and I began to attend the meetings less frequently. As I was still receiving many letters about treatment, I let many of the people who wrote know that this new group was functioning. By January 1967, the group managed to incorporate as Schizophrenics Anonymous International, with its headquarters in Saskatoon. The group published a monthly *SA Bulletin* and held both closed weekly meetings and monthly open meetings. Later, some of the original members began to do community education, presenting their experience to various groups in Saskatchewan who wanted speakers. They would start these presentations by announcing, "My name is such and such, and I am schizophrenic." Then they would outline the nature of their illness, what had happened to them while sick, and how they had gotten well or were getting well on the megavitamin program.

On one occasion two SA members were invited to a meeting in Lloydminster, Saskatchewan. This is a small prairie town near the border of Alberta and Saskatchewan, between Saskatoon and Edmonton. The local mental health group had arranged for that meeting and had also invited two professors of psychiatry from the medical school of the University of Alberta in Edmonton. A few days later, the two members of SA told me what had happened. As the two women had told their story to the group, one of the young professors of psychiatry had become very distressed and agitated. He stood up after their speech and accused these women of being frauds. He stated that they were actresses I had hired to imperson-ate schizophrenics. He could not believe that two women able to tell their story so well and coherently had ever been schizophrenic or that they could have gotten well just on vitamins. During the coffee break the SA members sat beside him and then told him details about their illnesses that they did not want to talk about in public. One of the women told me she felt sorry for that young psychiatrist and did not feel any anger toward him. She decided she must really let him know how ill she had been. When the group reconvened, the professor stood up and apologized for his outburst. This little epi-sode indicates the extreme degree of disbelief current in academic circles then that schizophrenia could be treated successfully by the use of megavitamin therapy. Unfortunately the same disbelief still permeates psychiatric academia in Canada today.

The group published a little booklet, "This is Schizophrenics Anonymous," which outlined the principles behind their activities. These paralleled those of Alcoholics Anonymous. It contained the following headings after the introduction: (A) What is Schizophrenics Anonymous? (B) The SA Recovery Program. (C) Vitamin B-3 Therapy. (In this last section the use of this vitamin is described, references are given to our book *How To Live With Schizophrenia*, to a treatment manual describing the use of vitamin B-3, to my book *Niacin Therapy in Psychiatry* and to Gregory Stefan's book, *In Search of Sanity*. In the early 1960s no other literature on how to use vitamin therapy was available.) (D) The Suicide Problem. (This is one of the earliest references to this problem, which until then had been discussed only in relation to the psychotic depressions.) (E) A Final Word.

In June 1967 the Reverend John Ralph McDonald submitted his thesis in partial fulfillment of the requirements for the degree of Master of Social Work at St. Patrick's College of the University of Ottawa. His title was "Schizophrenics Anonymous. An Experiment in Group Self-Help." Reverend McDonald concluded his thesis with the words, "Perhaps most essential to the continuance of SA will be its relationship to professionals. It is the author's opinion, as well as the experience of the first unsuccessful SA groups, that professional understanding and involvement are essential. Dr. Hoffer has had nearly 2 years of experience in this area fulfilling a role that seems quite different from the traditional concepts of a group therapist. He has been guided by principles in his relationships to the group, perhaps the most basic of which is that the group is a self-help group and survival depends on its members rather than on his direct involvement. Still he has an essential, supportive, challenging and indirect involvement".

The experience of two and a half years of Schizophrenics Anonymous seem to support Felix Cohen's observations concerning AA, namely that its principles can be applied to the treatment of a wider range of psychiatric disturbances. In an age when the outpatient approach is viewed as the desirable form of treatment for as many victims of mental illness as possible, organizations of this type may have a very important role in fulfilling a deep fellowship and consequently therapeutic need of those who find themselves in the still very stigmatized social position of being 'mental hospital out-patients.' The last sentence of the above would make an appropriate end for this project; however, in coming to the end the author is reminded of the phrase that became an identifying mark of SA members. It reflects the courage and determination with which they face one of life's most devastating illnesses, as when greeting a friend, be he schizophrenic or not, they state cheerfully: 'Greetings and hallucinations: Who are you today?'

Father McDonald made the point that professionals have to be supportive and involved. This is correct. They have to be involved in providing the type of treatment which allows patients to get well. As long as the patients remain sick and only controlled on tranquilizers, whether in or out of hospital, they will not be able to interact in any group. But when they are treated correctly, they can successfully run their own groups. The support must come in helping them become normal, not in running or directing their lives for them. This, ortho-molecular treatment can accomplish.

XV

LEAVING INSTITUTIONAL RESEARCH

I have already described how in 1950 I came to my position as Director of Psychiatric Research, Department of Public Health with the Province of Saskatchewan. In 1955, I was appointed assistant Professor of Psychiatry (Research) at the College of Medicine, University of Saskatchewan, in Saskatoon. This appointment coincided with the expansion of the medical school's offerings into the full four-year program required to become a medical doctor. In 1960, I was promoted to Associate Professor of Psychiatry (Research). The inclusion of the word "research" in my title meant that I had a minor teaching role and a major research role. I gave many clinics to third- and fourth-year medical students, but I gave very few formal lectures. My professorship played a secondary role to my research directorate, which provided 10 percent of my income.

By 1966 it had become apparent to me that I could no longer remain in either of my two positions with a clear conscience. Looking back, I see the first major event driving me towards this conclusion was the unexpected rejection of my proposal to set up a psychiatric research institute on the campus of the University of Saskatchewan. Before Dr. Osmond left Saskatchewan in 1961 for personal reasons, we had discussed the formation of such an institute. The logical place would be on campus, near the College of Medicine. Dr. McKerracher was in agreement with the idea. I was then Chairman of the Committee on Scientific Affairs of the Canadian Mental Health Association (CMHA), Saskatchewan Division. I approached the CMHA for financial support. They also thought my idea was a good one and agreed that they would try to raise $100,000 to initiate the institute. I then spoke to Premier T. Douglas, with the permission of the Minister of Health and of Dr. S. Lawson, director of Psychiatric Services Branch for the Saskatchewan government and my immediate chief. Premier Douglas also thought I had a good idea. He promised me the Government of Saskatchewan would invest $100,000 if I could get a commitment from the Government of Canada in Ottawa that they would commit the same amount. These three pledges added up to $300,000, not much today but very significant in those years. A year or so later I was in Ottawa and arranged to meet with the Minister of Health. He soon agreed to my proposal, telling me to pass on to Premier Douglas the message that if Saskatchewan were to submit a proposal with their pledge of $100,000, Ottawa would match it. Soon after I came home I went to meet Premier Douglas, with Dr. H. Osmond. The premier then ordered his Minister of Health to immediately place the money in the next budget.

The president of the University of Saskatchewan, Dr. Spinks, was also in favour of the institute. Dr. Spinks was my next door neighbor in Saskatoon. When I first presented the proposal to him, he immediately agreed that it was a good idea, but added that as a matter of protocol he would have to place the matter before the College of Medicine for its approval. He did not think there would be any serious problem attaining it. But at a meeting held in 1966, the proposal did not pass muster with the medical faculty. Professor A. Bailey, Head, Department of Neurology argued that having such an institute on campus would be detrimental to the Department of Psychiatry because it was likely that it would receive much more international attention than the latter and then the Department of Psychiatry would have difficulty recruiting residents. It had never occurred to me that there might be any reason for antagonism between the proposed institute and the Department of Psychiatry.

Neither Dr. McKerracher, who was by now the Chairman, Department of Psychiatry, nor other members of the Department made any effort to counter this argument. Furthermore, by this point the Department of Public Health had also lost interest. Premier Tommy Douglas had recently left the province for national politics. He had been a great champion of improved psychiatric care. When he left, the Psychiatric Services Branch lost the influence it had had with the government and it now became simple for the new deputy minister of health to provide such lukewarm support for the proposed institute that the College of Medicine realized they would not have to face an irate government if they blocked it. At the end of a subsequent meeting to the one described, Professor L. Horlick, Chairman, Department of Medicine, told me confidentially that there was no chance enough of the faculty would support the idea. I then told him I would make plans to leave the University and he thought this might be a good idea. The next day I wrote to Dr. Sam Lawson recommending that the institute was dead. The government had already spent $25,000 on its architectural plans—all wasted.

By this time, I was also feeling increasingly frustrated by indirect attempts to censor our group's work. Our most important discovery had been a new and better treatment for schizophrenia, using megadoses of vitamin B-3 with additional vitamin C. Despite our positive results, we were under indirect but increasing pressure from both the Saskatchewan government and the University of Saskatchewan to stop publishing our findings. Yet, the only way by which doctors learn about new treatments is by reading about them in the medical journals. If we could not publish, no one but us would know that schizophrenic patients had a much better chance of getting well if they were treated with certain vitamins as well as with drugs. In this situation, my two options, to either fight my superiors constantly to meet my obligations to the sick, or to give in and stop communicating my findings, were both unacceptable. The College of Medicine's hostility to our findings was not effectively countered by Professor McKerracher, who had become ambivalent about our work. The warm and encouraging support I had experienced for 15 years was no longer present. The flood of criticism and opposition conveyed to them by Canadian psychiatrists was more than he could bear. The tension came to a head one afternoon in 1966 when I was making my weekly report to Dr. McKerracher. Over the previous year I had been meeting with him every week in order to keep him informed about our research. I knew he was receiving a lot of negative comments about our work and I thought that by meeting with him in this way I could keep him informed of the fact that while he was receiving criticism, I was receiving support from a different group of scientists and doctors, including eminent individuals such as Linus Pauling, a double Nobel Laureate, Sir Julian Huxley, Dr. Nolan D.C. Lewis, Dr. Joe Tobin, Director Psychiatric Research, Bureau of Neurology and Psychiatry, Princeton, New Jersey, Dr. Heinrich Kluver of the University of Chicago and Dr. Bernard Rimland, founder of the American Infantile Autism Society (see Chapter Nineteen), as well as from the members of the committee on therapy of the American Schizophrenia Association (this group is discussed in detail in Chapter Seventeen). During this meeting, Dr. McKerracher remarked that I wasn't very popular with Canadian psychiatrists. I was astounded by this statement, not because it was not true, but because he had made it and thereby identified himself with the Canadian establishment. He did not say, "Abram, I am very sorry you are not very popular with Canadian psychiatrists, but I will continue to support you." I responded angrily that had I wanted to win a popularity contest I would not have engaged in psychiatric research. This exchange marked a major fracture in our relationship.

That night I did not sleep very much as I thought about what had happened. I was pretty certain that the break would become more severe and that my position would become more and more difficult and untenable. I could not understand why McKerracher had not taken a strong position in support of our work. When Dr. Manfred Sakel had started his original work at the Budapest Medical School treating schizophrenic patients with insulin coma at 1927, he was given powerful support by the Professor of Psychiatry and Head of the Department, Professor Schaffer, against his many critics. This support certainly helped establish insulin coma treatment. Dr. McKerracher was very influential and powerful in Canadian psychiatry. Had he taken a strongly supportive position I believe he could have persuaded other professors of psychiatry to repeat some of the double-blind studies we had completed. But he did not and not a single professor of psychiatry in Canada to this day has shown the slightest interest in repeating our work. (A pseudo attempt was made by Professor H. Lehmann and Dr. Ban while the former was clinical director of the Douglas Hospital in Montreal and had a minor teaching role at McGill under Professor Ewen Cameron; see Chapter Five.) I had kept McKerracher fully informed of all our research, sent him copies of all our manuscripts before publication, and copies of all the minutes of our research meetings, many of which he had attended. I met with him regularly and frequently at work and we had many social contacts, playing bridge, playing golf, and on the many trips we made together. Not once had he tried to modify our views, interfere in the research, or even suggest changes in our program. For years he had been very pleased with our work and had often told me how well we were doing. By 1966 we had become known far and wide and were considered one of the major research organizations in North America. As I tossed and turned, examining what had happened, I wondered if I had been dreadfully wrong.

Were all the positive results we had seen in our therapeutic trials wrong, were we deluding ourselves, were our critics right? If so, then Humphry was as deluded as I was and it did not appear to me that he was. Humphry was a very good and capable clinician and he was not one to withhold his honest opinion about any matter whatsoever. During that night I also asked myself, "Why was I doing this research?" By morning the answer was clear. I was doing it on behalf of schizophrenic patients and not to please the psychiatric profession. I would have to trust my own senses, my own observations, not the beliefs of the critics. I decided that I would have to resign and start a private practice in Saskatoon. I would exchange two employers in whom I had lost confidence for a large number of patients. I expected I would be able to help most of them, and none of them would be in any position to censor my research nor my presentations to the public, whether scientific or lay. I would also be able to increase enormously the number of patients I could see and explore with them the various facets of nutritional and megavitamin therapy. I concluded that financially I would be no worse off, perhaps better, and I would not have to work any harder. I was already, as I have always done, working as hard and as long as possible. And I would have one more advantage, in that I would no longer have to submit dull and repetitive research reports each year, seven copies of each, in order to keep renewing our research grants, despite the fact that our research results were available in the literature for all to see.

It was not until mid-1996 that I discovered another reason why Dr. McKerracher eventually became so lukewarm and even hostile to our work. I am a member of the Lotte and John Hecht Memorial Foundation, Medical Advisory Committee. This foundation's mission is to support research into and promote alternative treatments of cancer. At a meeting convened to consider grant applications, Dr. Lorne D. Sullivan, Chairman, Department of Urology, Vancouver Hospital and professor of urology at the University of British Columbia in Vancouver discussed a new way of treating enlarged prostate glands with no blood loss and little discomfort. At the dinner he suddenly became aware of who I was after we had met briefly before the meal to shake hands. I heard him say in a loud voice, "Dr. Hoffer. He was my professor." Then he told the group that I was the cause of his only B in the College of Medicine at the University of Saskatchewan. He had attended my seminars on schizophrenia, in which I had described our views. When he wrote his psychiatric examination he was given a B. He had attained As in every other course. He went to see Dr. McKerracher and asked why, as he had gotten As in every other subject he been given a B in psychiatry. Then he added that he knew what answer McKerracher had wanted on one of the examination questions but that he did not agree with his view of schizophrenia since he had listened to me and found our biologic explanation much more satisfactory. Therefore he answered the question using my theories. Then he asked him again, "Why did you give me a B?" Dr. McKerracher replied, "Because of your attitude."

This anecdote led me to realize that McKerracher was not happy with the fact that we were teaching that schizophrenia was biochemically caused and that it could be treated with vitamins. His view had always been that the disease was a sociological phenomenon, that there was no effective treatment, and that the best one could do was train physicians and families to be kind and humane and do what they could to make life easier for the sick person, but without any expectation that they would ever get well. He held to this view even though many of his patients who went on vitamin therapy did recover. He never told me that he did not want me to contradict the views he taught, nor did he ask me to change my beliefs about schizophrenia, but this underlying difference must have been one of the main factors contributing to the coldness which developed between us.

By 1965 it had also become obvious to my senior research staff that the situation was not good and they began to leave. Dr. Ronald Heacock, in charge of biochemical research, left to take a position with the Department of Health in Ottawa. He had carried out some of the world's best research into the biochemistry and chemistry of adrenochrome and its derivatives. His work would be fundamental to recent research at the University of Manitoba, where a method for measuring adrenolutin levels in the blood has been developed. Dr. Neil Agnew, in charge of psychological research, left for a university in Ontario. Dr. C. Smith, deputy director of research, pursued and was given Dr. S. Lawson's job as Director of Psychiatric Services Branch, in Regina when it became available. He did not know I was planning to leave when he applied for and got that position. Miss M. J. Callbeck, head research nurse, also wanted to leave. I invited her to come with me into my private practice. This turned out to be an excellent idea. She was very helpful to me in my practice—she had worked with me since 1951, she was familiar with my style of practice and she was very methodical and careful, almost obsessive, all good qualities for a research person. I decided to make my move in the middle of 1967.

Of my two positions, it proved hardest to leave the research directorship, after I had worked so hard to develop our group's expertise. Only a clinician could really do the job that the research required, namely, to coordinate the various activities that drove the research forward: biochemical, psychological, and clinical. But very few psychiatrists knew anything about physiology and biochemistry and even fewer were interested in schizophrenia research. Within a few years after I left the research, the whole operation had settled down into two main areas, investigations of brain chemistry and sociological research. Clinical research activity disappeared from the unit and the research psychiatrists drifted into routine clinical work. In my opinion, neither sociological investigations nor chemical research of the brain has so far led to any useful treatment for the schizophrenias.

As far as my university appointment, as Associate Professor Research, was concerned, I would come to miss my occasional contact with medical students but I certainly never missed the professors of psychiatry. Only one, Professor F. Coburn, had shown any interest in using vitamins for his patients. But he left the matter of practical application entirely in the hands of his residents, none of whom bothered to really learn how to use this treatment. Even then, those of his patients who received vitamin B-3 had a much higher recovery rate than those not given the vitamin. Professor Keith Yonge, who later became Chairman, Department of Psychiatry, University of Alberta in Edmonton was always highly critical of our work and regularly lectured to his students about how ridiculous an idea it was that vitamins could help any patients.

Indeed, the pressure against the use of vitamins as therapy in medical schools was almost irresistible. This is illustrated by the following vignettes. In 1954 a young man became schizophrenic. He was a patient in the double-blind controlled study at University Hospital, Saskatoon. He happened to receive placebo and at the end of treatment was no better. He was therefore declared a failure and given a series of ECT combined with 3 grams daily of nicotinic acid. He then became normal, and entered first the ministry, then medical school. I had advised him to stay on the nicotinic acid for at least five years. After the five years had passed, he consulted me and wanted to know if he could now discontinue the nicotinic acid. I agreed that he could. Five years later while in medical school, third year, he came to my office very worried that he was becoming sick again. I had him do the HOD test and found very high scores. This did support his fear. I advised him to start back on nicotinic acid, 3 grams daily. He saw me again one week later feeling well again. His HOD scores returned to normal. He told me he was so anxious to get well he had taken 6 grams per day. He completed his training in medicine, became a psychiatrist and established a practice. But he never used nicotinic acid therapy with any of his patients. Before he graduated he was convinced he had been cured by the vitamin and even gave a major address on the subject in Los Angeles, to a large meeting hosted by a union in that city. But after graduation I can only assume he was no longer as certain and probably ascribed his recovery to good luck, or to chance. He advanced in his profession and at one point was president of a Psychiatric Association for one year. He is one of seventeen young women and men seen in my practice who recovered from schizophrenia, entered medicine and became practicing physicians and psychiatrists.

The second example of how medical schools can distort their students' thinking concerns a young woman who became severely psychotic. Her family had heard about my use of vitamins and she was started on them. She made a complete recovery. Her boyfriend encouraged her in her treatment. Later they married. He became a physician. By the time he graduated, he was convinced that the vitamins could not be of any value. He has been trying hard ever since to persuade her not to take her nicotinic acid. But members of her family who see me occasionally tell me that she is still on the vitamins and they all credit her recovery to the nicotinic acid.

On the subject of medical schools, I would like to acknowledge, however, the much warmer relationships I enjoyed with several members of the non-clinical division of the Saskatchewan school, particularly with people working in the Departments of Anatomy, Biochemistry, and Physiology. Professor Rudl Altschul, Head, Department of Anatomy, and I, as described earlier, had worked closely developing nicotinic acid as a treatment for hypercholesterolemia. Professor Serg Federoff did some of the early studies using cell cultures to study the effects of blood drawn from schizophrenics; we thought it might contain the "toxin X" that caused the disease. Early in our work we gave him a grant to make this research possible. He later became Head, Department of Anatomy. Professor Charles McArthur, Head of Biochemistry, and member, Saskatchewan Committee on Schizophrenia Research, remained an advisor and close friend after my departure. Professor Vernon Woodford, in Dr. McArthur's department, had actively worked with our research group on the development of the adrenochrome hypothesis of schizophrenia. Professor Duncan Hutcheon, Physiology, was the only member of the Committee who knew anything about adrenochrome at the beginning of our research and he did the original synthetic and toxicology studies with adrenochrome. These were essential before we could do our human studies.

Travel Highlights

Since 1967 marked the end of my career as Director of Psychiatric Research with University Hospital I feel it appropriate to review some of the trips I took in connection with that research that I have not yet described. Some of this travel also furthered the causes of the Huxley Institute for Biosocial Research and the Canadian Schizophrenia Foundation, organizations that will be described in detail in later chapters.

March 10 to 23, 1957. I have already mentioned Dr. Robert Heath's work a couple of times. On this trip (the same one on which I garnered the information on how to make pure adrenochrome) I visited Dr. Heath for three days. Professor Heath and his colleagues worked at Tulane Medical School in New Orleans. They had extracted a compound they called taraxein from the blood of schizophrenic patients. When injected into monkeys, this substance produced marked changes in behaviour. Taraxein's discovery was a direct offshoot of our adrenochrome work. Dr. John Weir, Medical Director, Rockefeller Foundation, had gone to New Orleans after visiting us in Saskatchewan in 1954, to make an onsite visit to Dr. Munro, who was working with Dr. Heath. While there, Weir told Munro and Heath about our adrenochrome work. After Heath heard about our research, he immediately contacted the Professor of Pharmacology at Tulane University for his opinion. I had met this pharmacologist in the early 1950s before he took that post, as he was a friend of Dr. McKerracher's. I had spoken to him about our hypothesis and plans for research, all of which he found very interesting. He remembered our conversation and was able to give Heath information that he could not otherwise have gotten without writing to me.

Sometime after that, Byron Leach, the biochemist working with Heath, awakened at night with an idea which excited him. He realized that if adrenochrome was made in the blood there might be an enzyme in the blood that catalyzed the oxidation of adrenaline to adrenochrome. He was so excited by the idea that he got up at 4:00 am, went to the laboratory, obtained a supply of blood and added adrenaline to it. Sure enough, a colored substance developed, but he did not know what it was. As he continued this line of inquiry, he found that the reaction was faster in blood taken from schizophrenic patients. He then extracted a protein substance, an enzyme, that would catalyze this reaction. When this protein was extracted from schizophrenic blood, it contained a bluish fraction which Leach isolated and later called taraxein. It was present in the ceruloplasmin of the blood. This last is a copper-containing oxidizing enzyme which does oxidize adrenaline. He published his results quickly and their appearance was followed by a major controversy. Research units rushed in to either confirm or deny. The American psychoanalytical establishment, which had by now captured the American Psychiatric Association, reacted angrily. They looked upon Heath as a traitor because he had been a trained analyst but had gone into neurosurgery and was now making claims about schizophrenia which if confirmed, would harm the analytical cause. Bob Heath had implanted electrodes deep into schizophrenics' brains, into the hypothalamic area, and had found wild irregularities, electrical storms, even though the surface electroencephalograms showed no abnormality. Soon after Heath reported the discovery of the new enzyme in the blood, I proved that the new substance he had reported appearing in blood due to the enzyme's activity was not adrenochrome. It was adrenolutin, which, biochemically speaking, must come from adrenochrome. Heath, in reporting on his taraxein studies, did not refer to our prior work, which John Weir had reported to him. Weir was really annoyed with this omission and his anger may have prevented Heath from obtaining any Rockefeller money.

Dr. Max Rinkel was chairman of the Northeast Psychiatric Association. The association had invited Bob Heath to report on his taraxein results and Rinkel then invited me to be one of the discussants. Marg Callbeck had already gone to visit Heath for a few months to find out exactly what he was doing and also to look into their research nursing protocols. After receiving Rinkel's invitation I decided that I would be a more effective discussant if I could see firsthand what Heath was doing as well as discuss with Marg her reactions to the research. En route, I stopped in Vancouver, where I had lunch with an English chemist, Dr. Acheson, who, as already described, gave me the information that led to our team's ability to produce pure, stable adrenochrome. From Vancouver I flew to Los Angeles and met with Dr. C. Kepner, who had been one of our volunteers in taking adrenolutin. I also met Dr. Gordon Alles, who told me about an amphetamine derivative he had made that had hallucinogenic properties. This compound later hit the streets as the well-known ecstacy, still very popular. I also visited Dr. S. Cohen, a psychiatrist who had been working with LSD and was part of the group that included Aldous Huxley, Al Hubbard, and several others. Later Cohen became editor of a little journal, *Mind: Psychiatry in General Practice,* to which I made many contributions. It was published by Atherton Press, a division of Prentice-Hall Inc, New York. I was on the board of consulting editors.

While in Los Angeles, I missed a chance to meet Linus Pauling. He had recently been given a very large grant from the Ford Foundation to pursue psychiatric research. In 1956 the Ford Foundation announced a one time 15 million dollar grant for all psychiatric research in North America. I did not think I had much chance of getting any but I applied for a substantial sum of money nonetheless.

As events transpired, it became clear that the psychoanalytic influence on the selection process would be too strong to allow our research to be supported. Yet, Linus Pauling did get a grant from Ford. I was very curious as to what he was going to do with the funds. I therefore wrote to him, told him I would be coming through Los Angeles and asked if I could visit him. But once in the city, I got cold feet and did not go to see him. His stature was so great and I felt so inadequate. I have often wondered since what the outcome of such a meeting might have been.

Finally, I arrived in New Orleans. At Heath's laboratories the research staff showed me the EEG abnormalities in their chronic patients. I was impressed that they really had made an important discovery. These patients had been fitted with embedded wires that ran into the hypothalamic areas. These wires could be easily attached to the EEG apparatus. The patients usually wore caps to cover their wires. An amusing incident once arose from this research. Final certification examinations for psychiatrists were being held at Tulane. One of these chronic patients was being examined by a candidate. During the examination the patient reported that he had wires running into his brain. The applicant assumed that this was one of the patient's delusions until the patient whipped off his cap and showed him the wires. The student was shocked. Nothing more was said about it. As a psychiatrist, I can imagine that student's surprise.

From New Orleans I flew to Boston for the neuropsychiatry society meeting. Max Rinkel was a gracious host. Bob Heath read his report to a full hall and then the discussants got up one after another to comment on his presentation. I believe I was fourth on the list. I had prepared my paper on the flight to Boston. The gist of my comment was that his work was very important and that when a serious attempt would be made to confirm it, it would be. For the next few years a controversy raged about Heath's findings, and eventually died. In my opinion no serious attempt was ever made to duplicate his findings, despite the fact that American psychiatrists were eager to prove him wrong—the biochemical view of schizophrenia was anathema to the analysts who were in control of the American Psychiatric Association. I cannot remember whether his presentation and my comments were ever published. I believe that had Bob Heath given our adrenochrome work the same kind of support I gave his taraxein work we both would have been much better off. But it was already clear by this time that anyone who seriously considered the adrenochrome hypothesis could expect no grants from the NIMH colossus. A further significant barrier to our work's acceptance, beyond the philosophical differences with the analysts, was that the biochemical research and technical expertise needed to examine our hypotheses further was not available at the time. I suspect to this day that taraxein is an unstable fraction of ceruloplasmin and that as an oxidizing substance, it plays a role in the conversion of adrenalin to adrenochrome and subsequent indoles.

September 1 to 7, 1957. Humphry and I attended the International Congress of Psychiatry, held in Zurich, Switzerland. This conference was the most important Humphry and I ever attended together. It was organized to honor Eugene Bleuler, who had written a most influential book on schizophrenia which became the American bible on the subject after it was translated into English. His son, Manfred Bleuler, was chairman. The latter's orientation had become much more psychological than his father's. This meeting was memorable because it included the first international meeting on the theme, "Chemical Concepts of Psychosis," chaired by Max Rinkel and co-chaired by Carl Jung. Both Humphry and I presented papers on our work. The proceedings were published in 1960. Another memorable event at this gathering was the establishment of the Collegium Internationale Neuro-Psychopharmacologicum (CINP), a scientific organization that serves as a meeting ground for clinicians and scientists studying the biochemistry, pharmacology, safety, and therapeutic efficacy of neuropsychiatric drugs. Humphry and I are both founding members. The CNIP has become a very large and successful international organization; participating countries also have their own local branches. We also were able to visit briefly with Dr. Carl Jung. And we met many of the psychiatrists who later were in the forefront of promoting biological psychiatry.

After the meeting in Zurich, we went to Stockholm and called on Dr. Tiselius, the Nobel Laureate. He had discovered how to separate molecules from one another using a special apparatus. In Stockholm we were wined and dined by the large company Kabi, one of whose scientists, Dr. B. Melander, had been working with Bob Heath. Kabi had extracted ceruloplasmin and early studies had found it therapeutic for schizophrenics. No one knew why. I have since speculated that this enzyme may assist not only in the conversion of adrenaline to adrenochrome, but also in the production of less toxic compounds from adrenochrome, such as adrenolutin. Unfortunately, Kabi wanted a pure product and the more they purified ceruloplasmin, the less active it became. It appeared to me that in their zeal for getting a pure product they were inadvertently removing the active principle. As a result of this ineffective approach, interest in the use of ceruloplasmin quickly died. We then flew to London, where we attended a meeting of the Royal Society of Medicine.

New York April 21 to May 2, 1959. This trip included a meeting of the Macy Foundation held at Princeton Inn, in Princeton, New Jersey, Abramson in the Chair. I had been very impressed with one Dr. Harold Abramson ever since I had studied his book, *Electrokinetic Potential*. This was an elegant classical text used in the PhD program at the University of Minnesota; in it Dr. Abramson discussed colloidal chemistry, the properties of surfaces, and so on. The material covered was very mathematically oriented, very intricate, and very difficult. I discovered that the same Abramson now chairing this meeting was indeed the same man I had first met through his book. He had enlisted in the war and after it was over had taken medicine and later became a psychoanalyst. The meeting was very interesting and I met most of the investigators then using the psychedelic reaction in work with their patients. I also met Dr. Jack Ward of Trenton, New Jersey, who later became a key orthomolecular investigator and lecturer. Jack told me later that he had first become interested in niacin after my presentation at this meeting, in which I reported that niacin could reverse most LSD changes. He thought that if it could be that powerful against LSD it might be equally effective against schizophrenia. The meeting included a symposium on the use of LSD in psychotherapy. An outgrowth of our presentations was the book, *The Use of LSD in Psychotherapy*, edited by H.A. Abramson. I contributed one chapter to the book and participated in the discussions that initially conceived of, then planned, that project. The book's publication was sponsored by the Josiah Macy Jr. Foundation, the conference's sponsor. Years later I discovered that this foundation was actually one of the CIA front organizations active during that period. Their real purpose was to study the properties of LSD as a potential tool for mind control.

April 23, 1959. I drove to Wilmington, Delaware with my friend Joe Tobin, director of psychiatric research at the Bureau of Neurology and Psychiatry in Princeton, New Jersey, for an informal meeting of directors of psychiatric research in North America. One of the main problems discussed was that analysts were now so powerful that it was difficult for these investigators to do their research. One director complained that he could not even order samples of urine from the patients because this was considered an interference in the doctor-patient relationship.

July 1 to 15, 1959. Humphry and I flew to Le Piol, in the south of France, to visit a small villa on a hillside where Mrs. Eileen Garrett presided over a group of about 20 people, including Francis Huxley. Eileen Garrett was President of the American Parapsychology Foundation. She spoke about the aura around people that she had been seeing from childhood. I wondered if she had an ability to see into the infrared spectrum. We had sessions every morning for a week, discussing the need to seek the scientific basis for unique phenomena such as ESP. I participated mostly by listening. Although interested, I was not comfortable with the topic and could not make any major contribution. I had been invited primarily because Humphry had suggested I should be.

The second week we spent in London. When I arrived, I did not feel well. I could no longer see clearly from my left eye. Instead, I saw a doughnut ring with a black center. At Humphry's suggestion I consulted an opthalmologist, a friend of his, on Harley Street. He examined me and told me there was nothing he could do about it, nor did he hazard any diagnosis. On the way home to Canada I concluded I must be having an unusual allergic reaction and began to take niacin and vitamin C more regularly. After about two months the problem cleared and has not troubled me since. I suspect I had a minor edema of the retina around the fovia, perhaps caused by a virus. In London I also met again with my publisher, Dr. Donald Johnson.

November 29, 1959. I was in New York City. Joe Tobin came in from Princeton to spend an afternoon with me. Joe told me he had received a grant from NIMH that he had recently applied for. The scientist who had visited him had told him the Institute wanted to give him the grant but could not do so if he insisted on working with adrenochrome. Joe swore at him and told him that whether he got the money or not, he would continue with his studies. This attitude must have impressed someone, since he got the grant. I had for some time suspected that NIMH had blackballed our research but this was the first proof that they had indeed done so.

XVI

PRIVATE PRACTICE AND RESEARCH, SASKATOON, 1967 TO 1976

As decided, I resigned from my two positions in 1967. Professor McKerracher was surprised by my move—at least he appeared to be surprised. I did not outline to him all the reasons for my departure. That was the last time I saw him. He asked me whether I would like to remain on staff at the university as a clinical professor but I declined. I told him I wanted a clean break from the medical school. *The Star Phoenix*, the local daily paper, wanted to interview me but I refused to talk to the reporter.

I had already rented the second floor of a wooden frame house on Saskatchewan Drive, a street running parallel with the Saskatchewan River. I was on the downtown side of the river, just across from our home on University Drive. The house was owned by a dentist who used the bottom floor. I had my rooms decorated so that they were pleasant, not the forbidding type of office often used by physicians. Marg Callbeck was nurse and receptionist, and I had a secretary. My daughter Miriam also did some typing for me for a few months. I was very busy with the American Schizophrenia Association and the Canadian Schizophrenia Foundation (to be described in later chapters) and with my correspondence with thousands of people from North America and elsewhere. Three years later I would move into the CN Towers, in downtown Saskatoon, as one of the earliest tenants of that new building.

I made the usual announcement in the press about opening my practice. My announcement was followed by a flood of referrals and by the time I opened, I was booked for a month. Marg Callbeck had been in the office at least two weeks before my opening in order to set up the filing system and to receive phone calls from referring doctors and interested patients. I did not accept walk-in patients. Everyone I saw had to be referred by their personal physicians. Once a person was referred, they could come back any time they wanted, for the rest of their lives. Early in 1967 I had also applied to City Hospital, Saskatoon, for staff membership. Another psychiatrist, Dr. B. O'Regan, had already established his practice and was on staff. This hospital did not have a psychiatric ward but it allowed Dr. O'Regan to admit his patients onto the medical floor. He had already arranged that ECT could be given there. My application was accepted.

Several years later Senator Sidney Buckwold told me what had happened when my application had been received. The medical advisory committee had turned me down because Dr. Kinnear, a pediatrician, had concluded that I would present a danger to the hospital. He had heard about the LSD research we had carried out and believed that I would continue that line of research at City Hospital. He was unaware that all LSD research had stopped by 1960. Senator Buckwold was then Mayor of Saskatoon and in that capacity was also Chairman of the Board, City Hospital. This was a hospital managed and owned by the city. As a rule, the board would rubber stamp any recommendation made by the medical advisory committee about hospital appointments to medical staff. This time Mayor Buckwold overrode the committee as was his right and saw to it that I was accepted. Hearing this story I for the first time became aware of how seriously physicians misinterpreted what we had been trying to do with our LSD research, that we were working toward a better treatment for schizophrenia.

I was not aware of the attempt by the medical advisory committee to shut me out when I began to practise in that hospital. On the first day as I walked through the building where I had interned from 1949 to 1950, I became aware of a powerful sense of relief. I was at last free of the oppressive air of the University Hospital with its antagonisms, its petty politics, and its staff who, with few exceptions, were interested in their jobs much more than they were in their patients. I was at last equal among medical colleagues who might not agree with what I thought or did but who at least maintained a professional attitude of respect. I was tired of the competition for status marked by the size of one's office, the number of doors one's keys opened, the size of the rug on the floor. City Hospital was staffed by private practitioners, private entrepreneurs who competed for patients but not for position or prestige. l was happy I had made the move.

As my practice developed, I generally had anywhere from one to four patients in hospital. They stayed in one of eight beds set aside on a medical floor for psychiatric patients. I was not worried that there would be major problems since Dr. O'Regan had already been admitting there for some time. But I was amazed at how easy it was to mingle psychiatric with medical patients, even without having the usual complement of psychiatric nurses, social workers, occupational therapists, and the like on the ward. These patients were looked after by the regular RNs. Nonetheless, it was my policy to tranquilize my patients as quickly as possible, using larger than average starting doses, in order to avoid any major crises in the hospital. An average stay for one of my patients lasted less than three weeks. Patients who received ECT had to stay longer, as they were discharged one week after their last ECT. In addition to treating my patients I would see other patients in the rest of the hospital in consultation.

I saw the entire spectrum of psychiatric patients, but I had a greater proportion of schizophrenics than did other private psychiatrists. I was known for my research in schizophrenia and doctors would send these individuals to me. In contrast, Dr. O'Regan was known for his interest in depression and a large proportion of his practice consisted of depressed patients. We covered each other—in his absence I would see his emergencies and his patients in hospital and vice versa. He did not use orthomolecular methods, but with my patients he would continue what I had ordered; I would not place his patients on my regimen but would care for them according to his instructions until he came back. My patients came mostly from Saskatoon and its surroundings areas but a few arrived from the rest of Saskatchewan. On several occasions I admitted patients from other provinces.

My patients recovered just as well in this general hospital as they had in the psychiatric ward of University Hospital. I did not find this surprising, as I had concluded several years before that of all the factors necessary to treat any patient, the most important was a sound therapeutic regimen of good nutrition, nutrients, and medication. For the best treatment, I felt, patients must have a place to live where they can be cared for, fed, and medicated, and they must be attended by trained personnel. Ideally all would be at an optimum level. However, the non-medical aspect of the regimen could be provided at a much more economical level than often provided and patients would still recover. Dr. Colin Smith, my deputy director of psychiatric research, working with Dr. D.G. McKerracher, had once compared the outcome of treatment at the University Hospital, which then cost about $80 per day, against the outcome of treatment at the closest mental hospital, which then cost about $25 per day. The difference in cost covered ancillary personnel. The outcomes for similar patients given similar medication was the same.

A few years later I conducted another study that examined this issue. It was never published. A new nursing home had been built in Saskatoon, along the style of a modern (vintage 1970) motel. Each occupant was provided with a single room and had access to a main lounge area and dining room. The home was managed by nurses and other trained people, and was owned by a man I had known for some time. It occurred to me that perhaps I could admit chronic schizophrenics from Canada and the USA into this home and treat them there. I was receiving calls from all over North America and a few from overseas, from desperate parents who wanted to bring their sons and daughters to me for treatment. It would cost them $25 per day to place their child in the nursing home, which was usually less than what they would have had to pay for similar facilities in their own area. I was interested in whether I could treat patients successfully with even less staff and facilities than were available in the City Hospital. The nursing home agreed to take these patients in on condition that I did not accept more than two at one time. I then arranged with Dr. Chris Kilduff to help me with the ECT which I intended to use there. Dr. Kilduff was Chief of Anesthesia at City Hospital, and I worked with him when we gave ECT there. We arranged to give ECT at the home three times each week. After the treatment Kilduff and I would stay until the patient was secure; the nurse would stay the rest of the morning.

We had no problems with the nursing home nor with the treatment itself. However I did run into difficulty with a bureaucrat from the Department of Social Welfare who worked in the division that controlled licensed nursing homes in Saskatchewan. One day Harold Livergant, President of Extendicare, Canada, told me he had received a threat from that individual that unless I ceased giving ECT in his nursing home he would lose his license. A few weeks later I received a letter stating that the government was concerned about the safety of the procedure. I immediately replied, pointing out that Dr. C. Kilduff, Head of Anesthesia at City Hospital, was giving the anesthetic. I also asked Dr. Kilduff to write to the government. Then I wrote to the Minister of Social Welfare, winding up my letter with the statement that it was his duty as minister to protect his public from the civil service. I heard no more and continued to treat patients in the nursing home until I completed my study a few years before leaving for Victoria, in 1976.

Over a five-year period, from 1967 to 1972, I treated about 100 schizophrenic patients from out of province. Most came from the United States. They had all been treatment failures in their own communities. Every one had had at least one admission to a mental hospital and the average number of admissions must have been over three. Some had been refused readmission to the original hospital that had accepted them, because they had proved too difficult to treat. I accepted all patients provided they were schizophrenic, agreed to come of their own will, as I could not hold them against their will, and so long as their relatives brought them and returned to take them home after treatment. I charged the going Saskatchewan rate for services, but after a patient went home, I did not charge for advice by letter or telephone. The nursing home had few problems dealing with my patients. On the contrary, the presence of young men and women, even though psychotic, added life to the home. After the patients began to get better they were often very helpful with their elderly neighbours. I can recall only one who ran away and eventually went home. Many patients' families stayed in contact with me for years after the treatment. One person still sends me a card every year.

My objective in this situation was to test whether orthomolecular therapy could be successful in an economical hospital with minimal personnel resources, for a group of very psychotic patients. I was not able to follow up these patients after discharge because they had come so far, but the "much-improved" rate at time of discharge was 50 percent. The main problem after they returned home was aftercare. It was impossible in most cases for families to find psychiatrists in their community who would maintain my program, i.e. continue the megavitamin regimen. In a few cases, other family members would not provide support to the patients. I had an alcoholic schizophrenic patient from eastern Canada. He responded very well to treatment when he remained abstinent. During his last stay in Saskatoon we had to send him home because he would leave the home, drink, and come back drunk. However his father would not recognize his alcoholism and, against my advice and the wishes of the patient's mother, would drink with him. I have never seen any schizophrenic patient improve while drinking. My guess is that that patient is still a chronic schizophrenic somewhere in Canada.

A few other patients also stand out in my memory of those years. One was a chronic deteriorated schizophrenic patient, dirty, unkempt, disorganized, with hallucinations and delusions. She arrived from one of the worst wards of the Spring Grove State Hospital, in Baltimore, where her care had been totally neglected.

Her teeth had rotted in her mouth and we had to extract them all and provide her with dentures. I placed her on the megavitamin regimen and gave her a series of ECT. One month later she was normal and able to fly back to Washington alone. However after she got back, her family was not able to find anyone willing to continue my program and she had to be admitted to hospital again. This time she was placed in one of the best wards of the same hospital. If she had been maintained on my program with the usual adjustments that have to be made now and then I believe she could have maintained her good state of health. I am convinced that if any person, no matter how ill, can be normal for even five minutes, it is possible for them to become normal forever, because those five minutes indicate that there has been no permanent brain damage.

Bob W. was another patient from the United States who had failed to respond to all forms of psychiatric intervention in the best hospitals. He came to Saskatoon for treatment on September 8, 1971. He was 31 years old and had been ill since his mid-teens. Looking at his history, I decided his case would well test my ideas about how to treat chronic patients.

Dr. David Hawkins, an orthomolecular psychiatrist practising on Long Island, had already started him on vitamins and he was heavily tranquilized. It was impossible to determine his mental state because he was so confused. He appeared to have a severe organic confusional state, somewhat like an advanced stage of Alzheimer's disease. I immediately started him on a comprehensive orthomolecular program which included tranquilizers, antidepressants, lithium, dilantin (after he had a few convulsions), vitamin B-3 in large doses, vitamin C in large doses, and other vitamins as needed. I also used clomipramine, the antidepressant, because it is the most effective drug for the treatment of obsessions and compulsions, from which this young man also suffered. (This regimen has of course changed over the years. As he has become healthier, Bob W.'s drug needs have dropped considerably.) One month later Bob was better and more stable. He was rational part of the time, but more of the time still very immature and psychotic.

When I first heard from his father, Bob was a patient of Dr. Moke Williams in Florida. Dr. Williams was interested in my treatment, but felt he could not provide megavitamin therapy without learning more about it. He flew to Saskatoon to see me, and spent several days observing how I treated my patients. Following that visit he became one of the early orthomolecular psychiatrists. Later he sat on the board of the Huxley Institute of Biosocial Research, at one point becoming its President.

I visited Bob at least once a week. One day when I arrived at the home, I found him sitting beside an elderly totally senile woman who had no idea where she was nor what was happening to her. Bob was sitting beside her and patiently trying to teach her how to play checkers. He had no idea that she was totally lost in a world of her own.

He had a few bad habits which he had probably acquired in the various hospitals in which he had been living. These included smoking excessively and stealing food from other patients' trays. This is typical behaviour of chronic mental hospital patients because staff usually feel too harried to attempt to work with these patients, to correct their antisocial actions. Staff members also often encouraged smoking as a way of rewarding what they considered desirable behaviour or of calming agitated patients.

After a few years, Bob was much better. I had planned on returning him to his parents by this time, but his father urged me to carry on with him. Nonetheless, I thought Bob well enough to leave the nursing home and live with a normal family. Fortunately I knew a Saskatoon family with three sons, two of them schizophrenic. Both recovered after treatment with me. This family was not well off financially, but its members enjoyed a stable, intelligent home life and they all knew a good deal about schizophrenia. They agreed to take Bob. I promised them that I would place him back in the nursing home at the first indication that his behaviour was becoming impossible. The family then moved into a new home which provided Bob with a room of his own. He became a member of the family. I still visited him every week.

In November, 1971 his father wrote to a friend about Bob: "I have a son who has suffered from schizophrenia from early childhood. He is now 32 years old. During these years, I have had him in the best recommended institutions and with the best doctors in the country. It is only during the last two years, where fortunately, I was able to have him under doctors practicing this new biosocial approach that he has made real progress and it has been quite remarkable."

In December 1975, Bob was examined by my colleague Dr. J.B. O'Regan. He wrote: "On examination, he appears considerably younger than his stated age. He has a flat, inexpressive face although at times he appears to be grimacing. His speech is confused and rambling. His affect is basically flat but at times inappropriate. He describes his moods as being very high or very low. He feels he enjoys life and that life is worth living. He denies suicidal ideas. His thought content showed some rather vague paranoid delusional ideas in regard to religion. However there appears to be no systematized delusional system. He denies having had any hallucinations at any time. His thought processes show thought blocking, circumstantial thinking and tangential thinking. At times he also showed punning and clang associations. He tried to be abstract in his thinking but tended towards concreteness. His sensorium is intact and there is no confusion. However both his recent and remote memory are very poor. His general knowledge was good and his intelligence seems to in the high normal range. His concentration was very poor. Diagnosis: Chronic Hebephrenic Schizophrenia."

For a long time, Bob would become quite disturbed for a few days before the full moon. During these days, his tranquilizer intake would have to be increased. For the past fifteen years, Bob has been fairly stable. He has not needed any ECT and has not been in any hospital. Just recently his current "adoptive mother" took him on a trip to Edmonton in the car. They were gone for two weeks. Bob enjoyed the trip immensely and presented no problem to her. Today Bob lives in his own little suite in a very nice home. His room is full of books and he keeps up with current United States affairs. He eats with the family. His main symptoms are his inability to distinguish reality from fantasy when he describes past events and his tendency to be paranoid in interpreting events which he has experienced. An event he describes as having happened 20 years ago will excite him as much as an event of two days ago. He appears to have lost his sense of time passing and the past, present, and future are combined. He has a peculiar sense of humor, which reminds me of night-club humor. I have often thought as I listen to him that he could make a good comedian. He will never be able to live alone but he could today live anyplace if he had someone to cook for him and look after his medication, so long as they could tolerate his few remaining psychotic features. I think that he would have been well long ago had he received orthomolecular treatment the first time he became sick in the United States. Fortunately for Bob, his family can afford to look after him. Had he been poor he would have been a chronic back ward patient in some dump of a hospital or more likely, have died long ago in a deserted street or alley. In 1996 he leapt to a new, remarkable level of improvement. He stopped continually telling stories from the past, and shares with others his love of reading. He has his enthusiasm for the British Royal family, and for a new favourite television show.

Other patients have benefited from my experience with Bob. While still in Saskatoon, Bob was very paranoid. For example, he would tell me that the children playing down the street were talking about him and making fun of him. He interpreted their laughter as being directed against him and he became obsessed over this imagined slight. Thinking about this, I suddenly realized that I had never seen a cheerful paranoid. Every paranoid patient I saw was angry or irritable or depressed. It then occurred to me that if I could free Bob from depression with an antidepressant drug, perhaps the paranoid ideas would also go away. Anafranil has anti-obsessional properties. I therefore started Bob on this antidepressant. To my delight, within about six months, Bob was freed of his paranoid view of the world. Since then I have started a large number of paranoid schizophrenic patients on the drug with equally good results. I think my observation was correct. It is impossible to be paranoid when one feels good.

Overall, my experience with treating schizophrenic patients in nursing homes at minimal cost has convinced me that the most important part of the treatment for these patients must be the orthomolecular component. There is no need for expensive homes with huge staff resources. All the other treatment components, including the doctors and nurses, are minor compared to the importance of using the right chemical program. But of course patients must have decent living quarters and warm, humane care. Looked at in light of the adrenochrome hypothesis, humane treatment is essential because it reduces stress. Stress increases the secretion of adrenaline and therefore adrenochrome production. Unfortunately schizophrenics today rarely receive more than token care since so many psychiatrists are content to leave them forever on tranquilizers, hoping that someday in the far future they will have the magic bullet, the perfect tranquilizer. Few have shown the slightest interest in using vitamin B-3 or any of the components of orthomolecular treatment which come closer to the magic bullet than any drug available today. But of course, this treatment cannot be patented and therefore will not ever be promoted by any drug companies. At the time I first began these memoirs, December, 1996, we were surrounded by information about three new magic bullets for treating schizophrenic patients. The first, clozapine is so dangerous that blood counts must be done weekly or biweekly. I have seen its effect on twelve patients. Only one has responded and for him it has been excellent. It costs several thousand dollars per year. The second, risperdal, is much safer and equally ineffective. I have given it to about a dozen patients. Two became much worse and the remainder did not like the side effects. This third, olanzapine, has just been released. I have started two patients on this drug. These new drugs will cost over $3,000 per year. Using niacin, the total cost is about $100 per year. My opinion in 2005 has not changed. These are very potent, very dangerous drugs and have to be used with extreme caution. They are very addictive and once a patient has been on them for a while, it is almost impossible to get them off.

In addition to allowing me to help many patients as I continued to refine my treatment protocols, my new employment situation left me freer to pursue my involvements in the Canadian Schizophrenia Foundation and the Huxley Institute of Biosocial Research. My work in these organizations meant that I travelled a great deal to attend meetings and seminars, and to give public lectures. I have given so many talks, in fact, that I have lost track of most of the places where I have been. For many years, however, I was careful to do most of my public speaking away from Saskatchewan. In Saskatchewan I spoke only to mental health groups or Canadian Schizophrenia Foundation (CSF) meetings. (The CSF will be introduced in detail in a later chapter.) I did not appear on radio or television nor address large public meetings. I limited myself in this way because the Saskatchewan College of Physicians and Surgeons considered advertising an ethical offence and defined any public appearance as advertising. This rule was originally introduced to prevent members from gaining an unmanageably large practice by using the public media. Doctors could place an ad on opening a practice and one could only run that ad on three occasions. The size and quality of such an ad had to be submitted for rigorous examination by the College, to ensure it conformed to ethical standards. An announcement could also be made if one moved to another office or location and again upon giving up the practice. I also saw it as wise to limit my speaking engagements in Saskatchewan so as to avoid the appearance of competition with any of my colleagues. Since moving to British Columbia, I have followed the same procedure.

The College has even frowned upon those of its members who seek to publish books. One of my colleagues in Victoria asked me one day how I had been able to publish my books. I was startled by the question and told him I had not had any difficulty. He then explained that he had written to the College requesting permission to publish a book he was writing and they had warned him that doing so would constitute public advertising. I then told him that I had never asked permission from the College to publish nor would I ever do so. In my opinion, I explained, doing so would give the

College an opportunity to usurp power and exercise far more influence than their public mandate to regulate their members' practices.

Highlights

October 26 to 27, 1968, Minneapolis, Minnesota. I spoke to a meeting arranged by Florence O'Leary; 450 people were present. O'Leary was the founder and first president of the Schizophrenia Association of Minnesota. This remains a very active group. Mrs. O'Leary had a very interesting history. She had received many diagnoses from over a dozen psychiatrists in Minneapolis. Eventually she heard about my work. She then visited each of the doctors she had previously seen to ask them to supervise her treatment with a vitamin program. They all refused. She decided to do it without medical supervision. One day in a health food store she asked the proprietor if he would help her with her nutrition and he agreed. She went on to recover on the program. She became so enthusiastic about it that she and her health food store friend counselled over 200 patients between them over the next few years. Later she moved to Los Angeles, where she continued helping schizophrenics. Even her car license plates read "niacin." Once she was charged with practicing medicine without a license. She brought into court a host of her supporters. The judge found her guilty, saying he had no choice, fined her one dollar, and severely castigated the medical association for having initiated the charges.

November 26 to Dec 16, 1970, Puerto Rico, with stopovers in New York City and Washington, D.C. In 1969, I was called by the head of M.D. Anderson Hospital in Texas, who started the conversation by asking me if I still believed what I had written some time ago about double-blind controlled experiments. He referred to the papers I had published: Hoffer, A: A theoretical examination of double-blind design. *Can Med Ass J* 97:123-127, 1967 and Hoffer, A: Double-blind studies. *Can Med Ass J* 111:752, 1974. I replied that I did and asked why he had called me. He said that he and his staff of mathematicians had been studying my paper for six months and they had concluded that I was right. He added that the National Cancer Institute was trying to force them to do double-blind controlled clinical experiments with their cancer patients and they were determined not to go along with this plan. He said that the National Cancer Institute would soon be holding a meeting in Puerto Rico and would I come, to let them know my views on the double-blind? Since I had headed the first medical group in North America to do double-blind controlled experiments I decided I was the logical person to be one of the first to attack it. My statements at this meeting are available in the literature: Hoffer A: Symposium on statistical aspects of protocol design. Discussion. Cancer Clinical Investigation Review Committee, San Juan, Puerto Rico, 224-229, Dec. 9-10, 1970. We then flew to Puerto Rico hoping to have a good tropical vacation. But five days out of the seven were terribly windy and it rained the entire time. We were able to go into the water only once or twice. I read my paper on double-blind studies. I do not recall how it was received. We were happy to leave for Miami. The M.D. Anderson Hospital's resistance to double-blind methodology is ongoing. A few years later I met a young surgeon who had trained there. He told me that refusing double-blind research was still their policy and was surprised when I told him about my involvement in the matter.

XVII

THE HUXLEY INSTITUTE OF BIOSOCIAL RESEARCH

Early in the 1960s I received a call from an American, Bernard McDonough. He told me his friend's son had chronic schizophrenia and wanted to know if I could be of any help. He had been advised by Humphry to call me. Humphry later told me that one day they were astonished to see a helicopter settle down on the grounds of the hospital complex in New Jersey where he was then working. Out had stepped Mr. McDonough. He was a self-made millionaire who had started out as a taxi driver, had taken law in night courses, and had gradually accumulated a large sum of money. He had even purchased a factory in which he had once worked. I believe he had been fired from his job there and vowed revenge. He had also purchased a beautiful property, Dromoland Castle, near Shannon Airport in Ireland.

I saw the young man McDonough was interested in helping in New York City at the Barbizon Plaza Hotel on Oct 22, 1963. He was then 22 years old and had been sick for six years. The illness had come on suddenly. He had been given 20 ECT and been in and out of many psychiatric hospitals for psychotherapy and tranquilizer therapy. He had been started on niacin 4 months before I saw him. Before he started he suffered hallucinations, his skin was deteriorated, and he had a very powerful schizophrenic body odor. When I saw him he was clearly schizophrenic, but no longer hallucinated, his skin had cleared, and he had lost his body odor. I admitted him to University Hospital in Saskatoon on November 7, 1963. On admission to University Hospital he was still hearing voices, his thinking was severely impaired and delusional, and he was very tense and flat, experiencing little emotion. He was diagnosed as a chronic schizophrenic. On the urine test he was strongly positive for the mauve factor our team had discovered (kryptopyrrole). He was given four ECT, and discharged December 11, 1963 on a program of vitamin therapy combined with the anti-psychotics stelazine and haldol, and a drug that counters their side effects, cogentin, all in small doses.

After this brief treatment with vitamins he was in many ways better, both as shown clinically and by the results of the HOD test, but he was very far from being well. I advised his family that they must continue to maintain their son on the program. At that time, seeing these results, Mr. McDonough said that he wanted to do something for schizophrenics in general. That comment led to the start of the American Schizophrenia Association (ASA), later to become the Huxley Institute.

Humphry and I had been discussing for some time the need for an organization for schizophrenics. Humphry had been corresponding with Miss Miriam Rothschild of London. In one of her letters to him she remarked that if an international organization could be created to look after the interests of schizophrenic patients, she would try to persuade her brothers to donate some money. When Mr. McDonough offered to help schizophrenics, it occurred to us that with his help we could start toward the implementation of her suggestion by organizing an American Schizophrenia Association. Mr. McDonough was interested and agreed to finance the venture. About that time, Mr. Cal Samra, an experienced journalist, also became interested in helping schizophrenics. At the time, he was unemployed and we suggested that he might, at a very low monthly salary, become the first executive director of the ASA, with its headquarters in Michigan in his own small bedroom. He agreed to join us. He invited a friend of his, a lawyer, to help us. We had our first meeting in New York City in his friend's apartment, where we agreed on a constitution and began to organize. Mr. McDonough became the chairman of our board, which included Humphry, myself and the New York lawyer. Mr. McDonough gave us a start-up grant of $25,000. Cal Samra became our first president.

The initial years of the ASA were very difficult. Our chairman, Mr. McDonough, was accustomed to having his own way with his companies and I believe he began to look upon the ASA as one of his companies. He and Cal Samra, our president, did not get along and Cal was subjected to a good deal of harassment. The chairman also used to call us unexpectedly any time of day or night, even me in Saskatoon. I suspect he suffered severe insomnia and used the night to conduct his business. Another factor was introduced by his friend's son's challenges. Mr. McDonough had been unable to find a physician in Virginia willing to carry on with the regimen I had recommended. The young man relapsed, and the stage was set for Mr. McDonough to develop doubts about our work.

Around the same time, the ASA saw a need to reach the public with basic, understandable information about schizophrenia. Cal Samra summarized his view of the function of the ASA in 1969: "It should never forget that its primary responsibility is to its predominantly lay membership. And as such, it ought never stop being concerned with the high costs of psychiatric care, the ineffectual treatments so many patients get, high readmission rates, premature discharges, inadequate insurance, etc.—bread-and-butter issues which a lot of professionals would prefer not to talk about and would still be ignoring had not the Newsletter called public attention to them. Let us applaud the psychiatric profession on to greater achievements, more effective treatments, higher standards and ethics, more humane fees. But let the Newsletter also function as the conscience of psychiatry."

In accordance with these goals, in our first year, 1965, we prepared a booklet, "What You Should Know About Schizophrenia," providing accurate information about the disease and its treatment. This may have been the first time this kind of information was made public. Until then, information about schizophrenia had been kept secret because of the tremendous stigma associated with having the disease and with having been in any psychiatric institution.

A number of American Psychiatric Association officials responded hotly to the booklet's publication. Letters started flying in every direction, many of them to Mr. McDonough who until then had thought the booklet just splendid. Some of these critics contended that the booklet would "result in too much public anxiety" while others, curiously enough, contended that it made people "dangerously hopeful".

After the booklet appeared, the chairman of our board was cordially invited to visit the National Institute of Mental Health in Bethesda. He was also invited to visit the Lafayette Clinic in Detroit, and he returned from both of these visits expressing all kinds of doubts about the need for the ASA, its public education program, and its plans to do research. A prominent psychiatrist at the Lafayette Clinic also expressed his opposition to the Association's public education program, though at the same time he was equally eloquent in appealing for a sizeable grant from ASA for a pet research project. After his visit to the Lafayette Clinic, Mr. McDonough sent a telegram to the ASA national office in Ann Arbor, ordering the executive director (Cal) to clear any further pieces of ASA literature with the psychiatrist at the Lafayette Clinic before printing them. By 1966 it had become clear that we could no longer work with Mr. McDonough.

Honouring our constitution and bylaws, Dr. Osmond and I called a special meeting of the board in New York. Mr. McDonough sent a business associate who was empowered to act for him. After a long, heated discussion, we moved that the chairman not be re-elected to our board. McDonough's representative made it clear that Mr. McDonough would resign from the board and the chair only if we approved a grant of $25,000 to a group who in my opinion did not have a project of any value. But if we did not agree, Mr. McDonough threatened to tie us up in court forever. With only $30,000 in our treasury, we had not the resources to combat his many millions. The chairman had donated $25,000 to get us started and essentially wanted to strip us of that money—but having donated it, he could not get it directly back without breaking the tax laws. If we gave it to the organization of his choice, we would be left with less than $5,000 in our treasury. Things looked pretty dismal. However, by this time I was determined that what we had started would survive and Humphry agreed. We accepted McDonough's terms and the meeting ended. Our subsequent grant to the Institute of Living, a private psychiatric hospital in Connecticut, was announced in our newsletter. On my flight back to Saskatoon I decided I would approach Ben Webster, a personal friend who took a lively interest in our work. A few weeks after my arrival home, I called Ben and invited him to become a member of our board and our treasurer. I assured him that we needed his expertise, not his money, because by then we already had a plan for saving the ASA.

In 1966, at almost the same time as this meeting regarding McDonough, the *New York Times* ran an account of our work. Details of how this article came to be written are given in Chapter Eighteen. As a result, Humphry and I received thousands of letters. I had my secretary type out a list of all the people who had written me and Humphry did the same. We sent this list to Cal. He then sent out an appeal letter which yielded a seven percent return that added up to about $70,000. With this money, we were able to save the ASA.

The ASA was the first organization created to fight for and try to improve the lot of the schizophrenic patient. Older organizations in the mental health field had focused on the plight of patients in mental hospitals but had no committed interest beyond this. After the ASA had been functioning for a time, the psychiatric establishment, which could not control us, helped organize the "friends of schizophrenics" movements in the USA and Canada. These groups did try to better the situation for patients but did not antagonize the psychiatrists by demanding they do a better job of treating. Their main aim was to provide emotional support for families of schizophrenics who did not expect their ill member would ever get well, to improve legislation affecting the mentally ill, and to persuade governments to spend more money on research. These were and are worthy objectives—but I have always thought that small sums of money spent wisely are much more effective than huge sums on research which merely plows the same field again and again. It is also better to use effectively what we do already know before setting out to consume huge resources in examining and re-examining what has already been established. A recent example of the type of activity I am criticizing is the spina bifida controversy.

It was established around 1985 that if pregnant women took small amounts of folic acid, a B vitamin, the incidence of this congenital defect would decrease by over 50 percent. Yet the massive resistance to this idea by the vitamin critics prevented this knowledge from being used until millions of new dollars had been spent merely to show that the original study had been correct. In the meantime, over 100,000 children have been born with spina bifida, which would not have been the case had every mother been taking tiny amounts of this vitamin. The US government finally ordered the addition of folic acid to flour, to begin in January 1997. In Canada this addition came into effect in 1998. In the field of mental health, we are still even farther from applying what we already know works, despite a proliferation of research grants and support groups for schizophrenics and their families. Today the only organization which fights for better psychiatric treatment for schizophrenics, i.e. for more recoveries, is the International Schizophrenia Foundation, formerly the Canadian Schizophrenia Foundation and a direct descendant of the ASA.

The ASA furthered its aims in a number of ways. We published a newsletter edited by Cal Samra and a medical journal, and formed a Committee on Therapy. The first newsletter was published in the fall of 1966, and invited people to join the organization. Two thousand members enrolled in our first year. That first mailing contained information about the growth of chapters in the US, about a film called *Schizophrenia—Shattered Mirror* released in 1966, and on literature for schizophrenic patients and families. It also included a book review of *In Search of Sanity* which volume described a recovery via the use of niacin. The newsletter published Volume 1, Number 1 in January 1967 and it came out quarterly thereafter. This issue announced the launch of a new medical journal, *Journal of Schizophrenia*, provided a comprehensive review of *How to Live With Schizophrenia* and described Schizophrenics Anonymous (to be discussed later).

The aforementioned *Journal of Schizophrenia* was published by Dr. Lee W. Cozan, Elias Press Ltd., P.O. Box 5095, Longport, N.J. 08403. Dr. Osmond and I were co-editors. The papers published in the first two volumes, appearing in 1967 and 1968 respectively, broke much new ground in the area of schizophrenia.

Dr. Osmond and I published one of the first studies showing that the suicide rate among schizophrenic patients was very high. Until then it had been thought that the suicide rate among depressed individuals was much higher than among schizophrenics. Since then, our finding, that the rates in schizophrenics are much higher than in depressed patients, have been amply confirmed.

Dr. B. Kowalson, a Winnipeg physician and very effective orthomolecular therapist coined the phrase "metabolic dysperception" for the schizophrenias in our pages, discussing diagnosis and appropriate treatment within a general practice. Her term accurately reflects the biochemical and perceptual aspects of this disease.

Many others wrote about various aspects of the biochemistry of schizophrenia, effective treatment, and some provided subjective accounts of the experience of having schizophrenia, a first in the literature. *The Journal of Schizophrenia* became the *Journal of Orthomolecular Psychiatry* in 1972, and then, in 1986, the *Journal of Orthomolecular Medicine*, which title reflected the widening scope of the material published.

Back to the newsletter, whose contents sum up the ASA's history very well. In July 1967, it reported that the ASA had been attacked by the American Psychiatric Association in its official newspaper. In this APA newsletter, a psychiatrist from the University of Michigan complained that it was "cruel to give out information to the public about schizophrenia and promising new approaches to the disease." Dr. Osmond accurately characterized the attack as a tasteless and inaccurate attempt to damage a small, new organization whose only aim was to benefit many gravely ill people and their saddened and often bewildered families. In the same issue it was announced that Dr. Linus Pauling had joined the Scientific Advisory Board of the ASA. He was already describing his work with vitamin C. His views were under vigorous attack by physicians and Dr. Roger Williams came to his defense with his strong views about the safety of vitamin C. He reported that the optimum needs of guinea pigs for vitamin C varied enormously and he suspected the same was true for people. He stated it was nonsense to regard ascorbic acid as toxic since many people had been taking 1 to 15 grams daily for years with no side effects.

The October 1967 issue of the newsletter reported a conference we were going to hold at Fordham University in the fall of 1968, co-sponsored by the ASA and the University. We had originally planned to hold this conference at an eastern medical school but after the APA ran their attack on our work, the school changed its mind and reneged on its agreement. The Fordham meeting was arranged through the help of one of its faculty members, Professor Joe Ryan. Father Ryan was an alcoholic priest. He started to take niacin and, to his amazement, migraine headaches from which he had suffered for many years disappeared overnight. He recovered so fast he considered the vitamin almost miraculous in its effects. For the next few years, he was very active in promoting the use of niacin in combination with attendance at AA meetings for the treatment of alcoholics. He was so enthusiastic about the vitamin that he began to be called Father Niacin, while he called me Dr. Niacin. One day in the late 1960s, a letter came to me that had been addressed to Dr. Niacin, Canada. It had gone to the dead letter office, which traced me. I mention this incident as a tribute to the post office and how it functioned many years ago.

At the time the ASA was formed, there were about six psychiatrists in the United States who had studied vitamin therapy and found it very useful in practice. We invited them to join us in forming a Committee on Therapy of the ASA. This committee held its first meeting January 21 to 22, 1967 on Long Island at the Brunswick Hospital Center where Dr. David Hawkins was in charge of the alcoholic ward.

The last 1967 newsletter reported the data the Committee collected in its first year. About 1,500 patients had received vitamin therapy that year; the overall success rate was 80 percent. The following psychiatrists participated in this large study: Dr. Willard E. Beebe, Detroit, Dr. J. Ross MacLean, Vancouver, Dr. David Hawkins, Long Island, Dr. Jack Ward, Trenton, New Jersey, Dr. Allan Cott, New York, and Dr. M. Galambos, Prince Albert, Saskatchewan. In addition, Dr. Osmond and I reviewed our cases in Saskatchewan. Other psychiatrists participated but did not list their results. They agreed with the general conclusion of the committee. Dr. Joseph Tobin, Eau Claire, reported he had been unable to find a single negative report regarding megavitamin therapy in the medical literature. Five of the members of our therapy committee were psychoanalysts who had once been skeptical of the niacin claims and became strong supporters after they began to use the treatment.

In April 1968, we announced to our members that the NIMH had granted $517,000 to Dr. J. Wittenborn, a research psychologist with Rutgers University for the study of niacin as a treatment for schizophrenia. We had high hopes that this study would be done properly and would demonstrate the value of the treatment.

The reasons this study got started are interesting. Bill W., co-founder of AA, had long been keen on seeing niacin studies started. (His contributions to the growth of niacin therapy will be discussed in more detail a little later.) He contacted many members, including senators, congressmen, and other influential individuals, and persuaded them of the importance of such work. They began to apply pressure to NIMH, until one day I received a call from Washington telling me the Institute was interested in doing some studies. I invited one of their appointees to visit me and he did. On the basis of that visit he recommended that they proceed. They then approached a research psychiatrist in St. Louis and asked whether he would be willing to be the project leader of such a study. He replied that he would be only on condition that I be invited to act as one of the advisors to the study. NIMH never spoke to him again. They then approached Rutgers and granted the money to Dr. J. Wittenborn.

Dr. Wittenborn reported his results in two papers several years later. His first paper, published in the *Archives of General Psychiatry*, delighted our critics and was used very successfully to destroy our credibility. He reported that of the patients his group had treated, they could not find any significant improvement in the group that had been given niacin. I examined their data very carefully and discovered that they had treated very chronic patients, the type that we ourselves had reported much earlier did not respond to this vitamin alone. Of course his study was not double-blind since no study with nicotinic acid can be double-blind. The flush gives the active compound away every time. In addition, a psychiatrist familiar with the study reported that some patients on placebo realized they were not getting the same product as some on the active vitamin. They went on their own to local drugstores and began taking the vitamin. In a second paper, titled "A Search for Responders to Niacin Supplementation," Dr. Wittenborn corrected his first report. He found that when he examined separately the less chronic patients from their series, he saw exactly the same response rate as we had. He sent me a reprint on which he had written, "I am sorry for my previous mistakes." The critics of orthomolecular psychiatry, led by Professor Morris Lipton and the National Institute of Mental Health (Dr. L Mosher) used the first Wittenborn paper as one of their main pieces of evidence against our work but totally ignored the second. I believe Dr. Wittenborn destroyed his research career when he published his second report. Had he not done so he would have remained a darling of the National Institute of Mental Health.

In July 1968, at a meeting in Washington DC sponsored by the ASA and its Greater Washington chapter the ASA announced a $100,000 prize to the discoverer of a schizophrenia cure. We called it the Dixie Annette Award after a young California woman who, after 19 years of illness, took her own life. In making the announcement Mr. Samra said, "Dixie Annette's tragedy is, unhappily, all too frequent. Every year thousands of young Americans afflicted with schizophrenia disappear into our mental institutions. And every year our mental institutions discharge thousands of schizophrenics, often as sick as they were upon admission, and many of them kill themselves or fall into other terrible misfortunes." No one ever applied for this award.

The major news item in the July 1968 issue of the Newsletter was on Dr. Linus Pauling's report to *Science* on orthomolecular psychiatry. This report had been widely covered in the major news media. It alerted the world of science to the new interest in using vitamins as therapeutic agents and not just for deficiency/disease prevention. It also generated a tremendous amount of hostility from the medical profession, who did not consider it proper for a person not a medical doctor to comment on medical matters, no matter how brilliant and creative he might be. Members of the medical community went so far as to accuse him of senility. None of his detractors attempted to accurately duplicate his studies. To the medical world, Pauling's Nobel prizes meant nothing.

Dr. Pauling's first public rebuttal of the medical attack on his work appeared in that same newsletter. He stated, "My associates and I have carried on research on the molecular basis of mental disease for 12 years. For 10 years I have been aware of the opposition of many psychiatrists to the idea that patients might benefit by having a supply of vitamins and other nutrilites different from the recommended for the 'average' person. There is a danger associated with most drugs and other forms of therapy, such as electroconvulsive therapy. A physician has the duty not to impose this danger on a patient. The situation is different, however, for ascorbic acid, nicotinic acid, nicotinamide…They are nontoxic; they are cheap; and they have fewer side effects. I believe that a physician who refuses to try the methods of orthomolecular psychiatry, in addition to the usual methods, is failing in his duty as a physician."

In the same issue Fannie prepared an excellent report on the value of using the HOD test for diagnosing and treating patients. In the October, 1968 issue Fannie presented the arguments in favour of a Bill of Rights for Mental Patients, describing some of the problems faced by patients which could be prevented or resolved by an enforceable Bill of Rights. In this article, we were ahead of the times. Only recently have attempts been made by patient groups to achieve something like what we were proposing.

In the first 1969 issue, our editor, Mr. Samra, reported the efforts made by the psychiatric establishment, then controlled by psychoanalysts, to prevent publication of any views critical of mainstream psychiatry. We also told our readers of the NIMH announcement of the formation of a new Center for Studies of Schizophrenia, I believe in response to our existence and as part of their attempt to suppress our work. Dr. Osmond commented, "It is good to know that NIMH should now be taking schizophrenia seriously as an entity in its own right. This may not be a coincidence, since it will be recalled that very early in 1964 we all felt that by having a foundation devoted to schizophrenia, we would arouse much greater government and public interest. It looks as if we were on the right track." Dr. Walter Alvarez, formerly a senior gastroenterologist with the Mayo Clinic in Rochester, Minnesota, reported how his syndicated medical column, read by roughly 40 million people, had been removed by some newspapers following complaints by psychoanalysts who were hostile to his embrace of nutritional psychiatry. In the April issue the newsletter reported the formation of the Schizophrenia Foundation of Saskatchewan, with Irwin Kahan as executive director and myself as president.

Two new features made their first appearance in the July 1969 issue. There were aimed at educating patients about their illness and about their rights as patients. The first was an article in the "Living With Schizophrenia" series. I still run these in our journal when they are available. Reading the stories of patients who recover using vitamins, even when previous treatments had failed, provides encouragement to patients still struggling with their illness. The second was a piece about what families should be looking for in treatment.

Humphry provided most of its content. He stated that the first responsibility of the hospital is to do no harm, the second, to do some good. He showed how the senses everyone has could be used to evaluate the institution. "Your eyes will tell you whether the hospital is built on a human scale. Your ears will tell you whether the hospital is quiet, even in the cafeteria. Your nose will tell you whether the hospital is clean. If the hospital smells bad, it does not pass the test. Your feet, your touch, and your taste can also help." The old mental hospitals were huge, overcrowded, noisy, smelled awful, and discouraged recovery. Modern psychiatric wards do not have the same defects but our senses can still be used to determine whether proper care is being given. More information in this vein was given in the January 1970 issue.

The October issue reported that the Montreal group, led by Dr. Lehmann, had reported to the Canadian Psychiatric Association's annual meeting in Toronto, June 11 to 14, 1969 that they had corroborated our results. They concluded that "in this placebo-controlled cross-over study, nicotinic acid in a fixed dosage of 3,000 milligrams a day produced a statistically significant improvement in chronic hospitalised schizophrenic patients." These investigators, in the face of the criticism they received, quickly regretted publishing this conclusion and thereafter maintained that the treatment was not effective. We had suggested that niacin could be therapeutic because it bound or removed methyl groups from the body and thus decreased the production of adrenaline from noradrenaline, which occurs through the process of methylation. Ban and Lehmann then tried to test the idea that methionine would do what we claimed niacin did, namely remove methyl groups. They began giving their study patients 20 grams of methionine daily against only three grams of nicotinic acid. Their patients grew worse. As Linus Pauling later pointed out, this approach represented a thoroughly irresponsible research attempt, as it subjected patients to too much methionine; it is toxic in these amounts.

This Newsletter also summarized the excellent research carried out by Russell F. Smith in Detroit, who treated 507 alcoholics with niacin over a two-year period and found a 71 percent recovery rate.

We also had to announce the death of Bill W., a powerful friend of the ASA and of alcoholics. And we announced an award to Linus Pauling from the ASA for his signal contributions to the theory and practice of orthomolecular therapy. This issue further carried my report on the use of milieu therapy, namely, making changes in the psycho-social organization of the hospital. The psychoanalytic community claimed it to be very effective in treating schizophrenics. I pointed out that no research had ever established the truth of these claims. We also carried Dr. Kanner's statement in opposition to the claims made by Bruno Bettelheim, that parents made their children autistic. Dr. Kanner paid tribute to Dr. Bernard Rimland, one of the original member of the ASA board and a dedicated worker, author, and lecturer on infantile autism and other childhood diseases.

In April 1970 the newsletter reported Dr. David Hawkins' findings that of 160 schizophrenic patients followed over a two-year period, those discharged without any additional vitamin therapy were readmitted at the rate of 35 percent. Patients who took vitamins from three to ten months after discharge had a readmission rate of 25 percent, while of those who took vitamins for one year, only 16 percent needed to be readmitted. Dr. Hawkins presented these results to the Third International Congress of the Academy of Psychosomatic Medicine, in Buenos Aires, Argentina in January of 1970. I also spoke at the same meeting.

In April 1970 the ASA newsletter announced the formation of the Schizophrenic Foundation of New York, Mrs. Kay Fryer, President. After Mrs. Fryer's schizophrenic daughter died because she could not get proper treatment soon enough, Dr. Allan Cott asked her to take on this onerous job. Mrs. Fryer, a concert pianist and piano teacher, had never been president of anything before and thought it over the whole time it took her to walk the 17 blocks from his office to her home. "When I reached home," she later told me, "I knew that I was going to accept, that if I didn't I'd regret it. I knew that if there was any cause that I could ever be wholly committed to, this was it!" Later Kay launched the Fryer Treatment Center, which has provided orthomolecular treatment to an enormous number of schizophrenic patients. It is still doing so long after her death. I believe the city of New York ought long ago to have given her one of its major awards for the fine work she has done. The Center has treated large numbers of patients successfully and every recovered patient saves the state at least $2,000,000 over his or her lifetime.

In July 1970 we announced two major events. We had moved our headquarters from Ann Arbor, Michigan to New York City, and a new director, Melvin Mendelssohn, had replaced Mr. Samra.

Dr. Ross MacLean, a psychiatrist from Vancouver, B.C. and member of the board for some years, was elected President at the time. Cal wanted to go back to his first love, being an investigative reporter. I believe he was also worn out by the amount of work he had accomplished and by the difficulties with Mr. McDonough. Cal had been in the direct line of fire. He is an excellent journalist. It is a pleasure today to read the issues of the newsletter that he edited for so many years. Without his help, the ASA could never have gotten started.

Our move to New York had been mainly generated by the intense enthusiasm of Suzanne Mendelssohn, Melvin's wife who blew into our organization like a fresh breeze in the late 1960s. Her brother Jerome had been ill for 11 years, in and out of several hospitals, and was finally declared hopeless. Suzanne had finally arranged that he see Dr. Cott, who started him on orthomolecular treatment. The megavitamin approach provided him with some help. She was then vice-president with the Harold L. Oram Inc. advertising agency. In the face of our pessimism about our chances for creating long term financial stability, she quickly convinced us that with a proper fund-raising drive and a move to the big city we would be much more likely to achieve success. We agreed to her proposal, which included inviting Melvin to become executive director. The Mendelssohns made our move possible and launched us into national prominence.

Our New York offices were located at 56 West 45th Street, in Manhattan. Miss Mary Ellen Roddy was appointed office secretary. Upon our arrival in New York, we initiated a major fundraising drive with a meeting at the Gotham Hotel on May 20, 1970. Mrs. George Vanderbilt was the hostess. Special guest speakers were Dr. Walter Alvarez, Humphry, and I. In her invitation, Mrs. Vanderbilt stated, "The work of Drs. Hoffer and Osmond and their colleagues has already resulted in recovery for thousands of sufferers. Further advancements in this field can be expected to affect not only schizo-phrenics but victims of hypoglycemia (low blood sugar), alcoholism, heart disease, arthritis, cancer, drug addictions, retardation and senil-ity." At the cocktail party that concluded the evening, Mr. Donald C. (Ben) Webster, Chairman announced that the American Schizophrenia Association had reached $104,000 in its donations drive.

The October 1970 issue of the newsletter reported on a meeting held in Los Angeles, sponsored by the Food Employers and Retail Clerks Local 770 Benefit Fund and arranged by its secretary, Mr. Joe DeSilva, and the ASA. The scientific portion of this meeting was arranged by Dr. W. Coda Martin, Medical Director, 770 Predictive Medical Center, the Los Angeles clinic that served the union local's membership, and Dr. R. MacLean, President of ASA and Medical Director, Hollywood Hospital, Vancouver, British Columbia. How the ASA became involved with this union is a fascinating story, and the meeting held in Los Angeles was a dramatic one.

Joe DeSilva began organizing a union in 1937, when he was a buyer for a grocery chain. In 1959 he became one of the first union leaders to demand and get psychiatric coverage for the members of his union. For this he was attacked viciously in the Los Angeles Press; some articles suggested that he himself needed psychiatric treat-ment. Nonetheless, Joe negotiated a contract with the union's employers that stipulated that a small fraction of the members' hourly wages would be set aside and used to provide them with psychiatric treatment. He set up a psychiatric clinic with a full-time psychiatrist in charge. He was very proud of this clinic and he also became the darling of the APA. They saw him as the first of many union leaders who would one day insist that every union be provided with a similar contract. In 1964, he received the California Governor's Trophy "for the individual outside the field of mental health who has made the most significant contribution toward improving mental health in the State" and in 1965 he received the John F. Kennedy Peace Award in recognition of "28 years of service in the field of human relations."

Late in the 1960s, Joe's daughter became mentally ill. Joe naturally asked the psychiatrist in charge of the union clinic to treat her, which he did with the usual analytic psychotherapy. She did not respond and Joe became more and more worried and concerned. He had many conferences with the psychiatrist, but nothing helped. Eventually Joe, in desperation, decided he would have to learn all he could about mental illness. His interests had a biochemical slant. This may have been due to his close relationship with Dr. Martin. Joe had never had any training in science, and knew nothing about chemistry. Even so, he got hold of a book on biochemistry and mental health and began to read it every night, slowly and painfully, after a hard day's work. Each page contained many words he could not understand. He would underline each one of these words and the next day his secretary would type them out, look up each word's dictionary definition and type that out as well, for Joe to study that night. Methodically and slowly he plowed through that book until he came to the section dealing with pellagra and niacin. As he continued to read, he was suddenly struck by the similarity between his daughter's illness and the description of pellagra given in that book. He spoke to Dr. Martin about niacin. Dr. Martin had heard about our work but knew little about it. Joe found out how to reach me and called. After our conversation, he put the book aside and read no more. Armed with new information, he asked the psychiatrist in charge of the union clinic to place his daughter on niacin. The psychiatrist absolutely refused to do so since he "knew," as the APA had told him so, that niacin could not help and could be harmful. The two men got into a series of arguments and eventually Joe fired the psychiatrist. He then discovered that the psychiatrist had looked upon his position as a cushy job which allowed him to spend afternoons mainly on the golf course. I assured Joe by phone that niacin was safe and advised him as to how I was using it. But Joe was afraid that it might hurt his daughter. He therefore decided to take one gram of niacin after every meal for a month. He decided that if he survived the month, he would start his daughter on the vitamin himself. After a month, he felt fine and he then got his daughter to take the niacin. Within a few months, she was well.

After this experience, he became an enthusiastic supporter of the ASA and did everything he could to help spread the message that there was something that could be done for schizophrenics. Several Los Angeles psychiatrists learned of his efforts and informed the APA. This organization then made strenuous efforts to win Joe back into the ranks of their supporters, to no avail. Eventually Joe suggested that his union sponsor a scientific meeting of the ASA in Los Angeles. We agreed and arranged for the Committee on Therapy of the ASA to hold its annual meeting there. The purpose of the symposium, Mr. DeSilva wrote in the July-August issue of Local 770's official publication, was "to bring to the medical profession, to the mentally ill, and their loved ones, the light which had been shrouded by confused and unintelligible talk. We are then convinced and are even more positive now, that therapists can no more talk the patient out of his schizophrenia than it is possible to talk a diabetic out of his diabetes." This was strong talk from a former favorite of the APA. However the APA did not give up. They approached Joe and requested that they be allowed to send one representative to "balance" the views that would be given by the members of the therapy committee of the ASA at our meeting. They suggested that Dr. Morris Lipton would be willing to appear. Joe discussed the matter with Dr. R. MacLean and me and we agreed that we would invite Lipton, and give him the same amount of time that each of the other speakers would have. Dr. Lipton was Professor of Psychiatry and Chairman of the Department at the University of North Carolina School of Medicine, Chapel Hill, North Carolina. The meeting was held June 11 to 16, 1970. Dr. MacLean was chairman of the symposium. I was one of the speakers, as were Dr. D. Hawkins, Dr. Robert Meiers, Professor Harold Kelm, and Dr. M. El Meligi. Meiers was a psychiatrist at Twin Pines Hospital in Belmont, California. Kelm and El Meligi were psychologists. Dr. Kelm had worked with us on the HOD test and El Meligi had worked with Humphry in developing the Experiential World Inventory (EWI) test.

Just before the meeting started, Dr. Lipton asked Dr. MacLean for two hours for his presentation. He stated that since there would be several speakers describing their use of vitamin treatment and he was the only one being critical of the approach, he needed "equal time," to allow him to make a complete rebuttal. In other words, he thought he should be entitled to two hours while everyone else got one. His definition of equal time surprised me. For the first time I became aware of the *chutzpah* of the American psychiatric establishment. We turned him down.

When his one hour arrived, he launched a diatribe against the whole orthomolecular treatment program. In his speech, he outlined why he considered himself to be an expert on vitamins. He had earned his PhD in biochemistry before becoming a psychiatrist at the University of Iowa in the same department where Dr. Elvehjem and Dr. Wooley had done their work in identifying niacin and niacinamide as the anti-pellagra vitamin. Dr. Lipton told the large audience (about 1,500 people) that this association qualified him to comment, even though he admitted openly that he had never treated a single patient with vitamins. Later I looked for any papers he might have published on vitamins and I could not find any. Nevertheless, the attack he delivered became the basis for an APA Task Force Report published in 1973 which he helped prepare as the task force's chairman. Both his speech and this report were filled with similar lies, misinterpretations, and biases. The report was a document designed to destroy the orthomolecular movement, and as will be described later in my account of the HIBR's history, it had significant impact. I spoke after Lipton did and made what I considered to be a major attack on the views he had espoused. I challenged him to try the treatment out. I added that when I had read the paper wherein he claimed that thyroid hormone accelerated the response to tricyclic antidepressants, I had tried out his recommendation and had concluded that it did have some value. The basic challenge I delivered to him was to ask whether he had enough scientific integrity to test the treatment before condemning it. So far as I know, he never did so. At the evening reception, Dr. Lipton told me privately that if he saw even one schizophrenic patient get well on vitamins he would take the therapy seriously. Yet when I challenged him to open his eyes to the many who had been helped, he refused to do so. At the same meeting a young physician who had failed to respond to standard treatment had spoken about his own recovery on niacin. This physician later became a psychiatrist and eventually was elected president of one of the largest state psychiatric associations. He is still in private practice and well.

While in Los Angeles several of our speakers appeared on local radio and television. I remember one such appearance well. There were four of us—Dr. Allan Cott, Dr. H. Osmond, Dr. Morris Lipton, and myself. Of course we got into a fight, with Lipton taking an anti-vitamin stance. The interviewer favoured our side. It was clear then and is now that the APA had little concern about the state of treatment of schizophrenia, that its main consideration was the consolidation of power. The analysts had only recently gained the influence they had so desperately sought following World War II, and they were not about to yield to a bunch of upstart psychiatrists with crazy ideas about vitamins and no university affiliations. They considered Joe a traitor and did their best to destroy him. A few years later, Joe DeSilva left his local and started a vitamin distribution business.

In September 1971 we changed the name of the ASA to the Huxley Institute of Biosocial Research (HIBR). The ASA became a division of this parent organization. We had been discussing a name change for several years. The word "schizophrenia", we had found, made people very wary. Many potential contributors did not want to be associated with an organization mentioning this disease. In a rather strange way, the stigma associated with the disease spread to the organization conceived to help its sufferers. There had been the same stigma around cancer years before, but cancer can not be hidden as readily and its presence forced itself on the public in a way that schizophrenia could not. We had initially included the word "schizophrenia" in the ASA's name as a way of forcing this disease into public consciousness but had found this task more difficult than expected—and it is still not achieved. "Schizophrenia" has instead become a word used to criticize anyone who appears to simultaneously hold opposing points of view, which is a totally inappropriate use of this word. Of course, that meaning of the word is also inappropriate for the disease it names. Schizophrenics who need extra vitamin B-3 should be called vitamin B-3 dependent and patients who are sick because they are consuming foods to which they are allergic should be called allergic. What is common in both cases is that the sufferers have perceptual and thought disorders. Dr. Bella Kowalson's term for this was metabolic dysperception. Dr. T. Robie thought this was an excellent term and I do too, but it would take too much work to popularize such a term.

Suzanne Mendelssohn suggested that we use the word "Huxley". In his lifetime, the celebrated author and philosopher Aldous Huxley had been a strong supporter of our work, and his brother, Sir Julian Huxley, renowned British biologist and scientific humanist, still was. Laura Huxley, Aldous's widow, agreed we could use the Huxley name, as did Sir Julian, but he wanted the word "biosocial" in our name, since it represented his biological interest and Aldous's psychosocial focus. We agreed. Mrs. Huxley, a member of the ASA Board of Trustees, noted that "much impetus for the work of the Institute was given by the association of Aldous and Humphry Osmond and their investigation of psychedelic substances, consciousness expansion and the vitamin B-3. Dr. Osmond is a Co-Founder and Vice President of ASA." For the occasion, we also published a tentative statement of purpose that read: "More than 50 million Americans suffer from a number of severe illnesses which may be related to biochemical abnormalities. They include schizophrenia, alcoholism, drug addiction, learning disabilities, pellagra, memory loss and other degenerative diseases of the aging. In the course of their studies of human biochemistry, a growing number of research scientists—including Mark Altshule, Abram Hoffer, Humphry Osmond and Linus Pauling—have uncovered evidence that these illnesses may be linked by similar metabolic processes dependent upon nutrition...The Huxley Institute for Biosocial Research believes that we are now on the brink of a biological revolution that can be hastened by the development of orthomolecular medicine, as it has been termed by Linus Pauling. An increasing number of doctors are currently treating schizophrenia, pellagra, alcoholism and memory loss successfully with varying combinations of megavitamins, drugs and carefully controlled diet. By providing the optimum biochemical and nutritional environment for every person, the attainment of individual potential and social betterment can be maximized".

One of the more memorable meetings of the Huxley Institute was the last one we held in New York City. In our 1988 board meeting, it suddenly occurred to me that it would be very useful to us if the city's mayor, Mr. Koch, greeted the attendees of our annual conference. We had invited prominent members of government, such as the Minister of Health, to do the same at Canadian Schizophrenia Foundation meetings, and they had been pleased to help us. As soon as I got the idea I dismissed it as a fantasy, but I presented it to the board anyway. To my surprise, one of the members said that a business associate of his had once been a deputy mayor with Mr. Koch and he thought this man could approach the mayor. He later called his associate and eventually we contacted the Mayor's office. The administrator there wanted to have all the details of our meeting, who we were, what we did, and most important, I think, how many people would be present. We advised him we expected about 400 people, mostly from New York, to attend. The official then asked us to draft an opening statement which Mr. Koch could use. I learned later that one of the main reasons the mayor agreed to come was because his secretary had read our book *How To Live With Schizophrenia* and considered it very important.

I was chairman of the scientific part of our meeting. It had been my policy to always start our meetings on time, whether or not all the participants had arrived. I had found that in New York it was very difficult to start on time, at least with a full house, the usual reason being the attendees were held up by traffic. But members of our group knew that I ran a tight ship and usually at least 90 percent were present on time. That morning at 8:00 I went to the conference room to make sure everything was in order. At about 8:30 the mayor's advance man arrived and he saw no one in the hall. He became very agitated and told me that the mayor worked on an extremely tight schedule and would have to get away by 9:10 or so. I assured him that we would start at 9:00 even if only he and I were present. I was joking with him but I recall he did not see much humour in my words. However, a few minutes later the crowd began to pour in and by 9:00 the room was full, with over 400 people present. I met the mayor and some of his entourage. The meeting was opened by Mr. Ben Webster, Chairman of the Board. Mr. Disque Dean introduced Mayor Koch. He started his talk by pulling out the speech we had written for him, put down the paper, and proceeded to greet us on behalf of the city of New York. Then, to my surprise, instead of using the talk we had prepared, he asked whether anyone had any questions. My heart sank. To ask a New York audience whether they have any questions is to launch a mass community meeting. But the audience must have been sincerely interested in the day's agenda. Only two questions were asked, one dealing with the school lunch program. Then Mayor Koch said good-bye and I took over the meeting.

It went on to be one of our best, with many pioneers contributing rousing presentations on their work. I was very proud of that meeting.

The following day I was approached by a writer who asked me whether I would talk to him about our work. He said he had been commissioned by the *New York Times* to attend the meeting and prepare a report. He added that he had thought he would find a bunch of strange people, kooks, but to his amazement found that we were a sober group of physicians presenting obviously important work. He was so impressed he wanted more time with me to help him prepare his report. I replied that I saw no point in giving him that time, since if he wrote something favorable about our work, the

New York Times would not publish it. The *Times,* in my opinion, was still under the influence of their psychoanalyst advisors. The first time we had called a press conference in New York to present the ASA and Linus Pauling, the *Times* had sent one reporter only, after the publisher ordered their news department to do so. That order, in turn, had been sent because Mrs. K. Fryer knew the publisher and had used her influence with her. The *Times* had not wanted to cover that conference. The only reporter who ever wrote favourably on orthomolecular work in the paper's pages was John Osmundsen, when he was the *Times'* science writer. Generally, when it came to a discussion of vitamins, the *Times* consistently parroted the negative statements of the leaders of the US psychiatric establishment. The reporter assured me over and over that he had never been turned down by the *Times* when they had given him an assignment and he guaranteed that whatever he wrote would appear. He stated the piece would appear in about two weeks. With that assurance I invited him to our hotel and we spent about five hours going over the entire history of our work in detail. After several weeks, nothing had appeared in the *New York Times*. After several months I called him. He was apologetic, and immediately said that he had not been rejected but that the *Times* wanted some clarification and would I meet with him once more? A few months after that, on my next visit to New York, I met him and again answered all his questions. He once more assured me that his story would be printed. To the best of my knowledge, it never was. I was never shown what he prepared, but I have concluded that his story was favourable and for that reason was killed by a senior editor.

In 1971, the publication of the newsletter of the ASA (we had christened it *Schizophrenia* in 1967) was taken over by the Canadian Schizophrenia Foundation (CSF), which had been formed in April, 1969 and had its offices in Regina, Saskatchewan. Fannie Kahan became the editor of this new joint publication. The first issue was a little 16-page bulletin on rough paper that had little of the polish of the *Newsletter* which came later. By October 1971 the newsletter

(Volume 2, No. 4) carried the title "Canadian Schizophrenia Foundation" in bold letters, accompanied by a logo based on the chemical representation of an indole molecule. The contents did not include the same biting comments about establishment psychiatry that had characterized the earlier issues under the editorship of Mr. Cal Samra. Fannie had a different journalistic style. But it did carry more and more news items about a growing number of local foundations across North America.

The January 1972 issue described a brief presented to the Saskatchewan government by the CSF, requesting the establishment of an independent bureau that would assess the work of Saskatchewan treatment centers for the mentally ill. Nothing came of this. Dr. Colin Smith, Director of Psychiatric Services Branch and the Minister of Health, Mr. Walter Smishek, stated that the costs of opening and running such a bureau would be high and that there would be difficulty assessing the effectiveness of treatment.

The very idea of evaluating therapy has been very controversial for as long as I have been in psychiatry. During the entire tenure of my practice, no non-orthomolecular psychiatrist I have ever known expected any of the patients to really become normal. A standard psychiatric dictionary does not contain the word "cure". The first attack on the Canadian Mental Health Association, Saskatchewan Division from CMHA Toronto arose because someone from the Saskatchewan group had used the word "cure". None of the official statements from our research unit spoke about cures. We did discuss "one-" or "two-year cures" and these were described. Professor McKerracher had based a whole program of teaching general practitioners about the mentally ill on the premise that patients would not be cured, that they would forever need careful care and attention and that it was up to general practitioners to provide this since there were so many of them, and too many patients to be looked after by the psychiatrists, who were fewer in number.

At the time the CSF brief was submitted, the institutions in Saskatchewan had to file annual reports about their activities. The data included number of patients admitted or seen, number given various treatments, number discharged, and number who died. Never had I seen any statements about the number who got well, the number who were partially helped, and the number who did not get well. The public had to infer this themselves which they did very effectively by simply noting that there were as many readmissions as admissions in the mental hospital system and from seeing their own relatives and friends not get well. Such was the case across the board until the major antidepressants came along—these for the first time permitted doctors to successfully treat most of the patients with depression. But the government of Saskatchewan did not want to ask the hard question of their department—why did they not make more of the other patients well? I believe they had been advised by their psychiatrists that it was impossible to help most patients and a review of treatment outcomes would only embarrass the government. The response to our brief reminded me of an occasion when I was still a professor of psychiatry.

At a case conference I had suggested that we institute the equivalent of the post mortem. Surgeons have some pressure on them to be careful, since standing behind them are the pathologists who will soon let them know that they are removing healthy tissues. I suggested that a psychiatric post mortem would be similar. Every patient who had been treated in hospital and discharged would be studied in a case conference if they were readmitted. This conference would try to decide why that patient had failed to respond to treatment: was it due to lack of community support, patient non-compliance, or the treatment given by the psychiatrist? None of the residents or other professors made any response whatsoever. Only a clear silence hung in the air for several minutes until someone thought of something else to say.

The introduction of strong psychiatric drugs in the second half of the 20th century has made it essential to develop ways of evaluating the results of giving these drugs. Immense sums of money have been spent to develop scales that measure signs and symptoms before and after use, but these, too, still rigorously avoid telling us about recovery, about becoming well, becoming normal. In our research I used a different method of evaluating patients, which depended not only on symptoms but on performance. I considered patients normal if they were free of symptoms and signs, getting on reasonably well with their family, getting on reasonably well within the community, and performing the way they would have been if they had not fallen sick. This includes paying taxes. Very few schizophrenics on tranquilizers are able to pay taxes.

In April 1972, the newsletter announced the upcoming first annual meeting of the CSF in Regina. Our featured speaker was Dr. Bernard Rimland from San Diego, who was to speak about his studies of children. In the July issue, Bernie's speech was summarized. He reviewed the evidence that children's psychiatric diseases were caused by biochemical and physiological factors. He severely castigated psychoanalysts and psychologists who adhered to the backward theory that parents are to blame for their children's illness. As late as the 1990s, I have had parents tell me they were blamed for having made their psychotic children sick. Old ideas, no matter how wrong or distasteful, sometimes seem to take forever to die.

In the July issue, Dr. Max Vogel also criticized W.G. Coombs, Executive Director, Alberta Division, CMHA, for stating that we had claimed "cures" (that dreadful word again). Max stated that from his own large experience in treating over 2,000 patients, he was able to corroborate the therapeutic claims made for megavitamin therapy. In the October, 1972 issue I was very critical of the way hospitals were placing their patients on tranquilizers and returning them home before they were ready for discharge. This approach remains the present policy, pursued more vigorously than ever. My article of the time reads in part, "Instead of being looked upon as treatment centers, hospitals were looked upon as first aid stations where patients would be admitted if the pressure on the family became too great. The policy was to discharge patients as soon as possible even if they had not recovered...This policy would not have been that bad had tranquilizers not come along because fifteen years ago the mentally ill could not be held in the community. The tranquilizers made it possible to keep patients in the community while not doing anything about the basic disease. We are now beginning to see the results of 40 years of continuous medication on patients who still remain ill, have stood by while time has marched on leaving them as if frozen at a sick level and each year reducing the probability that they will ever get well…Thus my original concept of a community-based mental program was one where, as with the physically ill, there would be an adequate number of treatment facilities, out-patient clinics, hospitals where treatment would be given to cure the patient, etc. not merely to make it possible to hold him in a chemical straight jacket for the rest of his life." I would add here that recovery from schizophrenia cannot be rushed. It takes the body a long time to stop making excess adrenochrome and to clear the effect of this toxic compound after it has been present for many years.

In this issue we also featured excerpts from the new booklet the CSF had printed, called *This is Schizophrenics Anonymous*. In the same issue, Dr. W.R. Ayre, a Montreal physician, criticized the Montreal studies being done by Dr. T. Ban and Dr. H. Lehmann at the Douglas Hospital ostensibly to replicate our work (their studies are discussed in detail in Chapter Fourteen). Dr Ayre said, "Schizophrenics are diagnosed and sent out to the community on phenothiazines as though they are being discarded into the wastebasket." Dr Ayre reported that he had met with Hugh Pearson (a member of the board of the CSF) and with Ban and Lehmann. He said the pair admitted they had not followed the protocol we had used but were planning a further study in which they were going to attempt to replicate exactly the exact procedures which I had recommended, including dietary changes. Their intentions may have been good, but they never did carry out these plans.

On March 6, 1972, the HIBR hosted a conference in New York City on the theme, "The Crisis in Health Care For The Aging." We had planned an ambitious program; Sir Julian Huxley was our Honorary Chairman. Our 44 panel underwriters included Mrs. Laura Huxley, Mrs. John L. Lehmann, and Dr. Roger T. Williams. About 90 individuals participated on the conference advisory council and we had 60 co-sponsoring organizations! How Mel Mendelssohn was able to obtain the support of so many groups is still a puzzle to me. In my talk, I argued that chronic senility is a form of chronic malnutrition, referring to my experience with Hong Kong Veterans. In the concluding paragraph of my presentation, I said, "I am now running an experiment on myself. If I survive to 90, I will have some data. I am taking at least 30 vitamin pills a day—including 4 grams of nicotinic acid, 4 grams of ascorbic acid, 800 units of vitamin E, 250 milligrams of thiamin, 250 milligrams of pyridoxine, Vitamins A and D, some calcium, iron, and a mineral supplement. I now feel fine, but later I may not. I'll let you know in 40 years." At the time of this writing, 2005, I have almost completed this research. I am just past 87, and I am still getting on relatively well.

The January issue, 1973, reported that "Take 30," a popular national CBC TV show, had featured vitamins. In four presentations, doctors E. and W. Shute discussed Vitamin E, Dr. C.J. Reich, vitamins A and D, A. Hoffer, Glen Green, and Max Vogel schizophrenia and vitamin B-3, and Linus Pauling and Terry Anderson, vitamin C and the concept of orthomolecular medicine. The newsletter also ran a description of the book *Orthomolecular Psychiatry: Treatment of Schizophrenia*. This volume had been edited by David Hawkins and Linus Pauling, and would be published by W.H. Freeman of San Francisco later in 1973. I had conceived the idea for this book a couple of years earlier. We were having the annual meeting of the Committee on Therapy of the American Schizophrenia Association at the palatial home of Dr. Ross Maclean in Vancouver. As usual I was chairman by default, since neither Dr. Osmond or Dr. Maclean were interested in this particular role. Dr. David Hawkins was sitting on my immediate right. At these meetings each member of the committee would report on the last year's activities. Every innovation in treatment was considered important and in need of discussion. Thus, for example, if Dr. Allan Cott told us that he had added pyridoxine to his treatment program (as he did indeed once do) and that he saw positive results he had not seen before, this became a subject for further study. Many Committee members would repeat these studies and in this way consensus was rapidly achieved. Most medical research depends upon publications and then confirmation, but this approach can take many years. With our Committee's approach, the discovery process was markedly accelerated. During this meeting, as the various members were discussing what they were doing I suddenly thought, "How sad it is that such a large amount of valuable information is being passed around the table and yet will remain unknown to anyone not in the room." It occurred to me that we must begin to publish our findings. I immediately spoke up and suggested to the committee that we all sponsor a book which would contain the information being presented around the table plus much more. I asked David whether he would be willing to be editor-in-chief, promising that I would help. I suggested that the other members would also help. David was caught by surprise; he gulped and then agreed. Later it occurred to us to invite Dr. Linus Pauling to be co-editor. Dr. Pauling assented on the condition that he see and vet every manuscript. We of course agreed. The resulting book is, I think, one of the most important published in the history of medicine but also one of the most neglected. It sold very well to families of schizophrenic patients and produced small royalties for us all, but the medical profession simply ignored it. Only one favorable review appeared in the professional literature, by a physician from the Mayo Clinic.

In January 1974, The Huxley Institute and ASA / CSF Newsletters were combined. Fannie Kahan again assumed the role of editor of the new joint publication. At that point, I was President of the HIBR. The first of these joint newsletters contained my critique of a pamphlet written by Professor K. Pearce, University of Calgary, and distributed by the Canadian Mental Health Association. This article contained 11 statements about schizophrenia, most of which I strongly disagreed with, and still do. The fact that this article was even written gives away the role played by Canadian psychiatrists in suppressing the real story about this disease. Following is a summary of the misstatements that appeared in the pamphlet: (1) Schizo-phrenics live in an imaginary world; (2) The disease is triggered by stress; (3) Schizophrenics "adopt" the disease as a way of life so as to escape stress; (4) Tranquilizers get them well; (5) Side effects of tranquilizer treatment are minimal; (6) Psychotherapy is a useful treatment; (7) Orthomolecular theory states that sick people have only minimal vitamin deficiencies; (8) The biochemical theories which led to the use of vitamins for treating schizophrenia were wrong; (9) The placebo response is effective for treating schizophrenia; (10) Incorrect figures on the genetics of schizophrenia. I responded vigorously to these erroneous statements but was not surprised Pearce had made them. I first knew him as a resident in the Department of Psychiatry at the University of Saskatchewan, later as professor at the University of Calgary. I considered him to be an inadequate psychiatrist who fawned on his superiors and treated those under him like dirt. He did not like me either and once vetoed a request made by a group of Calgary physicians to have me lecture to them. He must have been afraid of the outcome were his colleagues to learn that schizophrenia was biochemical and would respond to proper vitamin therapy. I once took one of his patients on, a woman with schizophrenia who had become more depressed when her dog died. He concluded that she was depressed only because her dog had died, gave her a prescription to get a new dog, and sent her home. She followed his advice, but she did not get well until she was started on vitamins. Later I treated her daughter and her father, a rancher who was paranoid and also had high blood cholesterol. I started him on niacin. As a result his cholesterol became normal, the lipomas on his face and neck cleared, and his paranoid ideas vanished.

The April 1975 issue revealed more of the controversy between establishment and orthomolecular practitioners, as it included an exchange of letters between Dr. Alan D. Miller, Commissioner, New York State, and Dr. H. Osmond. Dr. Miller's letter, dated April 11, 1966, questioned Dr. Osmond as to whether he had really claimed that 75 percent of schizophrenic patients had been cured by niacin. Humphry replied that what had been claimed was that with acute schizophrenic patients, there had been a 75 percent cure rate when followed up at the five- and ten-year points, and he presented some of our follow-up data. Dr. Miller did not pursue the matter any further and New York State under his direction continued its new "enlightened policy" of kicking chronic schizophrenic patients out of hospitals and into the streets. He was staunchly supported by the American Psychiatric Association. The group today sings a different tune but has never found the courage to apologize and persists in blaming others for the current state of affairs.

In the July 1975 issue, Fannie described her visit to North Nassau Mental Health Center on Long Island under Dr. David Hawkins. The clinic treated all psychiatric patients, including alcoholics, and at the time of Fannie's visit, had seen about 12,000 schizophrenic patients. Dr. Hawkins told Fannie, "But the orthomolecular treatment works. Once they are off the addicting drugs, you treat them for their hypoglycemia, take them off sugar and sweets, overcome their resistance to AA, test them with the HOD test and pick up whether or not they have schizophrenia. If they do, you put them on megavitamins and probably a phenothiazine, at least at the beginning. And then the results are extremely good." Dr. Hawkins had been trained as a psychoanalyst. Psychoanalysts seldom saw more than 25 patients per year since the patients had to be seen regularly and frequently. After he started his orthomolecular practice he walked into his office one day and on the way in asked his secretary who the person in the waiting room was. She told him it was a new patient he had already seen several times. He then realized he was treating so many new patients he could no longer remember each one in detail, as was possible when giving psychoanalysis. That realization, that patients were recovering and thereby making room for new ones, left him firmly committed to the new psychiatry.

During the mid-1970s, a public debate between the College of Physicians and Surgeons and the public interested in megavitamin therapy carried on in Alberta. The January, 1975 issue of the newsletter had contained our first report of a problem generated by the Alberta College of Physicians and Surgeons in June 1974, when it declared that the use of vitamins was experimental. The registrar of the College announced to Alberta's patient population, "We are doing it for your own good." The College also insisted that patients getting vitamins must sign a consent form. The registrar explained, "We're only interested that a patient receiving megavitamin therapy be totally aware of the risk he takes." This kind of caution I considered commendable—if only the same degree had been applied to every drug used in the practice of medicine, since every last one is much more dangerous and toxic than are vitamins. The Calgary Branch of the CSF, under the leadership of Dr. Max Vogel and other board members, had protested loudly. (The CSF is discussed in much greater detail in the next chapter.)

Over 6,000 irate citizens signed a petition demanding the government not withhold coverage for vitamin therapy (health care in Canada is paid for by publicly funded insurance) and, after a meeting with the minister of the government, this request was granted. The government announced it would appoint a committee to look into the matter. The College was playing true to its historic role of trying to suppress new ideas in the practice of medicine. I can only assume its members were too lazy and ignorant to examine the literature carefully. The three members of the Joint University Megavitamin Therapy Review Committee consisted of Dr. E.E. McCoy, Chairman, Department of Pediatrics, University of Alberta, Dr. K. Yonge, Chairman, Department of Psychiatry, University of Alberta, and Dr. G.W. Karr, Associate Professor, Division of Pharmacology and Therapeutics, University of Calgary. I was not happy with these choices. Only one member had not expressed his opposition to megavitamin therapy in the public press before they were appointed. Dr. Karr had several years earlier issued a statement to the press announcing his belief that there was nothing to vitamin treatment, while Dr. Yonge taught his medical students it was a lot of bunk. Dr. Yonge and I had never had a good relationship and neither of us valued the other's ideas very much. I believe our conflict started when I refused to allow him to become head of research under Dr. Osmond at the Saskatchewan Hospital at Weyburn in the early fifties, after he had returned from his postgraduate training in England at the Maudsley Hospital. I so disliked the composition of this committee, that I announced I would not appear before it publicly. I expected that their conclusions had already been determined by their publicly expressed biases. However, after the committee got going, I was asked by Dr. Karr whether they could come and visit me in my office and I agreed to that. He spent two days with me going over the information I had and I gave him copies of some of the material I had available.

The committee began its work in mid-1975 and presented its report in December, 1976, to the Minister of Social Services and Community Health (Alberta). After the committee had completed its review of the literature, listened to briefs, and visited various institutions, including Dr. Linus Pauling's centre, they issued a report that was in general favorable to orthomolecular psychiatry. I concluded that in spite of the obvious bias of the committee the evidence had been overwhelmingly impressive and that they had had to change their position. Their report recommendations were actually encouraging: (1) "We, therefore, recommend that adequate financial support be provided for well-designed and controlled clinical trials of megavitamin therapy, as judged by a process of scientific peer review. (2) We recommend that strong encouragement be given to research into mechanisms underlying clinical disorders for which megavitamin therapy is now advocated on empirical grounds. (3) Therefore we recommend that collaboration between proponents of megavitamin therapy and other investigators, qualified in the field of clinical investigation, be encouraged in the design and execution of future clinical trials of megavitamin therapy. (4) We recommend that scientists in the fields of Nutritional Biochemistry and Clinical Nutrition use their expertise to meet the need for thorough evaluation of newer hypotheses regarding nutritional mechanisms of disease, including the evaluation of orthomolecular concepts. (5) We recommend that undergraduate education of physicians and other health professionals include more attention to the role of nutrition in maintaining health and to the critical appraisal of newer concepts such as those embodied in megavitamin therapy and orthomolecular medicine." There were many other suggestions, but one more I considered important: "(6) We recommend that qualified medical investigators who are proponents of megavitamin therapy be welcomed to carry out controlled clinical trials at hospitals under university auspices, in collaboration with other medical investigators not committed to the megavitamin hypothesis." Despite this recommendation, so far, not a single Canadian university has tried to repeat any of our group's earlier claims, nor to initiate new studies which would conform with the suggestions of this committee. Some of the claims made by orthomolecular therapists have been given very serious examination and all the claims that were made have been confirmed. These have to do with vitamins E and C, the so-called antioxidant vitamins.

Today, nearly 30 years later, the Canadian Colleges of Physicians and Surgeons seem little more enlightened, even though there has been a massive rise of interest in the use of vitamins in medicine, though not yet in psychiatry. The psychiatrists, bitten once by their too ready acceptance of analysis, appear to want not to make any mistake when it comes to vitamins and may decide to wait until a new generation appears before opening their narrow views.

The January 1976 issue discussed a clinic opened in New York by Kay Fryer in May 1971. Mrs. Fryer was a member of the board of the Huxley Institute of Biosocial Research and President of the New York Branch. There was a tremendous amount of interest in New York City in the new nutritional approach to psychiatry and medicine. Every meeting I addressed there was well attended. The few orthomolecular psychiatrists in private practice in the city could not meet the demand, especially given the large number of poor patients who could not afford to pay for their care. In many cases entire families became bankrupt pursuing treatment for their relatives, after their private health insurance had run out. Kay persuaded the board of the HIBR to help her open a clinic. At first the board gave her substantial grants to help pay for vitamins, since most patients could not afford even those. Later, the board persuaded Kay to place her clinic on an economically self-sustaining basis. It is still operating as of this writing, in 2005. The 1976 newsletter report stated that the clinic was seeing 50 to 60 patients per month and had already seen over 2,000 since opening.

The October, 1976 issue reported I had addressed the Canadian Medical Association Meeting in Calgary, June 1976. I had been invited to participate in a panel with Dr. Charles Hollenberg, from the Faculty of Medicine, University of Manitoba, as the main critic. I reviewed the results I had seen in treating acute schizophrenic patients, a 75 percent recovery rate compared to the usual 33 percent natural remission rate. I remember that Dr. Hollenberg was indeed critical, claiming that the results were inconclusive. This of course was not true since all attempts to reproduce following our methods had confirmed our findings and all research with different classes of patients and not following our methods did not obtain these results. To prepare his critique, Dr. Hollenberg had consulted the professors of psychiatry at his university. They had never researched vitamin-based treatment and had assumed that the APA could not be wrong. Based on what Dr. Hollenberg said, they were openly hostile to the use of vitamins. I remember distinctly his advice to the medical audience. He stated that no physician not on a university faculty should undertake any new treatment until it had been first vetted by the medical schools and pronounced efficacious. This was the first clear exposition I had heard of the view that university professors held of their non-academic colleagues.

The October 1976 issue also carried profiles of three physicians who had recently attended a CSF conference. Dr. Paul Finninger was on staff in a mental hospital in South Dakota. He had started using vitamins in 1972, but his program for treating chronic patients was destroyed by staff hostility. Dr. Finninger attended many of our meetings. The last time I saw him he had retired but remained active in community activities. He told me he had been taking 75 grams of ascorbic acid daily for the previous ten years and felt great.

Dr. Garry Vickar was also profiled. As a student in the College of Medicine, University of Manitoba, he was given a rough time by one of the psychiatrists because he was my nephew. I think this stiffened his back and made him more determined to pursue the vitamin approach. That skeptic was later charged with some type of fraud. Regarding orthomolecular therapy, Garry told Fannie, "When I had the opportunity to do it as a practicing physician, I discovered it worked. What I was taught [in medical school] didn't work but what I used [in orthomolecular practice] worked."

Dr. J.A. Yaryura Tobias was the third physician interviewed. Dr. Tobias was married to a Regina woman and was visiting with her family one summer when he called me, wanting to talk about the use of vitamins. I invited him to come to Saskatoon and sit in with me while I dealt with my patients. He told me later that he thought it was very strange that any psychiatrist would invite another to be with him in this way. Psychiatrists in general never permitted anyone but the patient to be in the office; even parents and other close relatives were excluded. For my part, I felt very relaxed about making this invitation. Over the years I must have had over two hundred doctors sit with me for anywhere from one to five days. Each one, without exception, became a practicing orthomolecular physician. Almost all had to face the harassment and opposition of their colleagues and regulatory bodies. Some lost their medical licenses as a result. Dr. Tobias spent two days with me and after that also became an enthusiastic orthomolecular practitioner. "With the new approach, I found I was doing much better here with my patients. At least people here said thank you, which sounds silly but in psychiatry it is very important because you rarely have positive feedback from patients." Dr. Ted Robie had made exactly the same point in his first letter to me over ten years earlier. He had written, "My paranoid patients have become my friends." Anyone familiar with paranoid people knows the great significance of this statement.

XVIII

THE HUXLEY INSTITUTE, CONTINUED

The newsletters of the ASA, HIBR, and CSF also contained a vast amount of material dealing with my ongoing research. The first ASA newsletter published in the fall of 1966, included an article titled, "A New Drug, NAD, controversy." In this writing, I described a treatment that had brought 13 out of 17 schizophrenic patients to normal or close to normal within three to five days. One had been ill in the mental hospital in Weyburn for 29 years. The story behind this article goes as follows.

In 1965, the director of research with Eversharp Corporation, in Detroit, Michigan, called me. He asked whether I would be willing to act as consultant to his company. They had been working with nicotinamide adenine dinucleotide, or NAD. This compound contains nicotinamide and is made from vitamin B-3. They had been working with a physician in Seattle who claimed that he had been able to help many alcoholic patients by giving them intravenous NAD. He gave the compound intravenously because this enzyme was destroyed in the stomach by the gastric juices and therefore would not be absorbed as such—only its components would be. Eversharp had discovered how to make enteric coated tablets containing NAD dissolved in some oil that could survive passage through the stomach and released the NAD in the small intestine where it would be absorbed in its whole form. I was never shown the complete composition of this product.

They had begun supplying the Seattle physician with these tablets and as a result had accumulated a lot of clinical data. However, it was disorganized and could not be presented to the Patent Office in its present form. They were hoping that I would be able to go over the clinical material and prepare it for them in such a way that it could be submitted to that office. I told them I would be in New York in about a month and would be willing to talk to them while there. We met in Bill W.'s room in his hotel on Lexington Avenue and spent the evening together, Humphry, Bill W., the Eversharp medical director, and I.

From the first moment I heard about this NAD research, I was very interested. I had been hoping for some years to be able to get some NAD, so as to test its therapeutic properties for my schizophrenic patients. I already thought that vitamin B-3 was therapeutic because it increased the formation of NAD. By this time, we also knew that NAD slowed the oxidation of adrenaline to adrenochrome. If this was true, the NAD might be much more effective, as in fact it later on proved to be. I outlined our research to the director and told him I would not be interested in helping them out with their work with alcoholics but that I would like to obtain supplies to test on my schizophrenic patients. After several hours of discussion we agreed on a proposal. Eversharp would provide me with ample supplies for what is now considered phase two testing. Modern testing consists of three phases: In phase one, the toxicity of the compound is evaluated. NAD had been used, was proven safe, and no longer needed to be tested again. In phase two, the compound is given in pilot trials to patients to test for optimum dose, duration of treatment, and for side effects. In phase three, the compound is subjected to double-blind controlled experiments in various centers. I proposed that I would do the phase two studies and that if the results were promising we would involve other orthomolecular psychiatrists. We agreed that there would be no release of information until phase three studies had been completed. Eversharp would pay the University of Saskatchewan about $500 per month earmarked for our research, and would provide some equipment our chemists would need. The director, an ex-Canadian, was very happy with this arrangement and we signed a contract. I also agreed to provide monthly reports.

I had several schizophrenic patients under my care in hospital at that time. As soon as the tablets arrived they were given to these patients, 1 gram three times daily. I did not know what to expect. But within three days I saw an astonishing response. Patients became normal in three to five days and remained well as long as they were on the NAD. The results were obvious to the nursing staff and to the research psychiatrists who were working with me. Each month I would send Eversharp a report. They became very excited. After several months, two representatives of that company came to Saskatoon and were able to see firsthand what was happening. After that I ran into some difficulty. I had started a large number of patients on NAD, based on the contract which stated that Eversharp would provide whatever I needed. But the supplies began to arrive more and more slowly, and soon I was faced with the problem of what to do with all the patients already on the compound. I spoke to the director several times. I could not understand what was happening and assumed they were having a problem making enough. However, one day the director called me from a pay phone near his office. He told me that the doctor from Seattle who had originated the idea of using NAD for alcoholics had now decided that schizo-phrenia treatment with NAD was his idea as well, and that if there was going to be any patent arising from our research he wanted in on it. They saw millions in profits for their company and for the Seattle doctor. They had therefore decided to squeeze me out by depriving me of supplies. As a result, my relationship with Ever-sharp, which had been worsening weekly, terminated. I sent them a final report, and told them I would no longer cooperate with them since they had broken the agreement to provide me with enough NAD. I also sent back their equipment, returned their last cheque, and told them to send no more money. Then I added that having completed the research as far as I could, I would be referring to my findings, not theirs, in a report I would read in New York at a meeting of the New York-based Carl Neuberg Society, a scientific group. This last statement led to a cloak and dagger affair.

Every week or so the director would call me from a pay phone and tell me how the officers of the company were plotting to prevent me from reading my paper at the meeting in New York. My reference to NAD made up a minor part of this report, but it was integral to my theory of schizophrenia. Then the company officially informed me that if I read my paper I would be breaking a trade secret. Later they sent a lawyer from Seattle to Saskatoon to see me. He was in the city for about three days and visited me several times. He tried to persuade me not to read the paper and offered to pay me, as I recall, $1,500 monthly if I would not. I liked him, we got along well. During these discussions I told him that they had broken their contract and that I had the right to present any paper I wished based on my research, that they could not censor what I would be saying. I advised him that by reading my report I would be putting my findings about NAD's efficacy as a schizophrenia treatment into the public domain, and that thanks to Eversharp's actions, further research with NAD would most likely be done badly by US investigators and that this poor research might suppress further research in this area for many years. I sent him away asserting my final decision to go ahead. Humphry agreed with me. I now sometimes wonder what would have happened had I accepted their offer to be bribed. I am certain they would have discontinued payments very soon and that our contribution to the schizophrenia therapy research would have been destroyed. Furthermore, I was convinced that after I published the original data on NAD, it would be confirmed sometime in the future, even if it might take up to 40 years. Meanwhile I was faced with many schizophrenic patients who had begun relapsing within a few days after we ran out of supplies. In anticipation of the problem to come, I had started them on vitamin B-3, but it did not work as quickly as NAD. NAD did in a few days what vitamin B-3 did over several months. My patients were soon as ill as they had been before they were started on the NAD. Later I was able to buy some pure NAD and try it out as a powder dissolved in water. It had some effect but was not nearly as good as the Eversharp preparation.

I came to New York a few days ahead of the Neuberg Society meeting and spent the weekend with Humphry in Princeton, in his room on the grounds of the mental hospital. The meeting was on a Wednesday at the Waldorf Astoria Hotel. On Monday I went back to my hotel, the Roger Smith on Lexington Avenue. I found a message waiting, asking me to call a Mr. Rose, from a legal firm which included Richard Nixon as one of the partners. I returned his call. He asked me whether I intended to proceed with reading my paper. I replied affirmatively. He then stated again that the company would consider this action a breach of their trade secret and that if I persisted in my plan they would get an injunction to prevent me from reading my paper. I replied that that would not deter me. Mr. Rose was aghast at my stupidity. He said that if I acted against the injunction I could wind up in jail. This statement immediately alerted me to the fact that I might be in serious difficulty. And I decided that if I had to go to jail I would prefer it be a Canadian institution, not one in New York City. I immediately called the lawyer who advised the ASA and told him briefly what was happening. He suggested I come to his office immediately. I arrived there at about 10:00 am. He worked in a large building on Wall Street, just across the street from the offices of the Nixon firm. The rest of the morning I told him about the NAD, our contract, and so on. He wanted to see the contract, but it was back in Saskatoon. I immediately called Marg Callbeck. She knew where I had hidden it. She obtained it and slowly read the whole document to a stenographer who worked in the lawyer's office. On consideration, the lawyer stated the matter seemed pretty serious, but that he would now negotiate for me. Early in the afternoon he called Mr. Rose to tell him that he was acting on my behalf and that he had advised me not to appear in their offices as they had requested me to do. This recommendation was a good one. I later discovered the Nixon firm had surrounded their building with process servers armed with my photograph. If I had gone anywhere near that building I would have been served. The negotiations proceeded for the next five hours. As the afternoon passed, my lawyer became more and more cheerful. At five o'clock, Rose's side capitulated. They pledged they would withdraw their threat of injunction, on the condition that I change one word in my paper. This I agreed to do, as the revision would not in any way change the essence of my paper. None other than the owner of Eversharp, a person in Los Angeles, had ordered them to stop the action.

My lawyer advised me to go into hiding until the meeting was over. He said that this law firm was honorable and would not break their pledge, but there was nothing to prevent the doctor from Seattle or even Eversharp from getting another injunction from a different judge. I called Bill W. and asked him to get me a room at his hotel, which he did. I then called Humphry in Princeton and told him what had happened. I asked him to go to my hotel the next day when he came to the city and bring me the clothes I would need for the meeting. I called the hotel and authorised them to let him in. Then my lawyer took me down into a sub-basement of his office building which led directly into the subway. Once I was surrounded by thousands of people I felt safe. My lawyer did not want to charge me for his day of negotiation, but I insisted on paying him $500. He had been most helpful.

Humphry arrived the next day. He found the whole affair very entertaining. To make sure he was not being followed, he told me, he had walked all around the Roger Smith several times. We spent that night in Bill W.'s hotel. From there we called Humphry's good friend John Osmundsen, science reporter for the *New York Times*. I told him what had happened and suggested he come to the meeting. I added that he might be able to report something like "Prominent Canadian Psychiatrist Arrested While Delivering Paper" the next day. John thought that might be very entertaining and promised to be there. The next day I read my paper and was not arrested. The Seattle doctor was present but made no attempt to talk to me. John was delighted with my paper and the next day a report on it appeared on the first page of the second section of the *New York Times*. This report probably launched the megavitamin movement. Later, John became Science Editor, *Look Magazine,* and he was listed amongst the Friends of the ASA in our first newsletter.

This visit to New York also included the board meeting described earlier, when we did not reappoint the Chairman of the Board and were left with $5,000 in our little ASA treasury. It had been a very hectic time. When I came home, I contacted the Canadian Patent Office to obtain information regarding the possibility of patenting the NAD I had been using as a schizophrenia treatment, but did not follow up with them due to lack of funds and necessary information. After my break with Eversharp, it was only possible for us to do a few further studies with another form of NAD, crystalline NAD, that did not work nearly as well.

Within a few days after the *Times* report appeared, I was flooded with mail. The first letters came from the eastern half of the USA and Canada. Then, as the days wore on, the mail began to come from the western part of the continent; then the trend jumped across the Pacific Ocean and letters began arriving from the far east. I must have gotten thousands of them. I could not answer them all personally, so prepared an information sheet which I sent back. For a long time I was receiving several hundred letters each day. I had to hire another secretary to handle the work. At one time I had two secretaries and one part-time worker helping out. Humphry was also flooded with these letters after our Chairman's departure. As mentioned earlier, many of the writers of these letters became the donors who kept the ASA alive after the loss of our Chairman's initial donation.

The *Times* report also generated widespread professional interest. A few US psychiatrists quickly tried to repeat our work—but in the usual way, without actually doing what we had done. I am still amazed at the facility with which physicians feel no compunction to repeat original work as it was done originally. This could not happen nearly as often in chemistry or physics. Our study was a pilot showing that NAD had anti-schizophrenic activity and that it was safe. It would have been confirmed by double-blind controlled tests later on if the company had not broken its contract with me. The first one to try to repeat was Dr. Nathan S. Kline, Director of Research, Rockland State Hospital, in New York State. I had initially met him in 1951 during my first tour of research centers and several times after at meetings. I had never been impressed with him as a research scientist. His main preoccupation was the development of a large computer system based in Rockland State Hospital to which everyone would send their data. When he decided to repeat the NAD study, he found he could not get any of the NAD that the company had given me. They properly refused to hand it out to anyone. I had warned them that it would be immediately tested on the worst and sickest patients in the mental hospitals and that it would not work in such chronic patients. Dr Kline then tried to make his own capsules. He ran a test on the most chronic patients in his hospital. He later described these patients as having been infected with chronic parasites and infections. I could only guess that these infections arose from the backward treatment given in the hospitals. In his papers, Kline had certainly made that observation about the source of such infections in criticising other mental hospitals' studies of their chronic patients. He also used our HOD test on these patients. When his report finally appeared, he had found no clinical improvement but when I looked at his HOD scores, it was clear that these showed significant improvement. The patients on placebo showed no change whatever, while the patients on NAD did. When I challenged him on this, he replied that he placed no value on the HOD test. I still do not know what happened to his patients, if anything. Later Dr. C.C. Pfeiffer tested the Kline preparation against the original preparation using a sophisticated electro-physiological method and found that the original company preparation had been active but that Kline's preparation had little activity. Thus Kline had "repeated" our study by (1) Not working with the same kind of patients we had; (2) Not using the same preparation; (3) in a backward mental hospital setting. We had worked with patients who were ill for the first time or had relapsed, and had given them the Eversharp preparation in a new hospital setting, with a high ratio of staff to patients. Only one of our patients was a chronic schizophrenic, from the mental hospital at Weyburn, Saskatchewan. After she had recovered, I invited the psychiatrist who had been treating her in Weyburn to examine her at University Hospital. He agreed that she was remarkably improved. We were even able to find a room for her in the community, but then we ran out of NAD and she relapsed. She never again showed any improvement, even on vitamin B-3, and died a few years later back in the mental hospital in Weyburn.

The second attempt to repeat was made in another hospital, again using chronic patients, again with negative results. As I had predicted, the NAD idea was killed by these two studies. Meanwhile, the American psychiatric establishment could not differentiate NAD from vitamin B-3 and assumed that Kline had tested vitamin B-3 and found it ineffectual.

The NAD we used cost $10 per day. I am amused while writing this to read in the last paragraph of the original newsletter report on the controversy, "Dr Hoffer expressed the hope that the confirmation of his work elsewhere would help bring the price down so that more extensive studies could be conducted at a more reasonable cost." I am amused because today psychiatrists think nothing of giving drugs that cost the state $5,000 per year while refusing to use vitamin B-3, which costs pennies per day.

This seems an appropriate point in the narrative to give tribute to one of niacin's great champions, and the man who inspired the adoption of the term "B-3", Bill W. I have at this point described several very important events which involved Bill W., the cofounder of Alcoholics Anonymous (AA). He welcomed me when I needed to go into hiding in his hotel and freely gave his advice when I sought his help with respect to organizing Schizophrenics Anonymous in Saskatoon. But he deserves much more attention in my memoirs than he is given in the recounting of these incidents because he played such a major part in both my research, and in the development of niacin as an alcoholism treatment. Our connection is also chronicled in more detail in the book *Bill W.* by Francis Hartigan, St. Martins Press, New York, 2000.

I met him for the first time in 1958 at a meeting in New York City hosted by Eileen Garrett, President, Parapsychology Foundation. He sat between Humphry Osmond and me. I knew about him thanks to my work on the treatment of alcoholics, including the role of AA. We were then studying a derivative of adrenochrome called leuko adrenochrome. It was a colourless substance and our studies showed that it was not a hallucinogen. It is described in detail in our book *The Hallucinogens*. Our preliminary studies showed that it had interesting anti-anxiety properties when taken sublingually. Several people who had not found any substance that would relax them tried it and some of them responded very well. We had three milligram pills with us. In this meeting, Bill appeared very uncomfortable and squirmy. Humphry gave Bill one pill. He took it and we continued to listen to the speakers. About 20 minutes later, Bill was thoroughly relaxed. He later told us, "Now I know what you mean when you talk about being relaxed." This occasion marked the first time he felt relaxed without the use of alcohol. We continued further studies with leuko adrenochrome, but eventually had to stop, as the drug company we had been working with wanted a product that had a pronounced effect on everyone, no exceptions. Unfortunately leuko adrenochrome seemed to have no effect at all on some people. We left Bill a supply but eventually we had no more and his tension returned. I then advised him to take one gram of niacin each meal. Two weeks after starting on the vitamin, he was free of tension and depression and he felt great. He continued taking it for the rest of his life.

By the time the leuko adrenochrome incident occurred, Bill W. and I had had many discussions about the Saskatchewan research. Nearly every time I was in New York I would spend an evening and/or have a meal with Bill. One day in 1965 he pulled out thirty files and said, "I want to show you my research." He told me that he had given niacin to thirty of his friends and colleagues in AA. He found that on the vitamin, ten had achieved normal mood and mental function within one month, and another ten within another month; the rest had not responded. I was very surprised and pleased. His data confirmed what I had been seeing when I treated those of my patients who were members of AA with niacin. The vitamin is the best treatment for the residual mood disorders many members of AA continue to suffer after achieving sobriety. Bill became enthusiastic and he handed niacin out freely to anyone who was not well. For example, he gave it to his gardener, who was suffering from arthritis, with great success. One day a member of AA who lived on the west coast called him, crying on the phone. He told Bill that his psychoanalyst had killed himself by flying his plane into a mountain, and that he was very depressed as a result, had in fact received a diagnosis of manic depression. Bill said, "Hang on. I will send you a jug of niacin and you must take it." His friend recovered. Another of his friends on the west coast with arthritis also benefited. This friend was a strong supporter of President Eisenhower. Ike suffered severe arthritis of his hands, which made his life very difficult. This man called me after experiencing recovery from his arthritis and wanted to meet me in Saskatoon. I was going to Los Angeles in a few weeks and we met there. He told me about Ike's arthritis and wanted to know whether niacin could help. I gave him all the information I could, but felt reasonably certain that the corps of physicians that surround any president would not even tolerate the idea that he might be helped by niacin. I heard no more about the matter.

As AA grew and established itself, subgroups formed in the organization. One of these was a medical association; its members were both physicians and AA members. Bill wanted to inform this association about the value of niacin. On their side they had been inviting Bill for years to address their annual convention, which they held in a motel near the Indianapolis speedway one week before the racing season started. Bill had decided some time before not to do any more public speaking as he was afraid he was being deified. But after receiving yet another invitation to the 1966 convention, he called to inquire if I would be willing to go with him and talk to the meeting. I agreed. Then Bill told the association that if they invited me he would speak to them. Of course they would. They would have invited the devil if this would bring Bill to their midst.

It was an interesting meeting. Bill spoke first. He was a marvelous, charismatic speaker, very clear and very convincing as he told the group of the many therapeutic properties of niacin. He emphasized how it could heal AA members of their chronic tensions, depression, pain, and fatigue, symptoms that in many cases, he pointed out, could lead to alcohol addiction in the first place. Then I followed with a more sober and less interesting talk about our research with the vitamin. At the end of my presentation, someone moved from the floor that they create a committee to investigate the claims Bill and I were making. They did and this committee soon reported back to the association. I thought the committee did a wonderful job. Normally any medical committee would look at the problem, read all about it and then many months, later report back. These three doctors cut to the quick. They immediately began to take the niacin themselves. They soon all felt much better, concluded that niacin was valuable, and said so. Their report started a new movement, that of introducing niacin into the treatment of AA members who were suffering from mood disorders. There was an unpleasant aftermath to these events. NIMH in Washington, DC heard about this meeting. It promptly persuaded the group to invite an NIMH physician, a junior psychiatrist, to appear. He did so at a special meeting of the association held about six months after our presentation, and a little later I was sent a copy of his talk by a member of the group. His talk heralded the medical attack on niacin and was full of lies and distortions. This young psychiatrist has since gone far and is now one of the prominent US professors of psychiatry. Bill was not deterred. He decided to distribute accurate information on niacin widely through all AA circles. With the assistance of Helen Wynn, he wrote and distributed his first communication to AA Physicians, and eventually a second. His third such communication was released after he died in 1971, by the orthomolecular physicians Ed Boyle, David Hawkins and Russell F. Smith. He soon ran into difficulty with the International AA Headquarters, which he had created many years before. The physician members of the board did not think that Bill ought to be meddling with medical matters like advising people to take vitamins, and they would not support him. The Huxley Institute of Biosocial Research gave him a small annual grant to cover the cost of preparing and distributing his important communications. They were distributed by the thousands. One Texas AA member printed many thousands and distributed them.

For the purpose of his writing, Bill wanted a popular and easily remembered name for niacin. I told Bill that this nutrient had been the third water soluble vitamin to be identified and he decided to call it B-3. This name has stuck. Whenever I use the word B-3, I remember him.

Bill W., now Mr. Bill Wilson, helped enormous numbers of alcoholics around the world and his name is still very potent. In Victoria I see a large number of AA members who know of my connection with him. They take my advice much more seriously as a result.

I will return now to the central theme of these chapters, the work of the HIBR. Throughout the late 1960s and early 1970s, the Huxley Institute was making substantial progress in establishing and financing itself. We had been bequeathed about $900,000 by a generous donor, which allowed us to significantly expand our activities. Until then we had been getting by, though it was an effort. I remember on one occasion I was called in Saskatoon by Mary Roddy, who administered our New York office; she was concerned that we could not meet the next payroll. I was upset and irritated, but after sleeping on it, called her back in the morning and asked for the names of the donors who had given us our most substantial contributions. She called back with a list of over a dozen. I have always found it difficult to ask people for money, but this time I had no choice. I called each person on the list, and explained to them what was happening. I was totally surprised by the friendly responses I received. Within the hour, I raised another $50,000 and this money allowed us to continue. These US donors were truly amazing. I do not remember their names now; they are listed in the Hoffer Archives in Saskatoon, to which I do not have ready access. I do thank them all, nonetheless. After we were given the large bequest, less money began to come in from other sources and the board members who had been contributing generously, also felt that now not as much was needed. At the same time, the psychiatric establishment was stepping up its efforts to destroy our work. The first major attack began in 1968.

In that year, I had received a letter from the president of the APA. (I had been made a Fellow of this organization in 1960. That year, Dr. Griff McKerracher had been elected its vice president and they had held their meeting in Canada. They then offered Canadian members the Fellowship as a tribute to Canada. Frankly, the honour had meant little to me beyond the fact that it increased my annual dues.) In the letter, the president wrote that complaints had been made that I was promoting a treatment that was unacceptable to the APA. He further stated that the APA's Committee on Ethics had instructed him to reprimand me and tell me to cease and desist. I immediately looked up the constitution and bylaws of the APA. According to these documents, any complaint against a member had to be investigated by one of their committees, which would then report its conclusion to the board, which would then take action. None of this procedure had been followed. I wrote back to the APA president demanding that the group follow their own bylaws and that, as required, they also let me know the identity of the complainant. He wrote back saying that the association was too poor to convene a committee simply to consider the complaint. I replied that we were not in any great hurry and were quite prepared to wait until their next annual meeting. Eventually they agreed that we would meet in Washington, D.C in December 1970. In all this correspondence, they did not divulge the name of the person or persons who had laid the complaint against us. I think they were surprised at my reaction. I believe they had assumed that we would mildly acquiesce in response to their first letter. But to do so would have compromised my work of letting the public know that there was something far better than tranquilizers alone available to treat schizophrenia.

Two days before Rose and I left for New York City and Puerto Rico, where I had other commitments including the presentation on double-blind studies to the National Cancer Institute described in Chapter Sixteen, I received a telegram from the APA. They said that our scheduled meeting would have to be postponed until the following day. Accommodating them would have meant not being able to meet my other commitments. I was incensed by their behaviour and promptly sent them back a wire to say that Humphry and I would arrive at APA headquarters at 9:00 am as previously arranged, whether they appeared or not. This we did, arriving early. We visited the library and spoke to the librarian. She was delighted to meet us, was very friendly, and told us our papers were in great demand.

At 9:00 am, the APA committee of five, including a lawyer, wandered in and after introductions we got to work. A microphone was set in the middle of the table. The legal representative opened by asking me if I was the Dr. Hoffer who had written a paper entitled "Five California Schizophrenics." (Hoffer A: Five California schizophrenics. *J. Schizophrenia* 1:209-220, 1967.) I admitted that I was that person. He then asked me the same question at least three more times, until I got fed up and retorted sharply. Then I made my opening statement. I told the committee that we did not accept the Committee on Ethics as the appropriate committee to consider any complaint against us when it was a scientific matter that was being debated. I insisted that we should be examined by the Committee on Scientific Affairs or the Committee on Therapy.

The chairman then tried to mollify me, adopting a tone I heard as the one used by professors to deal with junior, inexperienced associates. He said that we were all there primarily as colleagues in order to examine seriously the issue of whether our treatment worked. I replied that I would be prepared to meet with them all day if necessary, if the appropriate committee were present. The Chairman then said that the group of people assembled in fact wore two hats, intimating that they could also be considered a Committee on Therapy. I replied that as long as they accepted my rejection of them as the Committee on Ethics I would be willing to discuss the matter with them—they would have to use the other hat. Once that agreement was made, the Chairman soon raised the point that Dr. Nathan Kline, the psychiatrist in New York who had attempted to corroborate my work with NAD, had disproved our work. I had foreseen that they would raise this issue so I had written to Kline several weeks earlier and had asked him point blank whether he had ever done any work with vitamin B-3. He had, as described earlier in this chapter, completed a very poor earlier study with NAD, which is not vitamin B-3. He wrote back confirming that he had never studied vitamin B-3. When questioned I therefore told them Dr. Kline's "disproving" was not relevant and proceeded to read his letter to them. The committee was so ignorant of our work it did not know that there was any difference between NAD and B-3. We went at it in a very hostile way until noon. Then the chairman announced that they would recess for ten minutes and come back with their verdict. At the end of ten minutes the chairman told us that they had not been able to come to a decision and would let us know in two weeks. We have not heard from them since. Obviously their committee split and they could not resolve the internal conflict so they declined to communicate with us any more, probably with good reason. If they had ruled that our publications were scientifically sound, we could have claimed APA support. It was more prudent, and of course much more cowardly of them, simply to say nothing and to attack us in other ways, as they did in 1973 with Morris Lipton's report. If I had been practising in the United States, they could also have threatened to cancel my membership and this could have had a serious effect on my career. However, since I was a Canadian, they had no power over me whatsoever. Perhaps this is why I was able to take their charges rather lightly and stand up to their scrutiny with a defiant attitude. I looked upon the meeting as an attempt to exercise retrospective censorship, to expunge the scientific record, and that outraged me—I had no intention of letting such action come to pass. I found out later that the complaint had come from one or more California psychiatrists. On returning home I resigned my APA fellowship, bluntly saying I could no longer be a member of an organization that spent my money (the annual fee) to attack my work.

The next major attack on our work arrived in 1973, with the publication of the APA Task Force Report on Megavitamin Therapy.

Dr. Morris Lipton, the same man who had given a reprehensible talk at the HIBR scientific meeting hosted by Joe Desilva's union local in Los Angeles in 1970, chaired the task force that wrote this report. This report attempted to discredit our research by essentially misrepresenting it, on one detail after another. Any psychiatrist who read it would assume that niacin was a completely useless therapy for schizophrenia and that Dr. Osmond and I were quack doctors working within the misguided fanatic fringes of the scientific endeavour. The report was widely distributed to the APA membership.

Further hostility was directed against us via the agency of the NIMH. Shortly after the report appeared, Mr. McDonough arranged for a meeting of scientists from the NIMH with myself, Dr. Osmond, and Dr. Linus Pauling. Dr. Lipton, Dr. Seymour Kety, and Dr. Loren Mosher were present on behalf of the NIMH. At this meeting Mr. McDonough expressed his anger that we had not helped his friend's son. I knew that my treatment had helped, but that the young man had not received the follow-up support he required to avoid relapse, due to the fact that no doctor in his home region would agree to carry on orthomolecular treatment. I could not describe the case because I had been this young man's doctor and therefore would be breaking confidentiality. McDonough's speech, of course, served to heighten the animosity in the room. Morris Lipton then maintained that he was a biochemist because he had done research work in the laboratory where Elvehjem had proved that niacin was vitamin B-3. But he knew little chemistry and soon made a statement that even a first-year chemistry student should know better than to make. Pauling, the world's greatest chemist and two-time Nobel-prize winner, the first for chemistry, roundly berated him for his ignorance. Mosher was equally hostile. He told us that in his view, even if every psychiatrist in the United States came to adopt orthomolecular treatment, he still would not believe it had any value. Mosher was Director of the Schizophrenia Section of NIMH. Yet he did not believe such a disease actually existed, for if he had, he would not have been totally opposed to any form of chemical intervention.

The meeting did not resolve any of our difficulties and NIMH remained solidly opposed to everything that we did. Lipton told me privately that he would never publish any paper of mine no matter how good it was, and as Associate Editor of the *American Journal of Psychiatry*, he remained true to his word. In recent years, Dr. Mosher told one of my acquaintances that the only reason I had gotten good results was because I had carefully preselected only those patients who would have gotten well anyway. I know of no doctor so skillful that he or she could preselect the schizophrenia patients who will get well. Neither did his comments show any acknowledgement that we had done a double-blind study. None of us knew who was getting what treatment, and only one third of our placebo group recovered.

Such was the unreasonable and hostile nature of the criticism applied to our work. The Task Force report frightened psychiatrists and we could no longer induce them to join. The ones who had joined earlier continued to practice until they died or retired; the momentum of the movement was destroyed. This turn of events was exactly what the APA wanted and they succeeded, not in destroying us but in delaying the introduction of orthomolecular medicine for another 40 years. The APA was also very successful, whether they intended this outcome or not, in ensuring that hundreds of thousands of patients would continue to suffer the ravages of schizophrenia, condemned to a lifetime of taking ever more powerful and expensive drugs. I am left wondering, is any public organization ever punished for advocating views which needlessly suppress important information and harm so many people? The story of the HIBR versus the APA has a small postscript. In 1981, I was attending a meeting that coincided with an APA annual meeting at the same hotel. I went down for breakfast one morning and found that the only other person in the restaurant was Morris Lipton. I asked if I could join him and he assented. I told him what I thought of him and his report. He made no substantial reply. He could speak only of his daughter who was very ill.

The HIBR eventually moved to Florida for a few years to save money. In the early 1990s, both Ben Webster and I decided that we could no longer devote as much time as before and we quit the organization. The HIBR was dissolved several years later. In my opinion, the HIBR made an enormous positive impact on the development of nutritional and orthomolecular medicine in the United States and Canada.

The major contribution made by the HIBR was to provide information, both to the public and professionals. For instance, in addition to our many publishing activities, between 1963 and 1973 we ran a series of weekend meetings in dozens of US cities. Often these were initiated by one of the many local chapters of the HIBR. We would run an ad in the local paper inviting doctors to participate. They were charged a small fee for attending. Two of our teaching orthomolecular practitioners would attend. I was often one of them, as was Dr. Allan Cott, and Dr. C.C. Pfeiffer. These two physicians would each give three lectures over Saturday and Sunday morning. These would cover the entire field of orthomolecular medicine: nutrition, diet, the various vitamins, and how these factors are combined in a comprehensive treatment program. These weekend sessions were very successful and sometimes attracted as many as 30 physicians; probably 40 such meetings were held altogether. Many of the attending physicians later became part of a core group of orthomolecular practitioners and some became leaders in the field. We also held public meetings in many states, sometimes attracting as many as 1,500 people. Our newsletter was circulated widely, and our last meeting in New York City was an overwhelming success, with over 400 attending. But we could not continue. Meanwhile, the HIBR's expenses continued to mount, but our membership stopped growing. Thankfully, the CSF, now the International Schizophrenia Foundation, has ably taken on the HIBR's former role.

I, as former president, wish to thank all former members of the HIBR board, which at one time included N. Cousins, Mrs. A. Spanel, Mrs. A. Lehman, Mrs. K. Fryer, H. Osmond, C.C. Pfeiffer, Ben Webster (former Chair of the board), Disque Dean, M. Williams, and A. Cott. We did our level best with what resources we could muster. I thank them all for the many contributions they made to the activity of the Huxley Institute of Biosocial Research.

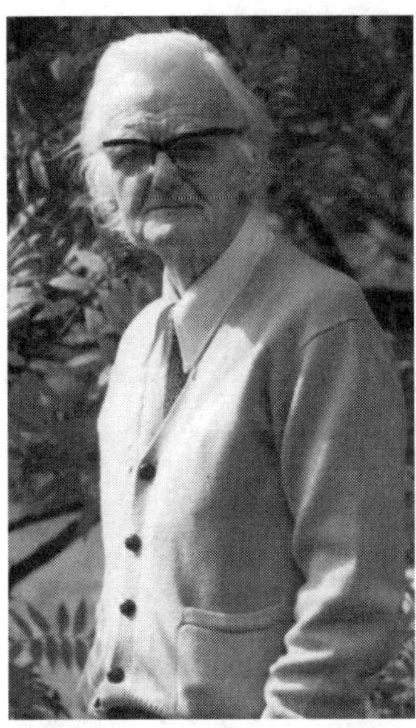

My friend and colleague
Dr. Humphry Osmond
(1917–2004) in the
mid-1990s.

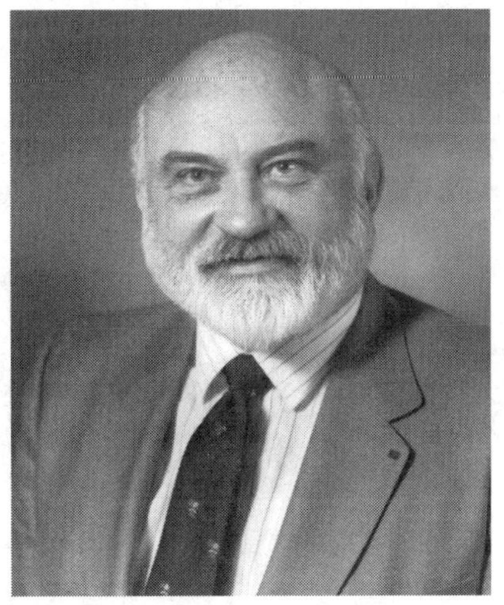

My friend and colleague for
many years, Dr. Hugh Desaix
Riordan (1932–2005).

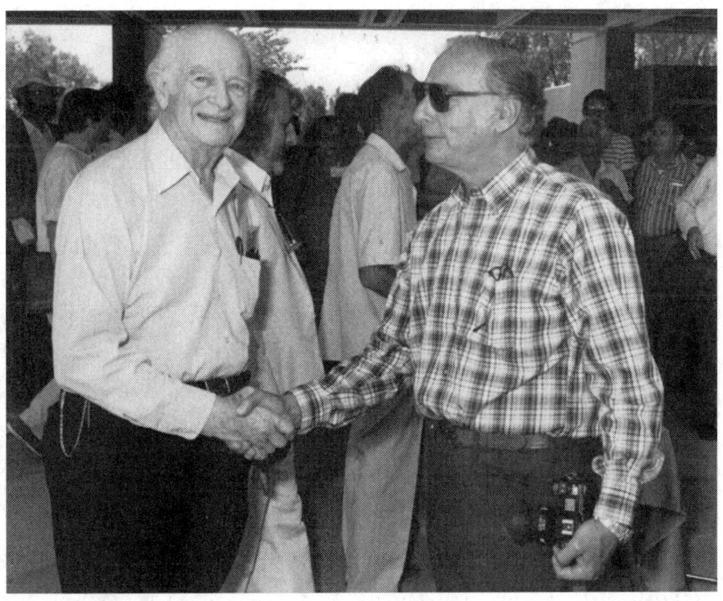

Linus Pauling is seen here in 1986 at the Beer Sheva
campus of Ben Gorion University of the Negev, in Israel,
on the occasion of the inauguration of the Hoffer-Vickar
Chair for Orthomolecular Psychiatry.

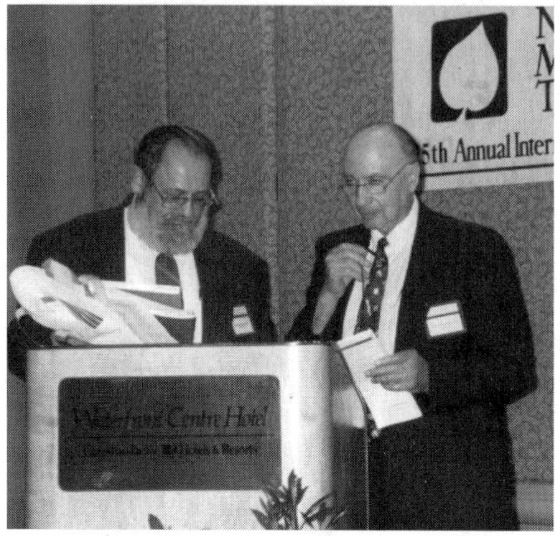

Here I am introducing Dr. Bernard Rimland, the autism researcher, in April 1996 when he was a speaker at our annual conference on nutritional medicine.

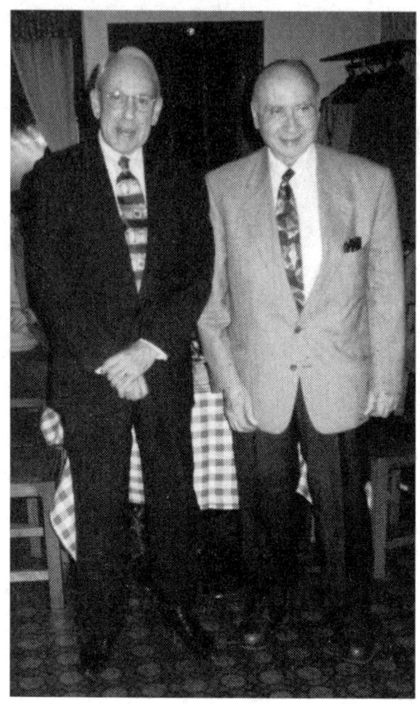

Standing by my side is Dr. William B. Parsons Jr., the author of the excellent book *Cholesterol Without Diet — the Niacin Solution* (1998). This picture was taken in November 1998.

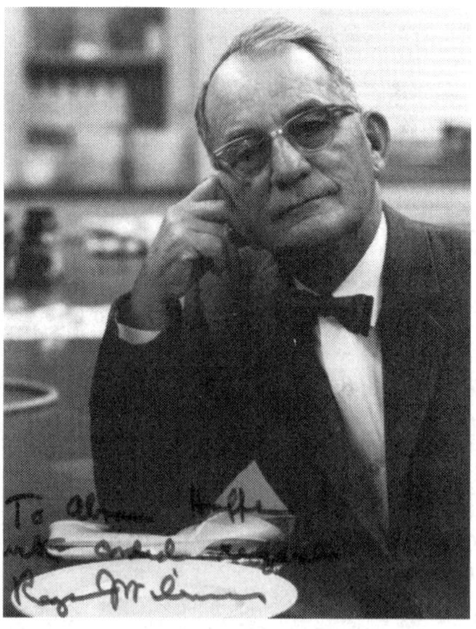

Dr. Roger Williams (1893–1988). Here the discoverer of the B vitamin Pantothenic acid and researcher into human biochemical individuality is shown in his 80s as professor emeritus of the University of Texas at Austin.

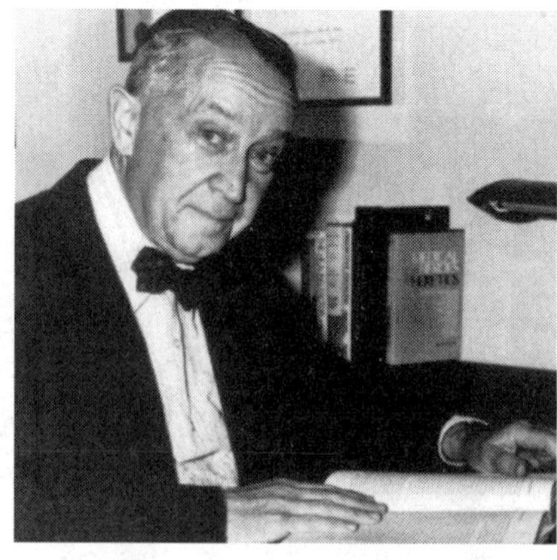

Irwin Stone (1907–1984), the researcher who introduced Linus Pauling to Vitamin C.

XIX

CANADIAN SCHIZOPHRENIA FOUNDATION

As the American Schizophrenic Association began to grow, I thought we should have an equivalent organization in Canada. After moving into private practice in 1967, I was free to help start such an organization. I and a lawyer friend applied for a Saskatchewan Charter and then for a loan from the Royal Bank of Canada for $1,500, which I countersigned. We appointed Mr. Irwin Kahan as our first executive director. He was free after having been fired from his job with the Canadian Mental Health Association, Saskatchewan Division, because the Government of Saskatchewan was annoyed with CMHA policy. The organization had remained critical of government policies with respect to the mentally ill. As I was chairman of their scientific planning division, and Irwin was my brother-in-law, they felt they could remove our influence from the CMHA, Saskatchewan Division, by buying the group off with the promise of a substantial annual grant of $50,000—the condition being that the organization must get rid of Irwin. This grant was ostensibly given to the CMHA to assist the group in operating their White Cross Center, a place where chronic patients could drop in. We looked upon the center as equivalent to a day care center for adults that relieve the load, at least during the day, on the nursing homes and other places that housed these patients, mostly chronic schizophrenics. The government's strategy was successful. After receiving the money and letting Irwin go, the CMHA, Saskatchewan Division, abruptly changed its policy and no longer attacked the government or criticized its lack of action in improving the conditions of patients. They still have not regained the stature they had early in their history when they were working on behalf of the patients and not at the behest of the governments of the day. These developments increased my desire to create an organization in Saskatchewan that would not yield supinely to outside pressure but would fight on behalf of schizophrenic patients.

I invited a small number of people interested in schizophrenia to join me on the board of the fledgling group, including George Morris, from Yorktown, Saskatchewan, a successful and inventive manufacturer of farm equipment. I decided to start our financial drive through an appeal to the doctors of Saskatchewan. In my capacity as president of the Saskatchewan Schizophrenia Foundation I drafted a letter and sent a copy to every doctor in the province. I did not anticipate any difficulty but soon found myself in hot water. A psychiatrist from Yorktown, Saskatchewan, who worked for the Government of Saskatchewan, complained to the College of Physicians and Surgeons that I was engaging in advertising. I was summoned to appear before the College. They did not tell me what the charges were. Fortunately one of the members of the College administration was a friend. Dr. Chris Kilduff was chairman of the Department of Anesthesia at City Hospital and administered anesthesia for my patients who were being treated in the nursing home at that time. After my meeting with the College, he told me privately that if that letter had been signed by I. Kahan and not myself there would have been no action. I met with the College on June 21, 1969, at 2:00 p.m. I had prepared a presentation and brought with me some of the books I had published. I thought they were concerned with my use of vitamins to treat schizophrenic patients. When I arrived, I found that my writing and speaking activities were to be scrutinized as possible examples of unethical advertising. I pointed out to my examiners that according to the College's own guidelines on unethical advertising, one must take into consideration the information which is given, the manner in which it is given, and the motive behind the dissemination of the information.

I discussed my motive and pointed out that as a research physician my motive must be to publish findings, because no research is completed until the results have been communicated to scientists and physicians at large. I said that my motives were not personal gain or an attempt to take advantage of the profession. I also explained that in fact what had happened to me was not financial gain but instead increased difficulty, especially in my relationships to my colleagues, who did not take kindly to the newer information I was disseminating. I then discussed the manner of presentation—which focused on scientific discoveries, not self-aggrandizement—and showed them the journal *Schizophrenia*, as well as the *International Journal of Neuropsychiatry*. I also showed the books I had written, discussed my participation in scientific meetings, and explained that on those rare occasions when I appeared in the news, I never built myself up as a physician more competent than any other but did discuss the treatments I used. Here I referred to the corroboration of our nicotinic acid work coming out of Dr. Lehmann's unit. (At that time the initial reports were supportive and Dr. Lehmann and Dr. T. Ban had not yet publicly divulged their remarkable opposition to the whole idea that vitamins might help schizophrenics.) I pointed out there had been no change in my financial income due to my activities and that 100 percent of my Saskatoon patients came to me by referral. I concluded that I was innocent of advertising.

Two of the members of the council examining me, from Regina, were extremely hostile and small-minded in their questioning and it was impossible to present any reasonable argument to them. They had come to the meeting with their minds already made up. The chairman was a bit better, but even he did not seem to understand the issues involved. At the end of my presentation it was quite obvious that I had not swayed my examiners but they were not prepared to take any action stronger than giving me a warning that if my activities continued along similar tracks, they might have to take action in the future.

A few days later I spoke to Dr. Kilduff who told me not to take the matter too seriously. The two Regina members were noted for their hostility, he said, and behaved that way no matter what was at issue. I said I had no plans to act in any way that would excite the College, but that I would not allow anyone to interfere with my right to publish papers or engage in private correspondence. He replied that the College had no intention of interfering in these matters.

Other than this bureaucratic interference, my letter gained much positive attention. The Saskatchewan Schizophrenia Foundation did receive substantial contributions from Saskatchewan doctors and we were soon able to pay off the bank loan. One of our major non-medical donors was Mr. Fred Mendel, Chairman of the Board and Owner of Intercontinental Packers, Saskatoon, Saskatchewan. His firm was the largest privately owned meat packing company in Canada. Fred and I were friends and I had taken advantage of his generosity to ask him for a contribution. As our coffers filled, we began to hold public meetings and to pursue the objectives of educating the public, especially the families of patients with schizo-phrenia, about the use of vitamins in treatment.

A year later we decided to go national and created the Canadian Schizophrenia Foundation (CSF). We folded the Saskatchewan Foundation into the CSF. We received our charter after an attempt by the Canadian Mental Health Association failed to block it. The CMHA was by that time controlled by Canada's top establishment psychiatrists, and it made representations to the Canadian government that it was already doing what we proposed to do. Of course the group ignored the major difference between their organization and ours, namely that we were advocating better treatment for schizophrenic patients through the use of an entirely new treatment while they were content to follow the official line put out by Canadian psychiatrists that tranquilizers were the only effective treatment. Their attempt to block our charter was defeated by Mr. D.C. (Ben) Webster, who knew the right people in Ottawa.

The Canadian Schizophrenia Foundation was formally established in April, 1969, with its head office in Regina, Saskatchewan.

The ASA had grown out of Humphry's discussions with Miriam Rothschild in England; she had recommended that we aim to eventually create an international association; in addition to spreading the work of the ASA in Canada, then, the CSF would establish a presence for our work in more than one country, as Ms. Rothschild had suggested. Miss Rothschild died recently. We were also lucky to have the CSF in place after the HIBR/ASA folded due to the hostility of the APA. The CSF took up the HIBR's role and as this chapter will recount, is today the International Schizophrenia Foundation.

Our major objective from the beginning, as with the ASA, was to provide accurate information about schizophrenia to patients, their families, and the community. We wanted to give the public accurate information about schizophrenia's causes, symptoms, and treatment, in such a way as to remove the fear of this disease and to provide hope that an effective treatment existed, if it was used promptly. We felt it critical to provide patients with names of physicians who were using the vitamin approach. Finally, we wanted to educate the Canadian medical profession about vitamin B-3 treatment—that it was available and easy to administer. There is nothing inherently difficult about providing orthomolecular psychiatric treatment, and at the time we started the CSF, many general practitioners were already doing so very effectively.

To meet our educational objectives, we have relied on both the written and the spoken word. As previously explained, in 1967 the American Schizophrenia Association began to publish the *Journal of Schizophrenia,* now called the *Journal of Orthomolecular Medicine* because our focus soon became much wider. The CSF took over the publication of this journal in 1969. Its readers are both laypeople and professionals and thankfully, over the years the proportion of professional readers has been growing steadily. We have also always published a newsletter, distributed to all members. This we saw— and still see—as a binding vehicle that maintains some unity and cohesiveness in the CSF membership.

The spoken word has been the communication vehicle at our annual meetings. The first was held in Saskatchewan in 1968 and we have not missed a meeting since. We used to meet in various cities across Canada but lately have been meeting in Vancouver in the West and Toronto or Ottawa in the East in alternate years. Only since 1999 have we seen an increasing number of physicians at these meetings. At the last two meetings, in fact, over 60 percent of the attendees were physicians. The main theme of our meetings has always been an exploration of the connection between clinical nutrition, ecological conditions and disease. We examined the schizophrenias first, but later it became apparent that orthomolecular therapy applied to all psychiatric disease. It was advantageous to start with schizophrenia since its clinical expression was so rich and varied. It was once said that if you knew the clinical manifestations of syphilis you understood all of medicine. In my opinion the same can be said about schizophrenia. Individual meeting themes have included crime, malnutrition and orthomolecular psychiatry; schizophrenia and the community; nutrition and behaviour; help for troubled children; treating and preventing health problems in contemporary society; and nutrition, the key to mental health. In 1990 we had one of the more successful meetings, when Dr. Linus Pauling drew over 1,500 people to his evening lecture. He was welcomed by the Government of British Columbia, the city of Vancouver, and the University of British Columbia. I have been chairman of every meeting and have spoken at most of them, highlighting the general theme of the meeting and talking about schizophrenia, its treatment and the problems associated with it.

Over the years, we have hosted numerous distinguished speakers.

Dr. Emmanuel Cheraskin, dean of the Dental College, Atlanta University of Georgia, had training in both medicine and dentistry and introduced us to the many decades of research he and his associates had carried out into the impact of nutrition on both disease and health.

Dr. Allan Cott (who died in 1992) was a frequent contributor who told us of his investigations into Russian fasting techniques for chronic schizophrenics, and the use of vitamin B-6 and dimethyl glycine for treating autism and other disturbances in children.

San Francisco-based Dr. Ben Feingold was one of the first allergists to publicize the fact that additives and chemically similar natural constituents of food cause hyperactivity and behavioral disorders in children. He presented his findings in 1979 to our meeting in Victoria, B.C. Before he presented these novel views he was a highly regarded clinical allergist in the United States; after, he became a pariah. But the mothers of the young patients who followed his dietary recommendations loved him because their children became well. He was a very passionate speaker. Once at a Toronto meeting he became so angry after listening to a scientist from the Hospital for Sick Children in Toronto who maintained that it was cruel to deprive children of their sweets, that he rushed to the microphone, grabbed it from the speaker, and lifted it as if to hit him. Sitting on that platform, I was amazed. His actions must have been effective, for several years later that scientist was endorsing his views. This incident proves that sometimes to get someone's attention you have to hit them first with a metaphorical two by four.

Dr. Glen Green, Dr. Max Vogel, Dr. Eric Paterson, Dr. Paul Cutler, and Dr. William D. Panton were the five most active ortho-molecular general practitioners in Canada and have all spoken at our meetings. Each of these doctors practised successfully for several decades and helped schizophrenic patients who were psychiatric treatment failures. All five conducted research which has been published in our journal. Dr. Cutler continues to make a major contribution in showing the importance of excess iron in the body as a factor in coronary disease and diabetes mellitus.

Ross Hume Hall, a professor of biochemistry at McMaster University in Hamilton, Ontario, provided very popular and stimulating lectures on the ways in which modern food technology has converted nutritious food into junk to a major degree. In my experience, I count him as unusual among biochemists because he understood clinical nutrition, that is, the effects of giving nutrients to real patients.

Dr. David Hawkins was an early member of the Committee on Therapy of the American Schizophrenia Association. He was the among the first psychiatrists to show that patients with both schizophrenia and alcoholism could be treated successfully with vitamin B-3.

As previously explained, he was co-editor with Dr. Linus Pauling of the enormously important book, *Orthomolecular Psychiatry*.

Dr. Michael Lesser was one of the early orthomolecular practitioners, a contributor to the journal, and a speaker at our meetings. He published several books describing his treatment protocols and he initiated a congressional hearing held many years ago into orthomolecular treatment.

Dr. Richard Kunin has been a major contributor to our meetings. He was the first to demonstrate that tardive dyskinesia is due to a deficiency of manganese, induced by tranquilizers and anti-psychotics. These drugs chelate with manganese and remove it from the body as they are excreted. The manganese deficiency, in turn, causes involuntary muscle movements, which may range from mild to grotesque. The addition of manganese to the therapeutic regimen, he found, prevents this side effect. He also showed that aspirin can moderate or prevent the niacin flush. The latter finding has been made again by more recent observers who seem unaware of or refuse to recognize his prior discovery.

Dr. Humphry Osmond was, of course, a frequent speaker during the first fifteen years of the CSF's existence.

Dr. Carl C. Pfeiffer was another major and frequent contributor to orthomolecular knowledge and to our meetings, as well as the writer of many fine articles in our journal. It is impossible to summarize quickly his many contributions, which range from the discovery that kryptopyrrole binds both vitamin B-6 and zinc and causes a multiple deficiency, to his studies of the schizophrenias, to his basic work with mineral and amino acid metabolism. He founded the Brain Bio Center, renamed the Princeton Bio Center. It was one of the foremost orthomolecular research and treatment centers in the world. Dr. Pfeiffer died in 1988. His work has been continued in London, England by Patrick Holford, BSc at the Institute for Optimum Nutrition, and in the US by Dr. William Walsh of the Carl Pfeiffer Treatment Center in Naperville, Illinois, and by Dr. Hugh Riordon at The Center For The Improvement of Human Functioning International, in Wichita, Kansas.

Dr. Hugh D. Riordan died January 7, 2005. We worked together editing the *Journal of Orthomolecular Medicine* (JOM), and on the board of the Canadian Schizophrenia Foundation, now the International Schizophrenia Foundation. Hugh joined the editorial board of the JOM in 1991, soon after publishing a book, *Medical Mavericks II*, then became Associate Editor in 2000. He began serving on the board of directors for the International Schizophrenia Foundation in 2003. In 2002, Hugh was honoured by the International Society of Orthomolecular Medicine with the "Orthomolecular Physician of the Year" award. He attended all our meetings and made major presentations which I always found enormously interesting and valuable. His productivity did not go down with age as it does for so many scientists and he contributed his column regularly to our journal, each time presenting very interesting cases. These anecdotes are very useful in teaching doctors how to apply orthomolecular ideas. He did significant research on histamine metabolism. This arose out of his interest in work developed by Dr. Pfeiffer, who classified some patients as having either too much or too little blood histamine. He also did studies on chelation therapy showing that it was a valuable procedure for many patients. His laboratory investigated food allergies and used a cytotoxic test for determining what foods disturbed particular individuals. But his main work had to do with the schizophrenic syndrome and with the treatment of cancer using non-toxic vitamin C chemotherapy.

Dr. William H. Philpott introduced orthomolecular psychiatrists to clinical ecology by demonstrating how allergen elimination diets could cure patients even of schizophrenia, and how re-introducing the foods to which they were allergic brought back their symptoms. Accordingly, consideration of the role played by specific foods and other allergens has become an increasingly important component of orthomolecular practice.

Dr. Bernard Rimland founded the Institute for Child Behavior Research, now the Autism Research Institute, in San Diego, California. He has been a stout defender of the view that infantile autism is a biological disease and is not caused by bad mothering, an idea which had become very powerful in North America. His massive investigative work has confirmed that vitamins are the most important component of treatment. In at least 17 controlled trials, vitamin B-6 has been found to be very effective in the treatment of autism, but must be supported by magnesium. He has spoken at many of our meetings and frequently published papers in our journal and others.

Dr. Harvey Ross was medical director at Gracie Square Hospital in New York, a private hospital in which Dr. Allan Cott treated psychiatric patients. Beginning in the early 1960s, Dr. Cott asked Dr. Ross to cover his patients when he was away. Dr. Ross was so impressed with the results he saw due to Dr. Cott's treatments that he joined his colleague as an associate. He went on to write several books on the orthomolecular treatment of depression.

One of our recent major contributors is Professor Harold Foster, University of Victoria. Professor Foster is a geographer who has examined worldwide the connection between the incidence of disease and soil composition and other environmental factors.

Of course, these speakers were able to educate professionals and public alike thanks to the diligent efforts of several people who worked behind the scenes.

Fannie Kahan, my youngest sister, and Irwin Kahan, her husband, worked as a team to run the CSF. Fannie had a degree in journalism and became the first editor of the CSF newsletter and later, managing editor of the JOM. She wrote many of our pamphlets, and published three major articles in our journal dealing with the criminally insane. She did a superb job acting as reporter, writer, and editor. Irwin was a social worker with the Saskatchewan Department of Public Health, Psychiatric Services Branch. In 1953, he became a member of our research team, heading up the follow-up unit. It was his job to stay in contact with schizophrenic patients who had been treated as part of our research, and help us to monitor their state of health through regularly interviewing them and filling in a questionnaire we had designed as part of that process. Later he became executive director of the CMHA, Saskatchewan Division, until 1967 when he was fired as a result of government of Saskatchewan machinations—the policy makers did not appreciate his pressure on them to improve the results of treatment for their patients. I believe that Fannie's writing was one of the other factors which so annoyed the Government of Saskatchewan. The CSF always felt free to call a spade a spade and made no attempt to spare the feelings of the government or its civil servants, the psychiatrists who were running its mental health services. The Canadian Schizophrenia Foundation depended on Fannie and Irwin for many years. Both received minimum pay because the foundation was always so close to being broke. Each year, we considered it a major triumph to have met our payroll.

Fannie died on December 21, 1978. Several years earlier, she had developed cancer of the breast. She was treated vigorously, and took large amounts of vitamin C and other vitamins. I was then not especially interested in cancer and did not advise her to follow the program I have developed since then. She responded to all the treatment she was given and at her last examination, by a medical friend of mine, was told she was free of cancer. However, a few months later we were horrified when a metastatic tumour was discovered in her spinal cord, one of the most vulnerable parts of the body. She died several months later.

Irwin carried on as General Director of the CSF at our head office in Regina. Our financial situation gradually got worse. At the time, the CSF was getting $25,000 annually from a Webster family foundation. But this was not enough to allow us to keep up with our expenses. In 1984, at a meeting of the board in Toronto, I finally reported that I saw no possibility of continuing our operation and recommended that we initiate steps to close down. After some discussion, Mr. George Morris quietly asked how much we needed. I replied that we needed an endowment of at least $500,000 so that we would have a stable financial base. He then asked us not to dissolve the CSF but to give him some time and he would see how he could help. A few days later he told me that he would give us $25,000 each year for five years, which would effectively double our financial base. He died before the five years were over, but arranged that his promise be kept. His generosity allowed us to survive and gave us time to make new plans for continuing our operation.

Two years after Fannie died, Irwin told me that he was going to retire and we would have to find a new director. I asked him if he would stay on until we found a replacement. He said that he would. I immediately began the search. I contacted a young woman who had arranged a large meeting in Vancouver which I had addressed. She had done a very competent job and I thought she might make a fine director. She was not interested, but told me about Steven Carter. Carter was then editor of the holistic health publication, *Alive Magazine*. He had his MA, had worked as a university lecturer, was a skillful editor, and knew the printing and publishing trade. He was not happy at *Alive*. We offered him the job. He accepted, on condition that we move our headquarters from Regina to Vancouver. He was gambling that we would survive, but needed to minimize his personal gamble by remaining in Vancouver. Our decision proved a wise one and Steven, who joined us in July, 1987 saved the CSF. He has proven an ideal director. He eventually advised us that it would be best for the CSF if we moved our headquarters to Toronto. The board agreed. The CSF opened a branch office in Toronto in 1990, then brought its headquarters to the city in 1992. After the move, the CSF became much more successful. Attendance at the annual meetings swelled, its literature list flourished, and the organization won international recognition and prestige. Essentially, after the move, the CSF has taken over for North America the function that was once served by the Huxley Institute, which collapsed in 1992. In 2003, we changed the name of the CSF to the International Schizophrenia Foundation, because our activities have become international in scope. The ISF is alive and well and ever more active in promoting better treatment for the mentally ill.

Among our most important contributions has been helping bring schizophrenia into public view. In 1960 it was considered unethical to discuss the disease with patients. Their families might be told, the patient, never. Dr. Karl Menninger, with whom I was very friendly and who himself began to take vitamins after he retired had written a paper condemning any psychiatrist who told his patients. It was his view that the news would be so devastating to the patient it would set him or her back. Today the majority of psychiatrists will discuss the diagnosis of schizophrenia—but many remain very reluctant to make it. I have noted a disturbing trend to label many patients as manic depressive or bipolar because this appears to be a more optimistic diagnosis and also permits the psychiatrist to try lithium in the hope it will work. Even more disturbing is a recent tendency to diagnose schizophrenic patients as having personality disorders and therefore not suitable candidates for any treatment.

Nonetheless, the profession has been forced to change. There is little doubt that the Huxley Institute and the CSF have been the main factors in forcing this change, since these were the first organizations to initiate a public discussion of schizophrenia and to provide informational literature to patients, families, and communities. No other North American mental health organizations active in the past 50 years, have provided any optimistic material, as these organizations have all focused on support of conventional treatment, using drugs only, and with this treatment it is not possible to be optimistic. Thanks to us, families and patients were no longer forced to turn to out-of-date psychiatric texts with their distressing pictures of demented patients for information. The HIBR and CSF also encouraged recovered patients to record and publish their personal stories. The best way for family members, doctors, and policy makers to learn what it is like to have schizophrenia is to read these accounts by patients who have recovered. I believe the CSF and HIBR have also contributed to the development of patient activism. Patients have become less acquiescent than when I started as a psychiatrist, and are demanding they be given the information to which they are entitled. Now, in most jurisdictions, they can even demand, and by law are entitled to see, the information in their medical or hospital files.

The British Columbia Ministry of Health, Mental Health Services Division, published a report, "Families Sharing The Caring" in 1993. It summarized the findings of the Task Force of Families of People with Mental Illness. Here are a few quotations from this report: "Relationships with professionals are a major source of anger." "Families want to be consulted and included in treatment." "Discharge is often premature, occurring before medication is stabilized and they would like to see discharge planning and a communication system that included family members." "Caregivers in many instances are being trained that schizophrenia is not a medical problem but the fault of the family. This education is outdated and outmoded. This must be changed." The educational process that HIBR and CSF started so many years ago is beginning to bear fruit.

We have not persuaded many doctors to become orthomolecular physicians, but there is a trend in this direction. The rapid increase since 1999 in the proportion of physicians who attend the CSF annual meetings indicates this trend is becoming stronger. Doctors have been fearful of coming to meetings or of giving vitamins lest they earn the censure of their colleagues and especially of the colleges of physicians and surgeons. I personally know several doctors who turned to orthomolecular practice who were then forced to give up their licenses. Some have become naturopaths, a field in which it is easier to innovate. I am convinced that when the colleges finally release their narrow definitions of "standards of practice," there will be a major rush by physicians to using vitamins as therapy. Doctors will be liberated when licensing boards return to upholding their original mandate, that is to ensure that their members are properly qualified. It is not their function to tell doctors how to practice—this is the function of the medical colleges. Once a physician has received a medical degree, he or she must be allowed to use their judgment as to how to treat patients.

The liberation process will need political help. In recent years, some progress has been made. In Alaska it has been illegal since 1990 for a licensing body to punish a doctor for using alternate medical procedures unless that body proves that what the doctor did was harmful to the patient. So far, one Canadian college has been deprived of its power to harass its more innovative members. In 1996 the Government of Alberta passed Bill 209, which ordered: "A registered practitioner shall not be found guilty of unbecoming conduct or be found to be incapable or unfit to practise medicine or osteopathy solely on the basis that the registered practitioner employs a therapy that is non-traditional or departs from the prevailing medical practices unless it can be demonstrated that the therapy has a safety risk for the patient unreasonably greater than the prevailing treatment."

In the United States of America, twelve states (Alaska, Colorado, Georgia, Indiana, Massachusetts, New York, North Carolina, Ohio, Oklahoma, Oregon, Texas, Washington) have passed legislation similar to Bill 209. The governments undertaking these changes have aroused the anger of their state licensing boards. But the blind resistance to innovation these boards hold is one of the main reasons for the high cost of modern health care. There is nothing cheaper than getting patients well. I know personally of 17 and men who became schizophrenic in their teens, were treated properly with orthomolecular therapies, recovered, and went on to become physicians and psychiatrists. All are practising successfully. One became the chairman of the department of psychiatry of a medical school in the United States, another became president of a psychiatric association. But each patient treated only with tranquilizers will, over their lifetime, cost the Canadian publicly funded provincial health insurance and other social service plans around $2,000,000. These 18 men saved their communities $36,000,000 over 40 years or $900,000 each year. They also pay taxes and, by helping others get well, further improve the physical and economic health of their communities.

X X

A MOVE TO VICTORIA

In 1972 Rose and I began to think about a move from Saskatoon. I was 55 years old, and felt it was time to plan my retirement. Rose did not like Saskatoon and I did not like the idea that I would have to fight the weather six months out of each year forever. Saskatoon winters are singularly unattractive and difficult unless one is a complete winter outdoors type. I thought that it would be too difficult to retire first and then make a move, because by then I would be older, less capable of enduring the stress of the move, but most important of all, would not have time to establish roots in the new place. I had heard of too many people who retired, moved, and were very dissatisfied with their new life in a strange environment. I also hoped that once I moved I would have enough time to establish myself in the medical community and that this would enhance the move toward orthomolecular medicine. Family ties did not hold us in Saskatoon, as our children were already scattered.

British Columbia was very attractive. Vancouver was too large and busy and I did not relish the idea of spending many hours each day driving to and from my office. Victoria was somewhat larger than Saskatoon but its small city appearance made it much more interesting. I had addressed a very large group there several years earlier, at a meeting arranged by the members of the local Canadian Schizophrenia Foundation. Another good reason for selecting Victoria, in my view, was that it did not have a medical school. I was by now all too familiar with the town and gown antagonisms in cities inhabited by professors from the medical schools and I wanted to avoid them. ("Town and gown" is a common university term that refers to the hostilities common between medical school professors and non-academically affiliated practitioners in the school's home city.) I knew that professors of psychiatry are very certain of their views, no matter how wrong they are, and that it would be more difficult for me to practise with nutrition and vitamins in a city they frequented. It is bad enough to be controlled by a College of Physicians and Surgeons which considers unethical any innovation in medicine unless it has first been vetted by the establishment, i.e., the professors, even if the newer treatments are safer and more effective. And professors are least likely to be interested in innovation because they seldom see patients except through the eyes of their residents. They are not driven to try harder by the failures of their most highly recommended treatments because they are not in personal contact with the individuals experiencing those failures.

In 1975 we decided we would move the following year. I wrote to the Registrar, College of Physicians and Surgeons, British Columbia to advise them I was moving and to get their application forms. I did not expect any difficulty in obtaining a license to practice in the province since I was a Fellow of the Royal College of Physicians and Surgeons, and my qualifications were impeccable. Later I went to Vancouver and met with the Registrar of the College. Toward the end of the conversation I asked him if he had any advice for me. He replied that he had—I should not seek out public attention by giving press conferences and so on. I was completely surprised by this statement and replied that in fact I had not ever given press conferences, that if my work appeared in the press it was most often due to presentations at scientific and medical meetings. I said that after I spoke on a topic, I was not responsible for what the press did with it. I finally added that I had published many articles and some books and that I would continue to do so. Before I left, I invited him to come to my office in Victoria after I had established my practice and observe what I did. He said that he would. Late in 1976 when my office was busy and everything was working well, I called him and reminded him of his promise. He spent an hour with me, seeing my treatment of one or two of my patients. Later he told me he had seen nothing at all wrong with the way I was working my practice. He complained about several other doctors whom he did not name who were using vitamins and engaging in activities the College did not approve of, such as giving public speeches. I also applied for and received staff privileges at the Royal Jubilee Hospital and the Eric Martin Institute, now called Eric Martin Pavilion and the psychiatric ward of the Jubilee Hospital.

We planned to move in August of 1976. A few months before, the British Columbia legislature had honoured Dr. Linus Pauling. When I saw that news item, I wrote to Premier David Barrett to congratulate him and his government. Later, when I knew when I would be in Victoria, I wrote him again and asked if we could meet. We eventually did, in the provincial legislature's restaurant. He was very interested in orthomolecular medicine, but said he could do nothing about the medical profession's refusal to look seriously at the work. He said the government was having enough problems already with the profession over the financial relationship. (Publicly funded health insurance means that the government provides doctors with their pay according to guidelines negotiated by the two sides.)

Margaret Callbeck was also looking to retire in a warmer and more gentle place, and she decided to move to the Victoria area as well, so she could remain as my office nurse until her retirement.

Moving presented us with major problems. We had accumulated so much material. When I left my jobs with the Saskatchewan government, I had taken with me the clinical research records which had accumulated over the years. I had not believed that they would be preserved if I left them at the University Hospital. The records covered the original work with the hallucinogens, the early double-blind controlled experiments, the early work dealing with the discovery that niacin lowers cholesterol levels in the blood, and a large volume of correspondence with many people all around the world. I had over 30 boxes of material stored in my basement. I approached the Saskatchewan Archives Board and they proved to be interested in obtaining this material. I donated the records and data to the archives. In return I received a tax letter for all the material I had accumulated between 1967 and 1976. The Hoffer Archives are now available for inspection by *bona fide* research scientists, who need permission from me to see these papers. I shipped another 60 or so boxes of material to the Archives in 1989, when we moved into a smaller residence in Victoria. They will also obtain the last of my records one day.

Before leaving Saskatoon, I inserted a simple notice in the *Star Phoenix* to announce my departure. I also arranged to leave a large number of clinical records with Dr. B. O'Regan until they had been stored the requisite ten years, after which he was to destroy them. In Victoria I had purchased a condominium for my office. I did not want to be at the mercy of any landlord with respect to rents and so on. I planned to start seeing patients in mid-October. Marg supervised the office move. I inserted the usual notice in the local paper, and sent a notice to all physicians in Victoria. The *Times Colonist* daily newspaper also ran a small item about my imminent arrival. I assume that some of the Victoria members of the CSF gave them the information. By the time I opened my practice, I was already booked two weeks in advance.

In 1989 the pressure of various circumstances brought us to move into a new townhouse in Victoria; this move proved to be an excellent decision. However, I forgot to take with me a heavy piece of stone art which had been given me as a gift by a Mexican artist. Three years later I suddenly remembered I had left this piece of sculpture behind. Its history was dramatic. Early in 1960 I had received a letter from a businessman who lived in Mexico City. He described his son's schizophrenia and asked for treatment advice. A year later or so I went to a meeting in Mexico arranged by the Institute of Neurology. I was invited to present a summary of my work. I then arranged to visit this man and his family, and I examined the son. A few years later, the young man came to Saskatoon and I saw him in the University Hospital to monitor his treatment. Then he went to Japan where he studied the art of sculpting raw rock under the tutelage of a master sculptor. He had completed this piece in Mexico, then personally taken the long trip to Saskatoon via Vancouver by train to deliver it. In Victoria, I placed it in our backyard, in a spot where we could see it from the house. Later I planted St. Johns Wort which filled in the area around it. When I finally remembered having left this gift behind, I called the man who had purchased our house, drove there and found the rock still where I had placed it. With great relief I took it home and placed it in our patio, off the kitchen.

My Practice

As mentioned earlier, by the day I saw my first Victoria patient I was already booked up for two weeks. Gradually the number of referrals has increased and at the time of this writing, 2005, it takes anywhere from one to three months before I am able to see new patients. I make an exception for emergencies, as defined by the referring physicians. I usually see patients experiencing a crisis within three days.

I accept only patients who have been referred by another physician. This relieves the psychiatrist of the need to do a physical workup and it screens out patients whose basic issue is a physical problem that really does not need to be treated by a psychiatrist. The referring doctor remains the primary physician. In British Columbia, the patient needs another referral to see me if they do not come to my office for six months or more. In Saskatchewan only one referral was ever needed. There are advantages and disadvantages to both systems. In Saskatchewan the referring physicians could lose control of the patient, who might remain under psychiatric care forever without being seen again by the referring physician. But the system made things easier for the patient and decreased costs to the province's health insurance plan. The British Columbia system provides for continuity of care by the referring physician, but increases the need for patients to request a referral after six months and increases costs to the plan. After the patient is seen, the specialist must provide the referring doctor with a consultation report.

Patient Interviews

I follow standard interview technique with my patients. The interview consists of three main phases. In the first phase the person who knows most about the problem, the patient, does most of the talking. He or she is guided and directed by the doctor by the judicious use of questions. During the second phase the doctor knows the most, about the diagnosis and treatment. During the third phase, both parties discuss what the diagnosis means and how the illness is best treated. A good interview provides enough information to allow me to establish a provisional diagnosis and to determine whether any laboratory testing or further interviews are needed to establish the diagnosis. If relatives accompany patients, they may be present at the interview if this is what the patient wants. It is valuable to have relatives present if patients are young or very disturbed. Patients are often stressed by an interview with a stranger and will forget much of what went on during the discussion. Relatives can be helpful in this regard too, by reminding the patient of important information in the days following the interview. After I have established a firm diagnosis and answered all of a patient's questions, I write on a prescription paper what I have suggested they do. I list medications and nutrients, and describe why I am recommending each one. I usually give patients a prognosis as well. I predict about how long it will take to get well, or to be much better. If they have cancer I discuss with them quality and duration of life issues. I never guarantee success and always point out that most of the work of recovery will have to be done by the patient. Nor do I guarantee failure. A woman with metastasized cancer came to see me three months after she had been diagnosed. She had been told she could not be treated successfully by conventional means and that she only had a few months left. She had always wanted to take a cruise but had also been told this would be impossible. After I interviewed her and placed her on a vitamin regimen I advised her to plan for the cruise. She came back to see me three weeks after returning from that vacation. It had not been the greatest of successes because she had been too weak to take some of the shore trips. But she had already won the odds against the advice given her. As she was getting ready to leave she stopped and said that she wanted to tell me something. She explained that she always wanted direct answers to her questions. At the end of her last visit to her oncologist, as she was leaving, he had volunteered, "Mrs. … I want you to know that you will never get any better." But she had not asked him whether she would or not. Apparently he believed that it was his job to be brutally frank and to remove any hope she might still have. I believe that no patient should leave the doctor's office feeling worse than they did on entering the office. There is always hope, if not for recovery, at least for relief from symptoms. Patients want and need that kind of support, especially when they are dying. I was appalled when she told me of this incident. She was justifiably angry about the oncologist's words and decided she would never see him again.

Enough time must be taken in the interview to obtain all the information needed and to outline the treatment. This can vary from several hours to a fraction of an hour. An efficient physician can obtain the information in a much shorter period of time, while a dithering, unsure one might need many hours. I think that the provincial insurance plans, which pay for service based on amount of time spent, penalize the efficient and reward the inefficient. I have seen patients who had already consulted twelve different doctors over several years without getting the correct diagnosis or treatment. In one case I made the diagnosis while the patient was walking into my office. She had pellagra—all the typical symptoms were present. None of the other physicians, including three professors of dermatology, had even considered this as a possibility. Thousands of dollars and much time had been wasted. I needed to see her for only a fraction of an hour and she went on to recover with the help of vitamin B-3 and other vitamins. In my opinion, there would ideally be a standard fee for initially seeing and advising the patient and after that a fee scale dependent upon the time needed for that patient to recover. The faster the patient recovers, the greater the fee. With each visit the fee should be lowered until after a certain time perhaps there should be a very low fee, not based on time, for patients like chronic schizophrenics who have an inherently low recovery rate, or for providing support for patients with cancer who are terminal. Such a fee schedule would adequately reward the physician for seeing patients and provide a bonus for doctors who catalyze a better recovery rate. A doctor who cures a patient after one visit and charges $10,000 is doing a better job than another doctor who treats that same patient five days per week for the next ten years and only charges $50 per visit.

I see patients Monday to Thursday only. I generally see five patients in the morning, between 9:00 and 12:00. One is a new patient. I see between four and five in the afternoon, between 1:30 and 4:30. One of them is new. However it is often necessary to see more patients than that when an emergency case is referred to me. If a cancer patient is referred I see them within a few days rather than have them wait several months. The provincial medical insurance plan sends me my profile yearly so I can compare my practice against that of the province's other psychiatrists. I see many more patients than does the average psychiatrist in British Columbia but not as many as are seen by general practitioners. The same was true in Saskatchewan. I earn somewhat more than the average psychiatrist but on a per-patient-seen basis I cost the provincial public insurance plan a lot less.

Diagnosis

I can use the American Psychiatric Association Diagnostic and Statistical Manual (DSM) now in its fourth edition, but will not unless I am forced to. It provides an awkward scheme which makes diagnosis altogether too complicated. And since using this manual does not lead to specific treatment recommendations, I see no point going through the process of diagnosis according to its guidelines. In this manual, no matter the name each one is given, all the schizophrenias are treated with a combination of drugs, based upon trial and error. All mood disorders are treated with different drugs again, based upon what works, i.e. trial and error. For practical purposes the main diagnostic categories I use are (1) the schizophrenias; (2) the mood disorders; (3) the addictions—drugs, alcohol; (4) children with learning and/or behavioural disorders; (5) adult personality and behavioural disorders; (6) organic disorders—Alzheimer's, strokes. Since opening my practice in Victoria, I have had an increasing number of patients referred to me who are suffering from different physical diseases. Since 1978, I have seen about 1,350 patients with cancer. But these patients always also suffer from a mood disorder, such as anxiety and/or depression, often as a result of having to come to terms with their illness.

Follow Up

I see patients every month, sometimes every two weeks, until I think they can continue to carry on the prescribed treatment with little supervision. Schizophrenics require the longest follow up, since recovery may be very slow. At the time of writing, I have about 500 chronic schizophrenics in my practice, who are seen at intervals ranging from every month to every two or three years. Usually I will see patients who have reached stabilization every two or three years if they are still on medication or if they are taking anything I have recommended that requires a prescription. Thanks to the safety of orthomolecular protocols, that is frequently enough to allow me to adequately monitor the effects of any prescription medications included in the total treatment. Patients also know they are free to call me if they have any concerns about possible side effects. In most other cases the patients decide when they should come back. In 1994 I published a ten-year follow-up in the *Journal of Orthomolecular Medicine* on 27 chronic schizophrenic patients, "Chronic schizo-phrenic patients treated ten years or more." Seventeen were well.

The Psychiatric Hospital

I have been associated with hospitals from the beginning of my psychiatric career in 1950 until I refused to renew my application for staff privileges at the Eric Martin Pavilion in 1993. From 1950 to 1954 I was at the Munroe Wing, General Hospital, Regina,

Saskatchewan. Until 1967 I worked at the University Hospital, now Royal University Hospital, in Saskatoon. Then I joined the staff at City Hospital with additional privileges at St. Paul's Hospital. I was at the Eric Martin Pavilion from 1976 until 1993. The general nature of the care offered at these institutions did not vary much. I am convinced that quality of care is determined by the doctors. If the doctor provides high quality care, so will the nursing staff. If the doctor is indifferent and does not care, so will the nursing staff. I have always had good relationships with nursing staff. I have seldom referred my patients for psychological consultations, considering these a waste of time and money in most cases. I do not need a psychologist to tell me when patients are sick or are not intelligent. Social workers are very helpful. Hospital dietitians were seldom helpful and in many cases tried to interfere with my use of nutrients for my patients, probably because they did not understand the reasons for my orders.

On average, my patients probably stayed in hospital for the same length of time as those under the care of other doctors. However, once their treatments were fully developed, my patients had many fewer readmissions. I have reported this fact in many of my clinical reports to the medical press. My relationships with other physicians and staff have generally been cordial, not close. Others have tolerated my use of nutrients, considering it idiosyncratic, but have made no attempt to discover why I was giving patients high doses of ascorbic acid or the B vitamins. I think I have been tolerated because many staff members had peculiar interests of their own. One prominent member of staff at one of the hospitals where I worked was an aggressive anti-abortionist. He frequently wrote letters to the local press on this topic. Another believed in the presence of satanic sects in the city. Another espoused the efficacy of pounding on pillows to relieve aggression. Several would never use ECT on principle. Many hospital staff members, I'm sure, considered me just as bizarre as I thought these individuals to be. Of the middle-of-the-road eclectic psychiatrists I worked alongside, several asked me about niacin for their own use after their GP recommended it to them. A few asked me to give a patient a consultation from time to time, usually because the family or the patient had demanded this. They would then continue giving that person vitamins, but they never started any other patients on them of their own accord.

I liked working at the Eric Martin Pavilion because having staff privileges there allowed me to provide continuity of care to my patients. The hospital's medical library was in the same building as the Pavilion and this too was useful to me. But eventually I relinquished the association because the amount of work, including night calls, had increased and because the hospital's administration and organization seemed to be constantly changing due to pressure from the government to reduce beds and costs. The last year I was there, over half the psychiatric staff quit for similar reasons. After I left, my work load decreased and night calls, most of which had come from the nurses on the wards, vanished. I also had continued to take my rotation on the emergency service. Staff members had the option of not doing emergency rotations after age 65. I continued to carry my load until I was 75.

Practising without hospital privileges has been simpler but does sometimes slow the progress of treatment. My patients rarely require hospitalization, but if they do, they go to the emergency room of the Jubilee Hospital, admitted, and then treated by the psychiatrist on duty at Eric Martin Pavilion, usually in the same old style, using tranquilizers. These doctors also generally stop my patients' entire vitamin programs. As soon as my patients are discharged, they come back to me and start back on the vitamin regimen; given a choice, patients prefer to follow my treatment program. But they are often worse after a hospital stay, and we have to start all over again on moving toward recovery. Usually when they return to my office, they are also full of stories of how badly they were treated in the hospital or by the psychiatrist.

Victoria Physicians

A few physicians began to refer patients to me before I arrived in Victoria and by the time I first appeared I was already booked up. These physicians were simply being friendly with their patients, because it was almost always their patients who initiated the referral process. But after having seen the results of my treatment, a few of those physicians are still referring to me. Still, I would guess that over 90 percent of the referrals made to me are patient-generated. Many have had great difficulty persuading their doctors to let them see me and sometimes have had to apply a lot of pressure to achieve success. Often after the referral was finally made, the patient would no longer go back to that doctor, but seek out another one. I remember vividly one woman with a large ulcerated cancer of her breast who refused to accept orthodox treatment. One day, after she had seen her doctor, she asked him when she should come back. He rudely replied there was no point in answering this question, since she would be dead in one week. She and her husband, a ship's captain, promptly demanded that he refer her to me, which he was forced to do. She lived another two and a half years. Another woman had been ill for many years, was very grateful for the help her general practitioner was giving her, even though she did not recover. She read about the use of a particular fast that would help her determine what she might be allergic to. Without consulting her doctor, she did the fast, discovered what the problem food was, eliminated it from her diet, and became well. On her next visit, she enthusiastically told her doctor of her recovery. She expected that he would be equally enthusiastic, but to her surprise he responded coldly and began to argue with her. They got into a fight. She then asked him to refer her to me. He refused to do so. She then told him, "I will sit in your office until you make that call." These, of course, are extreme cases. Still, I have noted with some amusement the many strategies doctors have used to cool their patients' desires to see me. To try and avoid making the referral they have told them the following tales: (1) That I am dead. (The patient decided to phone me anyway and was astonished to find I was still alive.); (2) That I had retired; (3) That I would force them to go off medication and take only vitamins; (4) That I would charge a great deal as my services were not covered by the provincial health insurance plan. Thankfully, over the years it has become easier for patients to be referred and since 1995 more referrals have been doctor-generated.

I am also happy to say that I have seen a major shift in the medical profession's attitude toward my practice. In the 1980's, I tried to organize a nutritional section of the British Columbia Medical Association (BCMA). We needed twenty-five members before we could petition for official recognition of such a group from the organization. A group of interested doctors met once in Vancouver, but our momentum soon petered out. Several years later, another medical group was organized in Victoria, the World Health Research. I asked Linus Pauling to come for our first meeting and to my surprise he agreed. Pauling spoke at the University of Victoria to over 1,200 people. Not all who wanted to attend could get in. During the medical meeting, Bryan Pound, Chairman, gave me a lot of credit for the change in opinion that was occurring. I was involved with this group for three years, but then the meetings because less interesting to me as the membership's focus shifted from the nutritional approach toward stress management, relaxation etc. In 1994, I joined another group of physicians interested in nutrition and in 1995 I went to the first meeting at Dr. S. Malthouse's home. Since then this has become an active group.

Research in Private Practice

I started my research career in 1940 when I went to the University of Minnesota for my PhD. I continued to pursue research, but to a much lesser degree, during my medical studies between 1945 and 1951, until I completed my internship at City Hospital, Saskatoon. From 1952 to 1967 I was a full-time researcher. When I went into private practice I decided that I would increase my clinical research work because I would have a large number of patients to work with. My main and overriding rule in this work was to not harm patients and looking back on my career I think I achieved this objective. Patients, in fact, have always very much wanted to see me, so as to work with newer treatments which were safe and effective. They knew that vitamins were safe and they expected that they would be effective since I was using them. I have always been frank with my patients and outline for them any possible problems that may occur from a prescribed treatment except for those I considered based on delusion, such as the idea that vitamin C causes kidney stones. Needless to say, the majority of side effects I warn my patients of are caused by drugs, not nutrients.

I soon learned that it is impossible to carry out double-blind controlled experiments in private practice because patients do not like them and do not trust a doctor who does them. I have already described, in Chapter Eight how my patients lost confidence in me after I was asked to compare a new antidepressant with one of the older ones I had used for years and tried to compare them in a single blind study. A couple of years ago I ran another study with a new drug. It was an open clinical study, with both the patients and I knowing what they were getting. This time I completed the study without any difficulty. Some of the patients are still taking the new antidepressant and all participants remained on my patient roster.

I studied the impact of the orthomolecular approach with every patient who came to see me. I assumed that every patient had been properly examined and diagnosed by the doctors, often more than one, who had seen them, and that they had been given the best possible orthodox treatment and it had not helped them. It therefore made sense to place them on an orthomolecular program and study the outcome. Any improvement above failure would be a success. The results have been much better than mere improvement; the majority of my patients have become well, with a few exceptions. Of those with Alzheimer's, for instance, none have responded. I have not done follow-ups with most of my patients except for those with schizophrenia and cancer. With these two conditions I have tried to follow up each patient I have seen, some for as long as 18 years. I have published the results of my clinical studies with these patients in journals and in several books.

The British Columbia College of Physicians and Surgeons

Society has entrusted the medical profession with the power to police itself and maintain minimal standards of competence. Each province has its own college of physicians and surgeons, consisting of physicians who have been elected from districts into which the provinces are divided. The elected college then appoints permanent officers to administer its affairs. The chief of these is the Registrar. No person may practice medicine unless registered with the college. The college examines the person's educational certificates to confirm that the candidate has really been trained at the medical schools listed and has met all the requirements of the college. Thereafter the college no longer interferes in the physician's practice, unless complaints are lodged against him or her.

Since arriving in Victoria, I had avoided annoying the college by not appearing in public in British Columbia unless invited to speak to professional groups or small lay groups. I have also chosen to practise in such a manner that no one could ever charge me with unprofessional behaviour. There have however been a few incidents; in none of them do I consider myself to be at fault. The first involved a young patient with chronic arthritis who had not responded to any treatment, including vitamins. I then added penicillamine to his program. This had been used by others for arthritis and I was familiar with it since I first began to use it in 1955 for some of my schizophrenic patients. He began to respond and felt a lot better. However after I had not seen him for several months (he was under the care of his general practitioner) he called me and told me about the drug causing some side effects. I immediately advised him to stop taking it. Unbeknownst to me, he then relapsed and felt so sick that on his own, without consulting me, he went back on to the medication. He then had a serious reaction to it. His doctor must have complained to the College. They wrote me that I should not have used penicillamine. I could have argued with them on that point, but since I had advised the patient to stop taking it, they said, they would not take any further action against me.

I am also aware of two patient complaints against me. One was made by a woman I had never seen and the second by a schizophrenic patient I had seen 35 years ago at University Hospital in Saskatoon. The latter complaint was made to the College of Physicians and Surgeons of Saskatchewan. There may have been others which the college did not consider appropriate to pursue. Today, the Colleges must act upon every complaint, no matter how frivolous, causing an enormous waste of time and money.

The first complainant had been referred to me and I had sent her an appointment time. She did not acknowledge receiving it. A couple of weeks before the time she was to be seen I sent her another reminder and asked for confirmation. On my appointment slip I include a statement that patients who miss appointments without 24 hours' notice may be charged for the missed appointment. This is a legitimate charge to the patient. I send this notice to cut down on no-shows but I never send any of the actual no-shows bills. If later on such a patient requests a meeting, I do not see them until they have paid for the missed appointment, unless they can demonstrate that they had a good reason for not letting my office know of their impending absence in advance. When I did not hear from the patient I am discussing here, I cancelled her appointment and did not send her a bill. Later she complained to the College that I was billing her even though I had never seen her. The College asked me for details, which I provided. They then sent her a harsh letter, pointing out the frivolous nature of her complaint.

The second complaint I am aware of was equally immaterial but more troublesome. In fact, I received notice of this complaint from the Saskatchewan College with a brief note which was a sort of apology. They said that they now had to investigate every complaint, no matter its merit. The package included a copy of a letter from a woman in Winnipeg who claimed that she had discovered that the reason she had been ill for the last 35 years was because I had diagnosed her as having schizophrenia when she had never had that condition. She demanded an apology and stated that after receiving this apology she would consider what other measure she would take. Her letter was supported by one from her psychologist who requested that for the sake of her patient, I comply. The threat in the letter was clear and I promptly sent a copy to the Canadian Medical Protective Association for their advice. I assumed that this letter represented a new way of exploiting false memory syndrome. The psychologist needed to pin her client's illness on an event from the past and had selected this one. I am surprised she did not claim I had sexually harassed her client. She had also sent a copy of her complaint to the British Columbia College but of course they had no jurisdiction over what had happened before I was registered with them.

I had to obtain all the relevant records from Royal University Hospital in Saskatoon. I discovered that this patient had also been seen by Dr. B. O'Regan, who had diagnosed her as schizophrenic. With the advice of the Medical Protective Association, I sent Dr. Loewen, the deputy registrar of the Saskatchewan college the following letter:

Dear Dr. Loewen: Re: Miss C____

I have reviewed the admission, discharge and outpatient files from University Hospital on the above mentioned patient. Since I have no recollection of having seen this patient I must be guided entirely by these notes.

This patient was first seen in the out-patient department and a comprehensive handwritten report, dated October 10, 1964, was prepared by someone whose signature I can not make out. The clinical reports describing this patient on her two admissions i.e. between October 8 and October 23, 1964, and between February 11 and March 5, 1965, were prepared by Dr. R. Denson. The only reference to any contact I may have had with this patient is dated March 19, 1965 where I recorded that she was much better. I dictated this note one day after I sent a letter to Dr. Kobrinsky in Winnipeg. There is no other reference anywhere in the file to any other direct contact that I might have had with her. Since I invariably dictate notes after interviewing a patient, I don't believe I saw her on any other occasion.

I was then Director Psychiatric Research, Department of Public Health, Psychiatric Services Branch and Associate Professor of Psychiatry, College of Medicine, University of

Saskatchewan. Dr. R. Denson was a staff member, University Hospital and he also worked in the research division. He was a well-trained psychiatrist and later stayed in practice in Saskatoon and elsewhere until he retired recently. I had no reason to doubt his diagnosis then, nor, having reviewed this file very carefully, have I any reason to doubt it now.

The complaint against me is that (1) I, incorrectly, diagnosed her as being schizophrenic (2) That this has caused her anxiety and suffering ever since.

In brief: Ms C was diagnosed by a competent, well-trained psychiatrist at University Hospital and given a diagnosis with which I would not disagree. I can not recall anything about her nor whether I saw her once or more often since there are no notes to substantiate this. She was much better after each discharge after appropriate treatment for her diagnosed disorder.

It is now fairly standard practice for psychiatrists to discuss with their patients what the diagnosis is. I have been doing this for many years and have never run into any difficulty, even after having seen several thousands of schizophrenic patients over my professional career.

I cannot comment on the present mental condition of the complainant. However I can not recall a single clinical report where discussing the diagnosis with a patient has been determined to be the cause of all their misfortune or illness thereafter.

The Saskatchewan College of Physicians and Surgeons dismissed the complaint.

XXI

HOFFER-VICKAR CHAIR IN PSYCHIATRY

In the mid-1960s, Rose and I purchased a condominium in Grand Cayman and began vacationing there every January for about three weeks. My sister Marion and her husband Edward Vickar spent their winters in their condominium in Ft. Lauderdale. We would visit the Vickars either on the way to Grand Cayman or back, often staying for several days. Ed and Marion were very interested in Israel and were benefactors to Ben Gurion University. In January 1986, during one of these visits, Marion asked me to come to Israel with them. She explained that she and Ed had contributed to the library of social work and in May a plaque honouring them was to be unveiled. Half seriously and half in jest I told Marian that if they endowed a Chair in Orthomolecular Psychiatry I would come with them. To my surprise Marion was open to the idea and we discussed what it might lead to. Ed was also very interested, as was Dr. Garry Vickar, their son, an excellent orthomolecular psychiatrist. Ed and Marion approached the university and they suggested that Professor Belmaker, a psychiatrist born and trained in the United States, would be the appropriate person to hold the chair. Professor Belmaker was interested and in February he assured Ed that he was familiar with molecular psychiatry. I made it clear from the outset that this was not to be a chair in psychiatry but had to be chair in orthomolecular psychiatry. The creation of such a chair would permanently enshrine orthomolecular psychiatry at the university and could not be ignored thereafter. The dean of medicine and the president of the university agreed to my conditions.

On May 21, 1986 we four arrived in Israel to meet with the President and Dr. Glick, Dean of Medicine at Ben Gurion University. Two days later we drove to Beer Sheva. I attended a seminar put on by the department of psychiatry and met several other psychiatrists. On May 31 we visited Dr. C. Belmaker and Mrs. Elaine Belmaker, also a physician, at the kibbutz where they lived. We were driven about and shown a good deal of Israel. On May 27, Ed, Dr. Glick, and I met for the final signing of the contract for the Hoffer-Vickar Chair of Orthomolecular Psychiatry. After some preliminary conversation, Dr. Glick suddenly announced that everything was great and ready to be accepted, except for one word. I knew immediately what that world was but listened to him attentively. He stated that the University could not accept the Chair if the word "orthomolecular" remained in it. I was very annoyed and abrupt and replied, "No word, no Chair." We were at an impasse and it looked as if all the original negotiations were wasted. The university's president was called and he suggested another meeting with the former founding Dean, Dr. Previs, who had originally agreed to our terms. We eventually worked out a compromise, calling the new position the Hoffer-Vickar Chair of Psychiatry, A Unit of Orthomolecular Clinical Research. Later that day we drove to Jerusalem by the Dead Sea and remained as tourists for a few days. I invited Linus Pauling to join us for the dedication of the Chair, to be held in May 1987, and he accepted graciously.

On May 18, 1987, Linus Pauling, Rose, my sons Bill, an antiquarian book dealer in Vancouver, and John, Professor of Medicine at McGill University in Montreal, and I flew to Israel on El Al. I was most impressed with their security measures. We joined Ed, Marion, Elaine, their daughter, and Sherry Sharfe, her husband, in Israel. Linus was very friendly and pleasant. He let Sherry know how much he admired my work by telling him that he had nominated me for the Nobel Prize.

On May 21, we attended a morning seminar. The room was crowded and 35 were turned away. Linus spoke first. Next, Garry Vickar discussed the application of clinical orthomolecular psychiatry. He was followed by Professor Belmaker whose talk was titled, "Folic Acid Supplementation in Lithium Therapy." John Hoffer then discussed the "Metabolism of Vitamin B-3," which presentation was followed by my speech on the "Treatment of Acute Schizophrenia." Bernard Rimland concluded the seminar with a presentation titled, "High Dosage of Vitamin B-6 in the Treatment of Autistic Children and Adults." Bernie and I have been close colleagues and friends since 1960. He is the founder of the American Infantile Autism Society and probably knows more about autism than any other person. Bernie had a cold and had a terrible time giving his speech. On May 28, we got the sad news that Arthur Sackler, the publisher of our first double-blind studies on niacin had died.

At lunch Linus was awarded the Ben Gurion Award, which honours achievement in science. In his thank-you speech to the university, he recommended that another Chair be created in orthomolecular oncology. I thought that was a great idea. No university, though, has yet moved to implement it.

After our morning seminar, a number of attendees who were refugees from Russia lingered on. Many of these individuals had sad stories to tell; one of these men particularly affected me, because we had a personal connection. In 1960 I had received a letter from the head of the Schizophrenia Hospital in Moscow. He wrote that in his unit they had been investigating the adrenochrome hypothesis with respect to establishing whether our ideas described real biochemical events in the body and that he would be sending me the collected papers for that year. This was very exciting news indeed. The book did arrive, in Russian, with English abstracts in some cases. One of my workers was able to translate the studies and it was clear that the Moscow group had corroborated our findings and did consider what I had done important. At the meeting in Israel that same psychiatrist introduced himself. He was unemployed in Israel, appeared very poor, and asked me if I had a research position for him in Saskatchewan. I was sorry that I did not and therefore could not return the hospitality he and his group had shown me. Meeting him brought back a stream of memories.

After I had read that book of Russian studies, I wanted to go to Moscow at the first opportunity. A year later, I received an invitation from the government of Czechoslovakia to participate in the first international meeting they were sponsoring since the communist takeover. This meeting was to honour Dr. Purkinje (1787 to 1869), a very famous research physician. I was one of two Canadians to be invited. They said that they were very poor but that if I could make my way to the border they would pick up all living expenses while in Czechoslovakia. This invitation gave me an opportunity I believed I could not afford to miss. With the approval of my immediate superiors and the government of Saskatchewan, I prepared to fly to Moscow and then on to Prague.

Rose and I planned on spending a few days in Moscow and after that a week in Prague. The cold war was still on and it was difficult for western scientists to exchange correspondence and reprints with workers from behind the Iron Curtain. I thought this situation ridiculous and did not hesitate to correspond with any scientist, anywhere. But I had been told that to enter Russia was not that easy and my passage at the border would be expedited if I had very formal letters of introduction written by distinguished officials. I therefore obtained such letters from the Premier of Saskatchewan, the Minister of Public Health of Saskatchewan, and the federal Minister of Health in Ottawa. The trip had to be arranged through Intourist, the Russian government-run travel agency which worked in close contact with the Russian Embassy in Ottawa. Intourist offered three different classes of tours. We selected the deluxe tour, which cost $25 per day Canadian—ridiculously cheap. We would be met at the airport by a limousine driver and a translator who was to be our constant companion while we were in Moscow. The charge included our transort in the limousine, our translator's services, the hotel, and all the food we could eat. We would not even need any money for Intourist assured us they would supply us with coupons for everything we might need in advance, to be doled out as needed. While all the arrangements were being made, I was amused one day by the visit of a young RCMP officer. He came to our house in Saskatoon and said that he had been informed we were going to Moscow. Then he became very embarrassed and began to talk about women. I assured him immediately that Rose was coming with me. He heaved a sigh of relief. His mission had been to warn me to be careful and not be seduced by a Russian spy.

Our flight to Moscow went well. We arrived at our hotel and were given a large suite, much too large. We had a bedroom, a large living room and ample closet space. Sitting outside in the corridor was a woman who kept the keys to the rooms. We thought that our room would be bugged, and had decided in advance not to say anything critical of the regime while visiting.

The next day our limousine and translator arrived to pick us up and we spent the day at the Schizophrenia Hospital discussing our mutual interests with the researchers there. They told me gleefully that a month before, Seymour Kety from the NIMH in Washington DC had been there. I gathered that they had not been very impressed by him and of course this pleased me enormously. All in all, I had a very interesting day. We toured Moscow for the next two days. The limousine driver took us wherever we wanted to go. When we drove by the University of Moscow, we discovered that our translator, a young woman, was a graduate in English literature. We had many interesting discussions which were very friendly, but of course we were very careful as to what we said. Moscow in winter was very cold and dreary. All the people wore black in various shades. Neither was there colour in the windows as in western cities. Strong, heavy-set women who worked with their brooms and shovels kept the streets clean.

During our last meal at the hotel, we had many food coupons left over and I did not want to waste them. I asked the waiter if he could use them. He became very indignant and told us that communists did not accept tips. Then on to Prague. We moved into a very nice hotel used by Canadians from the Embassy and consulate; the staff spoke English.

The meeting was well-organized and papers were delivered in three languages, including English. I attended all sessions faithfully. I was amused by some of the presentations. Communist governments then maintained that alcoholism did not exist in their states because of the perfection of the system. Yet several papers were devoted to the topic of alcoholism in Russia. Each speaker would start his presentation with an expression of sincere gratitude to the state and the communist system and how perfect it was compared to capitalism. Then they would present the main body of the research. The final statement would again provide proof of how superior their system really was. One of my colleagues from behind the Iron Curtain remarked that they had to live. His words reminded me that our group too had had to pay lip service to many in Canada and the United States who maintained that the double-blind method was so superior and that anecdotes, although usable, should be referred to disparagingly in any research paper.

After my presentation, my new friends Dr. Voytechovsky, who I believe worked for the Czech government's Department of Health and the two young Grof brothers, Stan and Paul, asked me if I would be willing to talk to them about our LSD research. They wanted to put on a special evening featuring a lecture by me that would not be part of the official program. They said that they were keenly interested in doing LSD work, but that the state would not permit them to initiate such studies unless a visiting physician spoke about the topic. I agreed and they arranged a meeting with a translator. I described our LSD work with alcoholics and how the psychedelic concept worked in practice. Later this group initiated studies of their own. They also corroborated our findings that adrenochrome was an hallucinogen in a double-blind controlled study. The two Grof brothers eventually came to North America and continued to be very productive psychiatric researchers.

The situation for professional people in Czechoslovakia was terrible. Taxi drivers made as much money as professors of psychiatry. Really, everyone was very poor and also very hungry. The citizens, we found, seldom had protein or butter, which were luxuries. Rose and I invited the Chair, Department of Psychiatry, of the university in Prague, his family, and the two Grof brothers to a meal at our hotel. It was a very fine meal with wine, and it was clear that our guests were ravenous. Yet the whole dinner cost only $25, including tip.

That we paid after discovering that Communist attitudes toward gratuities weren't unified. The first day we had gone to the dining room in Prague for dinner, the service was superb and the food good. Thanks to the lecture I'd received in Moscow, I did not tip. The second night the service was a bit more reluctant. Again I did not tip. On the third night it was almost impossible to catch our waiter's eye. Eventually, reluctantly, he seated us. I asked him what the hotel's policy with respect to tipping was. He suddenly became very warm and said that the staff's livelihood depended on tips as their salaries were so low they could not survive on them. I immediately gave him the tip for the previous meals and after that the service was superb.

This visit was very important as it resulted in the first corroborative study of the hallucinogenic properties of adrenochrome and made it possible for the psychiatrists in Prague to start their psychedelic studies.

We came home with mixed feelings. Everyone we had met had been unfailingly kind and helpful to us—and we felt very happy to be free of the oppressive atmosphere we had experienced in Moscow and Prague.

I returned from the sudden flood of memories and associations to a feeling of satisfaction that Ben Gurion University had just become the first institution of higher learning to accept the term "orthomolecular". The medical profession has so attacked Linus Pauling and this word he coined has long struck fear into any academics who hear it. As recently as 2002, I was invited to give a seminar at a university in northern Florida. This university had indicated it was keen on accepting a chair in orthomolecular psychiatry. But when the medical staff discovered I was to give the seminar, looked me up on the internet, and discovered my association with that word, I was de-invited, and the proposed chair never created.

Since taking up the new chair, Dr. Belmaker has to date (2005) published over a dozen reports in establishment journals dealing with various aspects of orthomolecular psychiatry. His studies have included investigation of omega-3 essential fatty acids as a depression treatment, the importance of inositol in treating anxiety and depression, and the finding that schizophrenic patients are high in homocysteine. High levels of this compound are associated with heart failure. Schizophrenic patients do not get cancer at as high a rate as non-schizophrenics, but they are more prone to develop heart disease. This particular illness pattern provides another possible corroboration for the adrenochrome theory of schizophrenia. My research has shown that adrenochrome inhibits cell growth, which could, in time, inhibit tumor formation, and that the compound is toxic to heart muscle.

I stay in touch with Professor Belmaker by e-mail, and we have a good collegial relationship. I am pleased to report that at the time of this writing, he is planning to conduct the first properly-done controlled trials intended to corroborate the research Dr. Osmond and I did in the early 1950s on niacin as a schizophrenia treatment. These will be the first such trials done at any university in the world.

XXII

OPPOSING MANDATORY RETIREMENT

We moved to Victoria in 1976 in large part because we did not want to live out our retirement years in the harsh climate of Saskatoon. I was fifty-nine and had always thought that at 65 I would retire. But when I reached that age I found myself busy, and my work too interesting to even think about retirement. There was no shortage of patients; the waiting list to see me was long; the patients I was seeing suffered from challenging diseases and most responded well to the treatment.

But toward the end of 1996, when I was 79, I was suddenly confronted with the reality that I would have to retire, not because I wanted to but because a coalition of the British Columbia government and the British Columbia Medical Association (BCMA) had, each for their own reasons, decided that all doctors over 75 should be turfed out of the medical services payment plan. The Canadian Constitution clearly states that there shall be no discrimination on account of age, which would make mandatory retirement illegal.

Like all the other provinces, British Columbia has a provincially sponsored medical insurance scheme. All British Columbia residents who pay the annual premium are entitled to "free" medical treatment including surgery, hospital costs, and some medication. Doctors working within that plan are assigned a billing number.

After patients are seen, the central plan is billed using an agreed upon payment schedule between the government and the BCMA. Every two weeks the plan deposits the payment into the doctor's account. If you do not have a billing number, you are not entitled to any payment. Doctors can practise privately, billing their patients directly, only under very strict conditions.

In mid-1996, Fran Fuller, my office manager, told me that a payment list I had just received from the government included notification that at the end of the year I would no longer be able to bill the government because I would lose my billing number. In September 1996 I wrote to the Ministry of Health and the Ministry Responsible for Seniors. The Ministry replied that the new Physicians Supply Measure was effective October 1, 1996. Section 6 states that effective January 1, 1997, a practitioner's entitlement to receive payment from the Medical Services Plan either through fee-for-service or alternate payments arrangement will be rescinded at the end of the calendar year in which the practitioner passes his or her 75th birthday. This meant that I would no longer be entitled to payment after Dec 31, 1997. But there was a possible escape. I could receive a two-year extension if need for my services could be established.

I was not yet ready to retire. I could have retired and lived comfortably the rest of my life. I also could have started to practise outside the plan, but this was inconvenient and would have prevented most schizophrenic patients from seeing me, as most would not have been able to afford to pay me privately. One of my patients, a very intelligent young man suffering from paranoia, whom I had been seeing regularly for many years, heard that he might have to pay. He asked me whether I would be willing to see him if he could afford to pay a much smaller amount on a regular basis. I assured him that I would but I had not yet conceded that I would have to adopt such a strategy. His question intensified my feelings of annoyance and indignation that groups who had never consulted me were attempting to force me into retirement.

I began to research the issue. I found that the question of mandatory retirement had even made its way into some medical journals.

Dr. Bill Trent[1] opened his discussion by quoting Dr. S. MacDonald, then 81 years old. The latter said, "Tell those people in Ottawa and elsewhere to butt out of mandatory retirement, I don't want anybody telling me I shouldn't be doing this. If you want to go on working and you have the health and ability, you should be free to do so." Another physician stated, "The majority of doctors want to practise as long as they can and keep themselves in good health in order to do so. They never expected the government would tell them they had to retire." Yet another doctor quoted by Trent argued, "It's wrong for anyone to demand that physicians retire until they are willing to say that lawyers, dentists and all other self-employed people must also retire." Doctors agreed that standard of care was much more important than the age of the doctor. The main groups supporting mandatory retirement were the governments and the doctors directly working for them. The prime interest of these groups was to control costs.

In 1996, the provincial governments of Canada were persuaded by their deputy Ministers of Health that Canada had too many doctors and that many of the larger cities, including Vancouver and Victoria, were over-serviced. They had accepted a formula which "proved" that the main factor driving costs up was the number of doctors practicing. Following this equation to its logical conclusion, if we had no doctors the costs would be zero. This does not mean that everyone would be well and not needing medical services. As a result, these governments were soon busy drawing up plans to reduce both the numbers of doctors coming into practice, and the number of hospital beds. They also discouraged nurses from continuing to work and did whatever else they could to decrease the size of the physician pool in Canada. Canada is currently experiencing a significant shortage of physician services. As I write this in 2005, it is difficult to believe that the "experts" could have been so wrong. But only British

---

1. Trent, B. Mandatory retirement: Should older MDs be forced to retire to make way for the new? *Can Med Assoc J* 1993; 149: 1697-1699.

Columbia undertook to make retirement mandatory in that year, when it passed the Medicare Protection Amendment Act.

The reasons for the introduction of mandatory retirement in British Columbia included a more selfish set, not explained in official communication. In 1997, I spoke to a man who had been on the original negotiating committee representing the government of British Columbia. He told me that at one meeting, the president of the BCMA had proposed his plan to dump every physician over 75 because the government had informed them that it would provide no more than 1.4 billon dollars per year for all physician services in British Columbia. The amount was not negotiable. But Vancouver and Victoria are very attractive places in which to live and practise and as a result, each new doctor locating in the province would decrease the size of each slice available in that 1.4 billon dollar pie. How would the BCMA maintain current standards of income for its members? Mandatory retirement became one solution. The government knew that the BCMA's suggestion was illegal, but they were tired of fighting with the organization and decided against their own better judgment to go along with the proposal. The BCMA president defended the actions of the organization in a letter to the *British Columbia Medical Journal*, published April 18, 1997. This letter expressed no concern whatever for what would happen to the doctors forced out, or to the patients who would have difficulty finding doctors to replace the physicians forced into retirement. (Neither was there any appreciation that the policy would help lead to a shortage of physicians and the long waiting lists we now enjoy.)

At about this time, I met Mr. Felix Reuben, President, Osugi Associated Consultants Holdings Ltd. During our first meeting he told me that he had admired my work for a long time. This of course was a great way to get started. He also had heard about the problem regarding my age and offered to help in any way that he could. This meeting was the beginning of our long, very helpful and friendly association. His legal advice and guidance made it possible for me to gain my exemption and later to reverse the illegal act passed by the provincial government.

On January 2, 1997, I applied for an exemption to the new law, which, if granted, would allow me to practice for another two years. The arduous task of preparing a brief to support my application for the special exemption began. Mr. Reuben prepared this massive and excellent submission, which took an enormous amount of time, energy, and skill to complete. The final application was contained in two books! I listed therein 523 of my published papers, now over 600, and nearly 18 of my books, now over 30. Most of the argument had to do with the legal problems and questions involved. It became obvious to us as we proceeded that the whole process was designed to make it almost impossible for any physician to obtain the exemption. The brief was submitted in April 1999 to the Medical Services Commission of British Columbia (MSC), a body charged with, among other things, supervising the government's payments to doctors. The following summary is based on that comprehensive report.

In the introduction we pointed out that British Columbia was facing a serious problem with respect to crimes committed by schizophrenics, that I specialized in the treatment of these patients and that I had under my care about 500 chronic patients. I added that most of them were getting on very well and were very seldom involved in any criminal activity. Physicians from Vancouver Island, from mainland British Columbia, and from the rest of Canada referred these patients to me, often because they had difficulty finding psychiatrists willing to take them on. For instance, Dr. H Barrydale Veasey wrote in my support that he had practised in the Victoria area since 1966 and that it had always been almost impossible to arrange for a patient to see a psychiatrist without a three- to six-month waiting period. Further, we explained, I was only one of two psychiatrists prepared to see emergencies within a few days. We also presented evidence that the use of medications alone was not adequate for these patients due in part to the serious side effects. We pointed out that the government's Medicare Protection Act, introducing mandatory retirement, had infringed on the Charter of Rights and Freedoms. Under the charter I and the unique population who sought my help were also legally protected. Below, I briefly describe the many areas we had to discuss in the main text of this document.

In general, it was our task to prove that my services were needed.

I pointed out that I was the only psychiatrist on Vancouver Island with expertise, skill, and long experience in using modern nutritional therapies for psychiatric illnesses as part of the entire treatment. If I were not to practise, doctors who depended on me due to the fact that the medical schools gave no training in these areas would be deprived of the help they sought, and their patients would be deprived of the increased chance of recovery that nutritional treatment provides. We added that a local holistically-oriented clinic, the Life Centre, wished to have me involved in patient care as a consultant. We pointed out that compared to other regions in British Columbia, Victoria was under-serviced by psychiatrists. I also explained that thanks to my effectiveness, I was able to see many more patients per year than the mean of all psychiatrists in British Columbia and thus saving the plan and society at large an enormous amount of money since each recovered patient saves the public about $2,000,000 over their lifetime. We were asked for evidence that my current patients would be denied access to care if I retired, and further asked to prove that appropriate acceptable care would not be reasonably available to my former patients. We faced a challenge in responding to these requests since the definitions of the terms "acceptable" and "reasonable" are variable. We pointed out that most psychiatrists find the use of drugs only for the treatment of schizophrenia acceptable and reasonable. However, very few patients treated this way reach my definition of recovery, which includes paying income tax. We explained that the vast majority of schizophrenic patients who have been ill for one year or less and who follow the orthomolecular program for up to two years recover. Orthomolecular care, we argued thus met my definition of "acceptable" and "reasonable.

We further enclosed letters of support from the 20 percent of the physician population of the Greater Victoria area who used my services, a petition signed by over 1,500 people with schizophrenia and their relatives and support persons, and other letters of support. A few patients were so worried they would be deprived of my services, they had insisted on signing the petition twice. Others reported to me that they would continue to see me if I lost my billing number, even though they would have to continue paying taxes for the benefit of other patients seeking help from other physicians, as well as compensate me.

The government also wanted proof that I had admitting and treatment privileges within a hospital. I had been on staff at the Royal Jubilee Hospital from 1976 until 1992, when I voluntarily resigned. Because of rumours spread by other staff psychiatrists that I had been forced to leave, I presented a letter from Mr. Ken Fykes, now OC, President Capital Health Region, confirming that my resignation was voluntary. He added that nothing would prevent me from reapplying and receiving admitting privileges.

Related to the issue of hospital privileges was the question of whether I possessed the skill set required to meet my role. I listed my qualifications and also quoted from a letter praising the quality of care I provided, written by Dr. V. W. Waymouth, of the College of Physicians and Surgeons of British Columbia.

I concluded this massive submission by stating that I was applying for a two-year extension of my inclusion in the billing plan, with the understanding that my submission of this application would not curtail my right to later apply for unlimited exemption, for so long as I had the ability and desire to keep on practising. I argued that in a free and democratic society, to work as long as I wished was my right, guaranteed by the Constitution of Canada and by the British Columbia Health Act.

I met with the committee of the Medical Services Commission of British Columbia (MSC) that considered applications such as mine on May 13, 1999. Also appearing on my behalf were Felix Reuben, consultant, Ms. Victoria Pitts, lawyer, and Salmond Ashurst, stenographer. Both Felix and I were certain at that point that my application would be rejected, but we had to go through the process in preparation for an appeal to the Supreme Court of British Columbia. Our determination to appeal was one of the reasons we had a court stenographer present. We believed that with a stenographer present, the civil servants representing the government would be more careful and circumspect in their statements and if they were not, we would have a permanent record of any illogical reasoning or hostile comments.

For the MSC, Keith Bennett, Chair, represented the public interest, while John Mullin and Dr. Deryck Smith represented the BCMA. At the outset of the hearing, Ms. Toms, a lawyer representing British Columbia's Ministry of Attorney General (the government body responsible for justice services) briefly reviewed the procedure followed by the MSC at administrative hearings of this nature. At the committee's request, she also acknowledged that I had raised Charter issues in the application, and indicated the panel's proposal to proceed as if it had jurisdiction to hear the application on its merits, since it had no jurisdiction on Charter issues, and to provide its decision within the limits of its jurisdiction.

The committee was provided with factual background through evidence provided at the hearing and as summarized in written materials provided by myself and another body, an Advisory Committee set up to review my application prior to the hearing and make recommendations on behalf of the government.

I sought the following declarations from the MSC:

1. That I be permitted to continue my enrollment in the Medical Services Plan.
2. In the alternative, that I be permitted to continue my enrollment in the Plan until the Courts had made their final determination in the case of Waldman v. MSC, a case whose outcome we had determined should be precedent-setting regarding my application.
3. That the MSC suspend enforcement of s: 13.1 of the Medicare Protection Amendment Act (which legislated mandatory retire-

ment) on the basis that it is contrary to s. 15(1) of the Charter of
Rights and Freedoms.

4. That the MSC suspend enforcement of s. 13.1 of the Act until the
    Courts have made their final determination in the case of Wald-
    man v. MSC.

I also requested that in the event the panel denied my application for
an exemption, that I be granted a stay of 90 days after the delivery
of the decision.

Dr. Alan Thomson summarized the position of the Advisory
Committee. They recommended against granting me an exemption.
The Advisory Committee, he said, based its recommendation in part
on the fact that my application did not include supporting recommendations from some individuals and organizations involved in
psychiatric services in the Victoria region. I knew that the detractors
of which he spoke violently disapproved of my methods, though
none had bothered to test them for themselves. Dr. Thomson also
indicated that the Capital (Victoria) Health Region had one of the
highest ratios of psychiatrists to population. Dr. Thomson further
provided the view of the committee that the evidence that the population I saw was special was not clear, (the government had sought
proof that my patients were a clearly distinguishable group) but he
acknowledged that my service was unique. The three-member board
appeared to be neutral or perhaps even friendly, especially the
Chairman, Keith Bennett, who was the main spokesperson. After
Mr. Bennett further questioned Dr. Thomson as to why he had
rejected my application, Dr. Thomson was cross-examined by my
counsel. Two questions elicited interesting replies. When asked
about the petition signed by over 1,500 people, Dr. Thomson said he
had not taken it seriously. There was a sudden look of shocked
surprise from the Chairman, as if to say "How can that not be
evidence, 1,500 petitioners representing the public?" When Dr.
Thomson was asked about the letters submitted by the physicians
who referred to me, he replied that he had not taken those seriously
either, since each doctor had not written an individual letter. I

suddenly was convinced, as I saw the reaction of the committee to these admissions, that we had a chance. Dr. Thomson's answers indicated he was so blatantly uninterested in the views of the non-medical and medical populations alike, that he could not have come to a balanced and fair decision with respect to my application.

At the end I was asked if I had any comment. I did. I spoke for about 10 minutes. I pointed out that I was providing a service that physicians found valuable, since they had not the time nor the expertise in my field needed to be helpful to their patients. I explained that if I were de-enrolled, 25 percent of my patients would be unable to pay for my services, and would therefore be denied orthomolecular treatment. Further, I pointed out, because orthomolecular psychiatry requires less psychotherapy be provided to the patient, I was able to see and help more patients in a year, than the average psychiatrist. I stated my firm belief that as a result I was providing a significant cost saving to the health care system. I also advised the panel that I had endeavoured since 1960 to recruit someone to join me in my practice. Since that time I had had 16 physicians join me for short periods to learn my method of treatment. All then returned to their own practices. I indicated that if there were even one psychiatrist in the area willing to do what I do, I would be happy to retire. A psychiatrist was needed, I felt, explaining that many general practitioners could practise as I do with regard to nutritional treatment, but could not take on the serious and chronic schizophrenic patients I am able to work with.

Because I was still fairly certain that we would lose and have to go higher, I became less cautious than usual and at the end I said to the Chairman that I needed not just the two years, the maximum permitted by law, but ten. To my amazement the Chairman immediately replied, "Dr Hoffer, you should have it." We had won. That afternoon I received a phone call from Miss Pitts. The MSC had approved my application; a few weeks later, their written submission arrived. We had won the first round. I was allowed to keep my billing number for another two years. But we were not going to stop with that. The British Columbia government had acted illegally in passing the mandatory retirement law in the first place. It had contravened the Charter of Rights and Freedoms, our constitution, and I was determined that we would have our day in court.

Mr. Felix Reuben went on to direct and carry out the plan of action that I and several other physicians initiated to appeal the retirement law to the Supreme Court of British Columbia. In order to prepare the strongest possible case for the MSC hearing, one that might have to be argued before the Supreme Court of Canada, Mr. Reuben and I had organized the Senior Physicians Society of British Columbia (SPSBC). We met for the first time on March 6, 1999. The officers elected at the inaugural meeting were myself, President, Dr. G. Thompson, Secretary Treasurer, and Drs. W. Downe and L. Kindree, directors. Dr. Alan Matthews joined as a director at the next meeting. Including our board, we had seventeen members. The group was incorporated on March 23, 1999 under the Society Act of British Columbia. We all agreed that the mandatory retirement law was ill thought out, had no practical value, ignored the financial loss, pain, and stress placed upon innocent physicians who happened to be over 75, and could create much misery in the lives of patients as well, due to British Columbia's physician shortage.

Our first main order of business after the MSC made its decision was to authorize Mr. Reuben to initiate proceedings by requesting the court to declare that Section 13.1 of the Medicare Protection Amendment Act is in breech of the Canadian Charter. He did so on May 28, 1999, on behalf of the Senior Physicians Society of British Columbia with The Medical Services Commission Appeal Panel and The British Columbia Ministry of Health and Ministry Responsible for Seniors as respondents. We also presented an affidavit in which I briefly listed the arguments that had supported my initial petition for an extension of my inclusion in the medical billing plan. We sent the court several pounds of material, the result of all that hard work by Felix. Our petition to the Supreme Court of British Columbia was at least partially successful; all members of our society became protected by the court's injunction of July 12, 1999, against the

British Columbia government. The court ordered by consent that "the operation of Section 13.1 of the Medicare Protection Act be stayed as against the following list of doctors, who are members of the Petitioner Society, until the hearing of the Petition, or until further orders of the Court." Unfortunately the protection set out in the Court's Order was not extended to non-members of the SPSBC. As a result of the Court's action the MSC notified all physicians by letter of the application process by which they could apply for exemption from mandatory retirement, but proceeded to use subterfuge in order to withhold knowledge of the Order and its available protection from new physicians who were reaching the age of 75. The SPSBC has had significant correspondence with the MSC in an attempt to get the MSC to notify those physicians who have reached the age of 75 that a Supreme Court Order exists that would allow them to continue their medical practice unencumbered, without having to apply for an exemption. Simple membership in the SPSBC would suffice. But the MSC would not even undertake to advise these physicians of the very existence of the SPSBC. As a result, individual physicians continue to be forced into retirement, not even aware of what the SPSBC has accomplished.

The SPSBC has also tried to persuade the BCMA to let its members know of the existence of the SPSBC, but we were unable to get an article about our group into the *BCMA Newsletter*. We had also requested a list of all physicians who were 70 years of age or older from the College of Physicians and Surgeons and they declined to give us one that includes phone numbers and addresses. Finally, we requested all our members to put up notices in their communities to help their peers find out about the existence of the organization. The SPSBC has further asked the provincial Ministry of Health and Ministry Responsible for Seniors to confirm in writing that Section 13.1 has been repealed.

Almost all the members of the SPSBC lost interest as soon as the battle was won and only the original five doctors who formed the board have maintained enough interest to attend the annual meetings and pay minimal dues. I have wanted to disband the society for many years, but the remaining members prefer to remain active, in case other issues affecting senior physicians should arise in connection with the College of Physicians and Surgeons, which has shown a serious bias against this group. The SPSBC is run out of my office by my secretary, Fran Fuller, a very capable administrator who does an excellent job of maintaining records.

My fellow doctors' concerns are justified. In a letter to me dated August 23, 2000, the Assistant Deputy Minister with the Ministry of Health advised the SPSBC that section 13.1 would be repealed, then added "That the Medical Services Plan [would] be asked to work with the College of Physicians and Surgeons to ensure that adequate provisions are in place to assess the competency of medical practitioners, particularly where there are reasons to expect a diminishment in competency, including effect of aging. The College of Physicians and Surgeons has been consulted about this matter, and is already involved in the assessment of competencies."

This advice to the College, which was readily accepted, was totally unnecessary as the College aleady had a very active program of competency assessment in place. The question of competence had never come up when the original decision was made to throw out all doctors over the age of 75. Clearly the government was still seeking the means by which to force older physicians out of practice. As indicated, the College was happy to receive this advice and soon followed it in a matter in which I was involved. The SPSBC did discuss this development as it indicated that the College was quite willing to take on the work the Medical Services Plan had been forced to stop by the Supreme Court, but we did not follow up in the matter with any action. Ageism is alive and well within the Medical Services Plan of the British Columbia government, the BCMA and the College of Physicians and Surgeons of British Columbia.

XXIII

Closing Reflections

Just as I had no intention of ever becoming a doctor when I was studying for my PhD in Agricultural Biochemistry, nor when I accepted my first job offer in a chemical control laboratory in a flour mill in Winnipeg, so I never had any intention of writing a book of memoirs or autobiography when I began to record the things that I did, the events I participated in, the trips I took, and the highlights of my career in psychiatry and in research and more or less kept the record up to date. I became aware that I had a terrible memory for faces, names, and events when I was 21, but not for ideas, hypotheses, and theories. I initially saw keeping a diary as a way to make review of important meetings and events more accurate, and easier for me. I had only my personal use in mind. However, about 20 years ago, I began to think that my family would be interested in what I had done and began to think about turning my records into a book. My first decision was to write an autobiography, but after I had written almost all of it, including much personal and family material, I decided that this was not what I wanted. I thank Miriam and John for helping me clarify what I was really trying to do.

I see this book as not really about me. It is about my research and what happened in my life on the way. It is a record of certain events which at the time they occurred were either interesting, frightening, or pleasurable; on looking back, they are all interesting, at least to me. The odyssey recounted in these pages was set into motion by a hypothesis involving adrenochrome and schizophrenia that I developed jointly with Dr. H. Osmond in 1952, based on an original hypothesis of his. Our hypothesis had all the attributes of a very good hypothesis. It was and is testable; that is, it can be falsified—but so far has not been. It has led to very important new questions and to my great pleasure has led to the recovery and improvement of thousands of patients who have been treated by orthomolecular methods. My personal and family life is equally interesting to me and my family and that is where I will leave it.

I will say that I have been given tremendous support by my family. My wife Rose was very patient and understanding and put up with the many years when we were very poor, and endured my absence from home in my last two years of medical studies, and later when I had to travel so much attending meetings, promoting better treatment for schizophrenic patients, and pleading for more money for our research. She may have been encouraged by her "knowledge" that I would one day get the Nobel Prize, while I assured her that it would never happen. I spent too little time with my children but I think they have forgiven me and have grown even stronger for that. They are marvelous, kind, and productive individuals, examples of the best in humanity.

The further support I received from women and men of medicine, science, and philosophy was fantastic and overwhelmed the attacks by our cynical critics. Many of these people are referred to in the text. The warm encouragement from individuals like Tommy Douglas, Griff McKerracher, Linus Pauling, Sir Julian Huxley, Aldous Huxley, Walter Alvarez, Eileen Garrett, Irwin Stone, Heinrich Kluver, Hugh Riordan, Emanuel Cheraskin, Tom Paterson and many others has left me with many warm memories. The support of these people made worthwhile the trials and tribulations of our research enterprise and has satisfied me that in the end, I made the correct choices. Perhaps what I have learned about the research process in medicine and the reactions of the medical professions to new ideas and information may be valuable to others. President Harry S. Truman coined the famous expression: "If you cannot stand the heat get out of the kitchen." In the kitchens of science, things can get pretty hot.

I went into research because I found it so interesting and exciting. My interest more than compensated for the many hours of drudgery and hard work involved in doing research science. My interest would also wax and wane and sometimes peak into something like a transcendental experience, the Eureka experience. My first such experience was not when I took LSD. It occurred on that evening in our little house in Regina when Rose was in the kitchen cleaning up after dinner and I was sitting at the dining room table (I had no office), and writing down the formulae of all the known hallucinogens (1952). Suddenly the indole nucleus leaped up at me as I looked at these compounds and I knew that I was on to something very important and powerful. That evening's work took Dr. Osmond's hypothesis one step further and it gave us the plan, the map which would guide me for the rest of my research career. The second peak experience occurred when our first patient, dying from catatonia at the hospital in Weyburn, suddenly recovered when we gave him a combination of niacin and ascorbic acid. The third peak experience came when we decoded the results of our first double-blind therapeutic trial and found that we had doubled the recovery rate for acute schizophrenia from 35 percent to 75 percent just by adding niacin and niacinamide to the treatment program current so many years ago. There were other such peak moments as well and they came along often enough to reinforce my interest. Over time, my interest and excitement became more and more secure, as I saw so many very sick schizophrenic patients, hopelessly ill according to the established medical knowledge of the day, slowly recover and be restored back to life.

Another dramatic story could be told by a patient who dropped in to my office in mid February 2005. Six years ago he had been told by two surgeons he would assuredly be dead in two years unless he had surgery for his huge sarcoma of the hip. The surgery would have involved partial removal of his pelvis and the operation alone assuredly would have killed him in less than two years. Instead he went orthomolecular. His pain was gone within a few months and he has gotten back to his work as a professional triathlete.

To give but one example of how satisfying my work can be, let me update you on Bob's progress. We have already met him in these pages. I saw him today. Bob, born April 15, 1940, became schizophrenic in his teens and after his father had had him treated in over ten mental hospitals, training schools, and the best and most expensive treatment centres in the United States, he came under my care in 1971. When I first saw him he was a typical deteriorated chronic schizophrenic patient with whom it was impossible to hold any conversation. Today we spent the visit discussing books he has been reading; he has a whole wall of books, which he has mostly bought himself. It took 20 years of treatment before he showed major improvement but since then it has been steady and significant. He shows very few, if any, schizophrenic features. His is another life saved and made worthwhile by orthomolecular methods, instead of a short heavily-medicated lifetime spent taking drugs which could not possibly have gotten him well.

As far as taking the less pleasant side of the heat is concerned, I will say that doing research is not easy, for if the research is to have any value at all it must explore outside what is currently known. As I have already shown, the establishments in any field do not necessarily take kindly to any really major innovations. The medical profession is more like a church than a truly scientific group of people. So if you want to go into research, be prepared. Success may not make you more popular. Know also that thinking is much more important than having all the fancy equipment in the world. The US National Institute for Mental Health, with all its vast resources, did not know how to make adrenochrome. In our research lab, working with very little equipment, we solved the problem. Original ideas are usually gleaned through good thought, and only later, when the arduous task of confirming or denying findings arises, does huge machinery sometimes serve the purpose. Finally, be wary of the advice given to you by your enemies and even more of that delivered by your friends. The advice given by destructively-minded critics is easily disregarded since it is obvious such people are not really interested in helping you, but in promoting their own point of view. What I noticed many times when I looked at our critics' suggestions closely, was that they were really interested in trying to get successful researchers—ones who were making a contribution—to take up the ideas they themselves had not yet been able to prove. The advice of friends has for me been much harder to evaluate because the people involved are really trying to be helpful. As director of psychiatric research for the Province of Saskatchewan, I had to learn to reject large numbers of freely-given ideas that would have deflected our focus from the problem at hand, schizophrenia. The most common bad advice I received from friends was to not continue what we were doing because it made us unpopular. It took me some thought and effort to reject this advice; I feel vindicated in this decision as I see that I have been very popular with patients who have been coming at a steady pace for the past 50 years.

It is my patients who keep me looking to the future. The researcher in me has also refused to retire. The adrenochrome hypothesis developed by Dr. Osmond, Dr. Smythies, and myself has not yet been fully explored. (The establishment has been reluctant to even have a look at it.) At this point, as I prepare to complete this volume with a glimpse at the future of orthomolecular medicine, I'd like to summarize the positive contributions, direct and indirect, of the adrenochrome hypothesis to date: (1) the development of psychedelic therapy for the treatment of alcoholism. McLean Hospital, affiliated with Harvard University, is planning modern studies of psychedelic therapy, nearly 40 years after we pioneered them; (2) an important addition to a growing body of knowledge about the effects of stress. We established that stress and the resulting secretion of too much adrenaline can lead to psychosis, if that adrenaline is transformed into a hallucinogenic indole in sufficient quantities; (3) the development of two simple and accurate clinical-psychological diagnostic tests for schizophrenia, the HOD and EWI tests; (4) the discovery of the mauve factor, kryptopyrrole, an excellent marker of oxidative stress and the possible presence of mental illness; (5) the concept of orthomolecular psychiatry and medicine, and the beginning of a new paradigm for vitamin use, the vitamins-as-treatment paradigm; (6) the safe treatment of cardiovascular disorders created by lipid disease.

These discoveries have helped lay the foundation for powerful changes in our overall approach to health and disease. Ever since I have been treating patients with the optimum doses of vitamins, I have predicted that one day society will recognize that one of the most important factors for maintaining health is the provision of the optimum amount of the basic nutrients needed by each person. Disease is the result of pathological changes in the body which either prevent it from properly fighting off infections or inhibit it from maintaining its own integrity or health. The origins of disease, in my opinion, are not genetic; no genes are bad genes. Any genes that are truly bad would destroy the individual before birth. I think that all diseases must be due to a defect in the nutrients supplied to that individual. If multiple sclerosis strikes at age 25, why were the genes supposedly at fault doing so well until then? If a person has been well until age 60 it is obvious again that genes cannot be blamed for an emergent illness. They were serving well. But they must have been abused through the intake of incorrect or inadequate nutrients (and what is correct and adequate is unique to each person) or by radiation or chemical injury. The problem is not in our genes, it is in the way we feed our genes.

I envision a future in which simple laboratory tests will be available which will advise which nutrients are lacking and how much of each nutrient patients need to regain and maintain their health. They would then continue to eat the most nutritious food available reinforced with those nutrients essential for them. This scenario is already in place to a limited degree. The United States government for instance, mandated in 1942 that flour milled in that country must be enriched with vitamins. This legislation was probably one of the greatest single public health measures ever introduced; it has prevented millions of people worldwide from getting and dying from pellagra. My vision has only been made stronger by the additional experience and information I have gathered over the years.

Currently I am investigating another offshoot of the adrenochrome hypothesis, the hypothesis of global sub-clinical pellagra. This hypothesis suggests that the question of enriched food is more urgent than ever. When animals broke away from vegetable life, they eventually began to move, and then to make sounds, which also involves movement. As a result, animal life found it more economic from an energy point of view to eat their nutrients than to make them. A plant needs only a place to grow, water, sunlight and the right minerals. It makes all the organic molecules it needs on its own. But it is so busy doing that that it cannot develop muscles and a brain. To conserve the energy needed to take these evolutionary steps past plant life, animals lost the ability to make their own vitamins. This must have happened many millions or even billions of years ago. The dynamics of the shift from plant to animal life were first clearly explained by Linus Pauling in 1968, in his seminal article in *Science*, "Orthomolecular Psychiatry."

Pauling had been profoundly puzzled by the fact that many patients needed large doses of vitamin B-3 and vitamin C before they became well. If these substances were so critical to health, he wondered, why would the body not produce them on its own? Pauling eventually realized that our loss of the ability to make ascorbic acid from glucose about 50 million years ago was advantageous from an evolutionary point of view. He showed that dropping the chemical machinery needed to convert glucose to ascorbic acid saved energy and therefore allowed it to be used for other purposes. But the change could only be advantageous if there were external sources of the vitamin readily available so that it would not need to be synthesized in the body. Such was the case when man still lived primarily in tropical areas, eating great amounts of plant foods. Since humanity has moved into more northern areas where vitamin C is not as plentiful in food, sub-clinical scurvy has been pretty well the norm throughout large populations of people.

With Professor Harry Foster[1] I have summarized the evidence that mankind is in the midst of similar evolutionary change in that we are losing the ability to convert tryptophan into nicotinamide adenine dinucleotide (NAD). Normally about 1.5 percent of the

---

1. A Hoffer and HF Foster. *Feel Better, Live Longer With Vitamin B-3*. In press.

tryptophan in our diet is changed into NAD. When you eat vitamin B-3 it is also converted into NAD. This is the anti-pellagra enzyme. If the vitamin cannot be converted into NAD, taking it will not prevent nor cure pellagra. But why does the body need two sources for making NAD? If the mechanisms for converting tryptophan to NAD were dropped, there would be two possible positive consequences. More of the amino acid could be converted into the very important neurotransmitter serotonin and its derivatives; secondly, at least some of the energy needed to make NAD would become available for other activities. But this change would be advantageous only if enough vitamin B-3 was available in the food. If, after the ability to make NAD from tryptophan is lost, the amount of vitamin B-3 in food is decreased, then the change that had been advantageous will become pathological.

Schizophrenia was first described around 1800. This date coincides with the introduction of modern flour mills which could at last make the perfect, pure white flour that the public demanded. Before that, the flour always contained some of the germ and bran in which the B vitamins are concentrated. After 1800, the amount of B vitamins, including vitamin B-3, consumed by the average person decreased significantly, except among those who liked whole grains such as whole wheat flour and brown rice. The rest of the population developed various manifestations of vitamin B deficiency, we argue, because the ability to make NAD from tryptophan was already decreasing. Foster and I estimate that over half the North American, and perhaps the world's, population needs extra vitamin B-3, ranging from 100 milligrams per day to 3,000 milligrams or more of niacin when cholesterol levels are high. The prevalence of niacin deficiency becomes clearer when one considers which conditions can be treated successfully by optimum amounts of the vitamin: arthritis (affects 20 percent of the population), mental illness (affects 5 to 10 percent of the population), blood lipid problems, and alcohol addiction. Our test for need is whether the patient becomes healthier when they are given this vitamin.

Once society has accepted that there is a real problem, there will be a mass movement towards whole, unrefined food consumption;

in addition, food processors will replace the vitamins that are now so routinely removed from food, and perhaps reinforce our foods with even higher levels. Everyone will easily obtain nutrients in the amounts needed by the average human to stay healthy, and doctors will recognize that some people require some nutrients in even larger amounts. That is my vision of the future. If our research of the past fifty years helps bring this future into being, I will be content.

Orthomolecular medicine will become the norm and the major diseases which plague us today will disappear. We will then also be spared the never ending, boring debates in the press about how to deal with the escalating costs of health care, lengthening waiting lists, and dangerous side effects of the drugs currently in use. Drugs, indeed, will become minor aspects of modern medicine rather than the major treatment and preoccupation of the medical establishment.

With our newfound health, we will be able to expand our exploration and mastery of the arts and sciences, enjoy time with our loved ones, and generally live more productive and happy lives.

October 1997

Dear Dr. Hoffer;

When you offered me the job as a typist and receptionist in 1977, you asked for assurance that I would stay for at least one year. I remember thinking, you might change your mind about wanting me to stay even that long. I never dreamed I would still be working with you over twenty years later, but I have never regretted accepting the job, and because of your graciousness in giving me credit for what I can contribute, I have been priviledged to feel useful in the important work you are doing. I have found working with you stimulating and rewarding, and I have always been been impressed with the dignity and courtesy with which you treat your patients.

It is also a real pleasure for me to share in the recovery process of so many patients, because you so obviously enjoy the positive results you see in your patients. Orthomolecular treatment has also been beneficial to me personally, for which I am very thankful.

I have continued to be awed by your courage and dedication in the face of so much - often vicious - opposition. A lesser man might have either sunk to the level of his enemies, or given up altogether; you have done neither. You have never forgotten what your battle is all about - the recovery of the patient.

You have always been extremely kind to me, and have always treated me with respect. During periods of difficulty in my life you have been a constant source of support and stability, an especially great comfort to me as I lost my own father at fourteen. For me, there have been many times when being able to come to work has been an oasis of calm, and I have always felt fortunate in this. You have many times had to be extremely tolerant and patient with me, and you always have been, for which I am extremely grateful.

On this, the celebration of your eightieth birthday, I would like to thank you personally, in print, not just in thought, for everything you have done for me, for your patients, for continuing to hammer away at the ivory towers of psychiatry and medicine for their sake, and for letting me share in your work in my own small way.

Thank you.

Love,

fran

Fran Fuller, my secretary.

Abram Hoffer is a man for all seasons, tireless in his efforts, thoughts and understanding of the plight of others. A friend in all times, good, bad or indifferent. Someone who had developed some goals early in life which kept broadening to my amazement, year by year, decade by decade. There are not many like him. I was flattered and humbled before him and it is a great pleasure to be able to express a few words at his four score anniversary. Some people take the extra step, but you only see it once in a while, not every day. The adrenaline pours in. This is the father of three with a wonderful wife. He was ready and willing 24 hours a day to step into whatever the gap or breach was. It is very hard to express in words and when you read about the poets who speak of the ineffable side of life, Dr. Hoffer comes as close as anyone I've seen to expressing the ineffable and making it stick. Let's celebrate this day. Let us send out our thoughts and prayers which we're always talking about, which work when you want them to work. Let's send joy to the Creator that we have been blessed with such individuals as Abe.

With never ending devotion,
Ben Webster

Donald C. ("Ben") Webster, the venture capitalist who was the founding chairman of the Canadian Schizophrenia Foundation

UNIVERSITY OF CALIFORNIA, SAN DIEGO

UCSD

BERKELEY · DAVIS · IRVINE · LOS ANGELES · RIVERSIDE · SAN DIEGO · SAN FRANCISCO

SANTA BARBARA · SANTA CRUZ

DEPARTMENT OF PSYCHOLOGY, 0109
OFFICE: (619) 534-3000
FAX: (619) 534-7190

9500 GILMAN DRIVE
LA JOLLA, CALIFORNIA 92093-0109

Dear Abram,

Happy birthday! I would like to take this opportunity to reminisce over the last 45 years since we first met. At that time we started two new approaches in medicine. The first was the role of aminochromes in schizophrenia for which you and Humphry were largely responsible. The second was what was known then as mega-vitamin therapy. Both of these received a hostile reception by main stream medicine. However, it is sadly true in medicine that most really exciting new ideas get a hostile reception by the orthodoxy of the day; think no further than Lister, Pasteur and Semmelweiss. It is therefore both pleasing and ironic to note that today it has now been established that aminochromes certainly occur in brain, that they probably have important functions there to do with synaptic plasticity and that they are involved in the pathobiochemistry of at least two diseases—Parkinson's disease and schizophrenia. After forty years in the official wilderness aminochromes are very much here to stay.

The second development is even more remarkable. The scorn poured by the orthodoxy upon adrenochrome was mild in comparison with the contumely lavished upon the outrageous suggestion that vitamins do more than simply prevent vitamin deficiency diseases and that people need to take more than the official RDAs of these vitamins to achieve optimum health. Forty years ago nothing was known about the role of oxidative stress in disease or that many vitamins are potent antioxidants. Again the situation today is radically transformed. It is now known beyond doubt that oxidative stress plays a key role in many chronic diseases, for example coronary artery disease, cancer, diabetes, cystic fibrosis, AIDS, Alzheimer's disease, Parkinson's disease and many others. It has also been established beyond any doubt that a proper lifelong intake of antioxidants and other phytochemicals is essential in order to help protect against the development of these diseases. The only debate today is whether this level of intake can be achieved by increasing the intake of fruit and vegetables or whether supplements are needed. Furthermore there is now a very large body of research under way in the bastions of orthodoxy into the ways that antioxidants can be used actually to treat on-going diseases. Prominent examples are myocardial infarction, ARDS, cystic fibrosis, AIDS, ischemia-reperfusion, organ transplants and many others in all of which very promising results have been attained.

In my new book *Every Person's Guide to Antioxidants* (Rutgers University Press) I describe the role of oxidative stress and of antioxidant therapy in all these diseases. The discovery that vitamins A, C and E are among the leading antioxidants in the body, and that vitamin B3 has an important role in recycling vitamin E, represents one of the most significant advances in medicine in our day. It also explains why the old "mega-vitamin" treatment program worked in so many cases. The concept that the only function of vitamin C is to prevent scurvy is about as sensible as the suggestion that the only function of gasoline is to prevent an automobile from standing still on the roadway.

Lastly I would like to congratulate you for not giving up forty years ago and in showing qualities of grit and determination by being largely responsible for forming the Orthomolecular movement, which allowed people to take the right amount of antioxidant vitamins during the dark ages when everyone else was not. This must have resulted in the prevention of untold thousands of cases of disease and of very many deaths.

greetings from your old friend

John R. Smythies M.D. F.R.C.P.

John Smythies, PhD, co-researcher and lifelong friend

To Abram, on Your 80th Birthday

I've known since I was very young that I am specially blessed. Born with a hole in my heart and not expected to live past two years yet surviving to age nine to undergo successful corrective open heart surgery, I was aware, early on, of my mortality. After the surgery, I grew to have a profound love of life and sense of mission. This love I discovered through music, literature, science, travel, dance, a wonderful array of mentors and friends, and as a teacher, husband and parent.

When I first met you and Rose in the summer of 1987, just a few months after my father's death, I knew that I was entering a new challenge but I didn't realize that this would become the most important work of my life. I am very grateful for having been able to give back so much to life because of you. Whenever I talk about wishing to continue my studies in literature and music, get my doctorate and return to teaching, my university friends remind me that I am making a far greater contribution through the work I am presently doing. You have been a constant anchor for me, an inspiration of love, commitment, integrity, courage, humanity and steadfastness. We both know the pain of loss and the joy of gain. Your support and acknowledgement of me are deeply appreciated.

When I ran into serious new problems with my heart a couple of years ago, I spoke to you about withdrawing from my work with the CSF. But since then so much new growth has developed with this great Foundation and orthomolecular medicine that I realize this mission is far from complete, and I find myself more committed to it than ever. I want you to know that I will continue to do all in my power to keep your vision alive and thriving. I look forward to working at your side well into the next century.

Thank you, Abram, for being so much to me and to tens of thousands of others. You are the greatest mentor a man could wish for. You are a major force in my life, a constant reminder of my blessedness.

I wish you a very Happy Birthday, in love and deep respect,

— Steven

Steven Carter, the Executive Director of the International Schizophrenia Foundation

November 11, 1997

What a pleasure it is for me to be able to share this photo of Dr. Abram Hoffer presenting his fascinating views at The 14th International Conference on Human Functioning, held September, 1995 in Wichita, Kansas. His topic, **_Schizophrenia: An Evolutionary Defense Against Severe Stress_**, was thought provoking and inspiring. This, of course, has been true throughout the odyssey of his professional life, which has provided me and so many others with not only inspiration, but also sound judgment and a profound capacity to observe and record for the benefit of humankind.

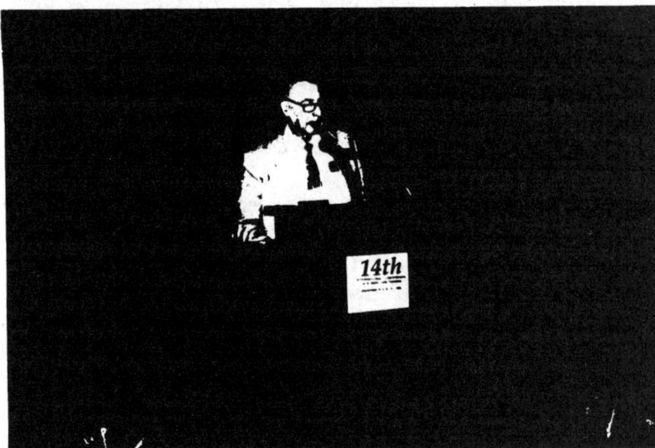

I wish Dr. Hoffer a very Happy Birthday, as he has become "40" again.

Hugh D. Riordan, M.D.

Dr. H.D. Riordan, lifelong friend and colleague

RICHARD A. KUNIN, M.D.
2698 Pacific Avenue
San Francisco, CA 94115
TEL 415-346-2500
FAX 415-346-4991
EMAIL rkunin@aol.com

6 November, 1997

Abram Hoffer
2424 Quadra
Victoria, British Columbia

Dear Abe,

Happy Birthday. I wrote a memento for the occasion of your family get-together but delayed mailing it so that I could search for some of the older pictures that I have put away somewhere. Damn!

I just talked to your daughter, Miriam. The sound of her voice and her compassion at my foibles brought up the deeper feelings of affection that I have always had for you and your family. The desire to complement those feelings with well chosen words can slow down my response time, however. I probably should never re-read anything that I write! I'd certainly get things off my desk a lot quicker. In fact, Abe, I promise you that I will not read this letter but will just get it off this instant. The main thing is that I treasure you as a mentor and friend and I celebrate with you the good fortune of your 80th birthday. That's a very lucky thing, as we both know only too well.

So let me wish for you that you enjoy each and every remaining day of your life as much as this one, where you count up all the blessings of 80 years of family, friends, career--and the life force, itself, and feel yourself buoyed up for the rest of this delightful journey through time and into eternity. You are in good company.

With love,

Richard A. Kunin, M.D.

Richard Kunin, president of Orthomolecular Health Medicine, USA

From Erik T. Paterson, Creston, B.C.

30 September 1997

I have a very restricted list of heroes. In no particular order, they are **Robert Bruce** — who gave everything that his people should be free in the face of appalling odds, **Isaac Newton** — who made the Universe accessible to reason, "and God said let there be light and there was Newton", **Charles Darwin** — who opened up the ascent of humanity to reasoned study against the opposition of extremely powerful forces for unreason, **Florence Nightingale** — who founded two major branches of Medicine, the nursing profession as we understand it to-day, and statistical epidemiology, and who was a major pioneer in founding Public Health, **Albert Einstein** — who showed that the Universe did not behave according to "common sense" — an arrogant human presumption — but by rules which were nonetheless reasonable, **Linus Pauling** — upon whose work **all** modern chemistry (and chemical related fields) is based, **Stephen Hawking** — who united the theories of Relativity and Quantum Physics, **Gerard K. O'Neill** — who invented the tool which gives an understanding of the realm of the ultra-small, and who opened the way for humanity to migrate into the Universe, and **Abram Hoffer** and **Humphry Osmond** — who created a paradigm of Medicine, Orthomolecular Psychiatry — later Orthomolecular Medicine, which will become prevailing in time.

It has been my privilege and honour to have met Pauling, O'Neill, Humphry Osmond and Abram Hoffer. Of these Abram has had the greatest influence upon my life in many ways.

When I was at school and university in Scotland I heard, through my father, of the pioneering work carried out by Abram and Humphry in Saskatchewan. I also encountered the strong prejudice against what they were doing — prejudice which still sadly continues to-day.

In practice in Creston in B.C. I became very dissatisfied with treatment given to mentally ill patients. I spent several days with Abram in late 1973. Those were exciting days, stripping from my mind preconceptions about the wisdom of my teachers. I tried for myself what I had learned from Abram, and my patients, when they stuck with my advice, became well again where my colleagues could not believe such a thing could happen.

Years of study followed, and are still continuing, guided by Abram, allowing me, like many other doctors, to extend the principles of Orthomolecular Medicine into other medical fields to help many suffering patients with many different illnesses.

As a result I have found myself in the role of the medical problem solver of my part of B.C. What happens is that a patient becomes unwell with some illness and goes to his/her doctor, but is unable to become well again. She/he is sent to a specialist of some sort who is unable to help. The patient then hears of me and comes to seek my help. I try harder, and, more often than not, I succeed. Financially it is not rewarding. Emotionally it is very rewarding indeed.

Abram helped my younger daughter overcome severe educational difficulties to become an Honour student at school, and ultimately gain a degree at university.

His advice has helped my wife with the long process of overcoming a long and debilitating illness.

Catastrophe struck me in 1996 when I developed Acute Myeloblastic Leukæmia. Abram's moral support was one of the many influences which helped me in my struggle to survive. Now, far along the road of recuperation, it is his advice which I am using to try to prevent a recurrence of my illness.

My grandmother died when she was nearly 102 years old, but still bright mentally. It is my hope, perhaps unrealistic, that I will surpass her in age and condition. If I do, one of the memories which will remain rich in my mind will be the friendship, support, teaching and influence of Abram Hoffer.

Thank you Abram for so much that you have given me.

Dr. Erik Paterson, orthomolecular physician

Freelance Communications

484 High Ridge Road • Stamford, Connecticut 06905 • area code 203 322-1551

Dr. Morton Walker
Creative Director

COMMUNICATIONS
SERVICES:

WRITING
Editing
articles
books
features
serials
speeches
theses
Ghostwriting
Economics
Medicine
Politics
Psychology
Science
Sociology

ADVERTISING
Copywriting
Layout
Public Relations
Radio Productions

PUBLISHING
Books
Brochures
Catalogues
Flyers
Pamphlets
Printing

RESEARCH
Clinical
Laboratory
Literature
Patents

REPRESENTATIVE
Invention
Literary
Organizations
Syndication

For fastest response, teleFAX (203) 322-4656

October 25, 1997

To you, <u>my cherished coauthor</u>, Abram Hoffer, M.D., Ph.D.,

In mid-September your daughter, Miriam, advised me of the "book of rememberances" in commemoration of your 80th birthday on November 11, 1997. This date is a glorious opportunity to remind you about twenty-two years of our writing together. As one author to another, I have a story to tell.

Our affiliation started in late 1975 when I contributed freelance articles to <u>Drug Therapy Medical Journal</u> and simultaneously was going through the parental agony of a son just recovering from schizophrenia. Two positive circumstances made life less of a burden then. I saw my son's progress by use of orthomolecular nutrition under the supervision of New York City orthomolecular psychiatrist Allan Cott, M.D. And, I was doing good work for <u>Drug Therapy Medical Journal</u>. The editor owed me a favor and I owed orthomolecular psychiatry.

My reward from the journal's editor, Rhoda M. Michaels, Ph.D., was agreement that she would publish two articles about the nutrition science side by side on opposing pages. I was to produce the copy and get leading authorities in psychiatry to contribute the opposing viewpoints. I did so! You represented orthomolecular psychiatry and James Bozzuto, M.D., Assistant Professor of Psychiatry, Department of Psychiatry, School of Medicine, University of Connecticut Health Center, provided strictly drug-oriented information. For instance, Dr. Bozzuto stated: "There is no substantial evidence that megavitamins offer any therapeutic effectiveness as compared to the standard agents."

As a ghost, I wrote the two articles. They were reviewed by the two contributors and accepted for publication by Ms Michaels. At the last minute, when I let drop to Dr. Bozzuto that the format was opposing viewpoints, he withdrew his name and information. He wanted no part of any kind of support for a "quack science"! Consequently, your byline was the only one to appear in the Journal's issue of August 1977, under the title "Orthomolecular Psychiatry in Theory and Practice." I provide a photocopy of that piece here.

As it turned out, yours became the most popular "quack" piece in the history of <u>Drug Therapy Medical Journal</u>. Letters to the editor were more voluminous than for any other article and the vast majority of them were positive. Physicians in drug-oriented medicine told of efficacious effects for patients for whom they recommended nutritional therapy. It was a revelation for the doctors and our giving exposure to the issue was confirmation that they had done well.

Well, Abram, you and I went on to publish several more articles together which culminated in Keats Publishing, Inc. coming out in 1978 with our landmark book, <u>Orthomolecular Nutrition: New Lifestyle for Super Good Health</u>, with a foreword by Linus Pauling, Ph.D. This was updated and reissued last year by Keats as <u>Putting It All Together: The New Orthomolecular Nutrition</u>. Then in 1980, for Keats, we coauthored <u>Nutrients to Age Without Senility</u> which has been reissued by Avery Publishing Group, Inc. as <u>Smart Nutrients: A Guide to Nutrients that Can Prevent and Reverse Senility</u>.

Merely through our affiliations together, Abram, I have become a better person. A certain uplift occurs for someone coming under your sphere of influence. That has been my impression and others have told me the same. You are a very special human being, and for that reason, when Stockholm's Karolinska Institute, in July 1997, allowed me to become an invitee to put forth a candidate for the NOBEL PRIZE IN MEDICINE OR PHYSIOLOGY, I provided the Committe with your name, location, and whatever qualifications I know.

Quite simply, I respect you and love you, Abram. Being a part of your life has made my own life better. And for this, I thank you!

Your coauthor and friend,

Morton Walker, DPM

Morton Walker, D.P.M., Editorial Director
FREELANCE COMMUNICATIONS

Morton Walker, medical science writer

William B. Parsons Jr., M.D.
8121 E. Del Plomo Drive
Scottsdale, Arizona 85258

October 20, 1997

Dear Friends,

In August 1955 Dr. Abram Hoffer gave a series of lectures on schizophrenia at the Mayo Clinic, Rochester, Minnesota. For years he had given large doses of niacin (nicotinic acid) to schizophrenic patients. His former Professor of Anatomy, Dr. Rudolf Altschul had suggested measuring cholesterol levels, predicting that they were being reduced. A brief, informal study showed him to be correct. On his last evening in Rochester, Dr. Hoffer shared this experience with Mayo's chief of psychiatry, Dr. Howard Rome.

On the following morning, Rome passed this information to Dr. Edgar Allen, consultant on the Peripheral Vascular Service at St. Mary's Hospital that month. His first assistant, Dr. William Parsons, was the only one sufficiently intrigued by the idea to confirm it, in the first systematic study of niacin for abnormal cholesterol values. His paper introduced niacin therapy to the medical world. It was the first successful drug for cholesterol control and is still the best.

Consider the series of coincidences leading to these developments:
- Altschul and Hoffer, driving to a meeting, shared their interests.
- Before becoming a psychiatrist, Rome was a board-certified internist.
- Rome was especially interested in drug therapy since Thorazine, a fairly recent development, was getting people out of mental hospitals. Thus he was a receptive listener.
- For years Allen and Rome had hunted ducks together each fall.
- These duck-hunting buddies were on their respective hospital services that month.
- Parsons was on Allen's service at the time of Hoffer's visit.

Niacin's ideal actions on all serum lipid values make it a designer drug. Despite lack of commercial promotion, its value is even today becoming better recognized. A major study showed that niacin reduced heart attacks, strokes and related events, cardiovascular surgery, hospitalization, and deaths. One can only imagine the number of major cardiovascular events and deaths it has already prevented, and the number keeps increasing.

IT WAS MEANT TO BE!

Thank you, dear Abram, for the inspiration to pioneer niacin for cholesterol control. I look forward to meeting you in person next week.

With the greatest respect and affection on the occasion of your 80th birthday,

Bill Parsons

Dr. W. Parsons, formerly of the Mayo Clinic

Autism Research Institute

4182 Adams Avenue
San Diego, California 92116

BERNARD RIMLAND, Ph.D., Director

(619) 281-7165

fax: 619-563-6840
www.autism.com/ari

September 29, 1997

Abram Hoffer, M.D.
379 Concord Ave.
Toronto, ONT M6H 2P9
Canada

Dear Abe

You are a <u>very</u> special person — a really terrific guy. There are very few people in the planet who even come close to you in terms of the positive contributions you have made to mankind.

Faced with massive opposition from powerful forces, you remain undaunted and simply continue your good work.

I admire you greatly and am proud to be your friend.

With respect and affection,

Bernard Rimland, Ph.D.

BRmo

R. Rimland, PhD

Abram Hoffer,

Eighty years ago, on November 11 1917. A young lad came into the world . One year later one of the greatest wars this world had ever seen, ended.. This youngster was to grow up and dedicate his life to the saving of people and to make a major contribution in the field of Medicine. Ab. as he is know to thousands of people around the world, is one of the most sought after speakers at International Conferences on Complementary Medicine.

In addition to this heavy load of speaking engagements and all the traveling that goes with it, he still finds time with his first love, that of helping patients facing life threating illnesses. One wonders how he keeps up with all the demands on his time and the stress that must go with it.

Recently I was talk to an old friend of mine from Saskatchewan. It seems she was a patient of Doctor Hoffer some fifty odd years ago. I told her that he was one of a very select number of Doctor's that advise the Lotte and John Hecht Memorial Foundation on Medical Programs and Issues. She told me of a poem she once heard.

Around the corner I have a wonderful friend,
In this great city that has no end,
Yet days go by and weeks rush on,
And before I know it a year has gone,
Yet I never see my old friends face,
For life is swift and a terrible race,
He knows I respect him just as well,
As in the days when I rang his bell,
And he looked after my Medical problems,

And now I am busy, a tried old girl,
Tried with playing a foolish game,
Tired with trying to make a name,
Tomorrow ,I said 'I would call Ab.'
Just to show that I remember him,
But tomorrow comes and tomorrow goes,
Around the corner-yet miles away.
There is a note in the paper,
That Ab. spoke again today,

And that 's all I get, and deserve in the end,
Around the corner a vanishing friend,
And may God forgive me in the end..

A patient's poem

3580 Cedar Hill Rd
Victoria, BC. V8P 3Z1
Oct 30-97

Dear Dr. Hoffer

I would like to congratulate you on your 80th Birthday! I would also like to tell you how much I admire you as you have pursued a career in medicine, the purpose of which has been to improve the general health of we human beings and especially those who are mentally ill.

While the psychiatric profession, as a whole subscribed to the theories of Sigmund Freud you reasoned logically that mental illness was the result of a persons body chemistry malfunctioning.

If I had met you, or known of your approach to treating schizophrenia 10 yrs. earlier, my daughter, Diane, may have well been spared the agonies of hospitalization and ECTs and experienced a normal childhood. (Her symptoms were so minor until she reached puberty.)

As it is, I am so thankful that we were put in touch with you when all seemed hopeless. I believe I mentioned briefly in your office how that came to pass and how we felt that it was an answer to our prayers because it was really a miracle.

My wife's Brother, who was in the Canadian Navy was on a two-year assignment to a U.S. Naval Depot in Charleston, S.C. One evening, he turned on the TV and it was announced that a Canadian psychiatrist by the name of (guess who) was going to be interviewed on the subject of schizophrenia. He turned to his wife (a Registered Nurse) and asked "Isn't that what Diane has?" Of course, in that day and age few would admit that it was "in the family." Well, fortunately, she phoned my wife (Italian) who confirmed that Diane did have schizophrenia. (We were living 3,000 miles away in California at the time). I still remember receiving a letter from them with a clipping out of the Charleston newspaper mentioning the 3gms. of Niacin and of Vitamin C. It must also have given your address as we began corresponding with you immediately. I recall how punctual your letters were. We would have a response from you within a week of mailing our letter.

We started Diane on the Megavitamins in 1966. After 5 months our local psychiatrist said he saw no improvement in Diane. However, Lil & I knew there was something changing even although not too obvious. We were able to reduce her medication Thorazine from 1000 mgms/dy to 300 mgms/dy. Also, there was a black substance which came out of her body which, after much scrubbing (even lightly with steel wool) left her skin pink like a baby.

Once again I wrote to you stating that our local psychiatrist was ready to give up on the megavitamins as he had seen so results. You responded with the most encouraging letter telling us to "stick with it & not to give up." Would you believe it was that very same week that I saw Diane's first significant improvement. I went to the Bathroom and wrapped on the door to ask her to pass out the deodorant as she did, she raised her gown to conceal her breasts (she was sponge bathing). I thought to myself "Praise the LORD, she had regained "modesty" which she had been taught in her youth.

It has been a rather tedious up till battle but by sticking with the MEGAVITAMINS as you suggested, we now have a lovely girl, anxious to please, and a good help around the house. I am so grateful to you for all you have done for me and my family.

Most Sincerely & Respectfully
Glenn Tamblyn

P.S. I tell Diane she has so much to be thankful for. With most illnesses, people seem to get worse as time goes by, but with your treatment she continues to improve each year. (She had her first "crush" on a man 2 yrs. ago so I think romantically she is going through her "teens")

A letter from the family of a recovered patient.

BIBLIOGRAPHY

To date I have published nearly 600 articles in the medical literature and over 30 books (including translations). The articles include original papers written alone or with coauthors, book reviews, editorials, and comments. The following is a focused listing of what I consider my most important publications. I have grouped the papers by topic. I consider my most significant contribution to scientific research to be the work I did with Dr. Humphry Osmond in developing the adrenochrome hypothesis and examining the various derivative ideas and findings that that hypothesis generated.

The Adrenochrome Hypothesis of Schizophrenia

The adrenochrome hypothesis is basic to all the research I planned and carried out. The main objective of any scientific hypothesis is to direct and focus research which will lead to new and valuable information. Hypotheses can never be entirely correct because they are always based on current knowledge. As new information accrues, the hypothesis itself will be subject to change. The following list of publications indicates how thoroughly and widely we reported our hypothesis and its ramifications. In these writings, we showed that all the conditions necessary for the formation of adrenochrome and similar compounds are present in the body, that adrenochrome is in fact made by the body, and that it is an hallucinogen.

Hoffer A & Osmond H: Paper to Dementia Praecox Committee, Scottish Rites Masons, New York. Given at the Canada Room, The Waldorf Astoria, New York, 1952. This paper was our first report on the adrenochrome hypothesis.

Hoffer A., Osmond H & Smythies J: Schizophrenia: a new approach II. Results of a year's research. *Journal of Mental Science* 1954;100:29-45.

Hoffer A: Experimental pharmacodynamics and psychobiology. *Journal of Clinical Experimental Psychopathology* 1956;17:376-377.

Hoffer A & Kenyon M: Conversion of adrenaline to adrenolutin in human blood serum. *Archives of Neurology Psychiatry* 1957;77:437-438.

Hoffer A. Adrenolutin as a psychotomimetic agent. In, *Tranquilizing Drugs*, Ed. Himwich HE, American Association for the Advancement of Science, Publ #46, Washington, DC, 1957.

Hoffer A. *Hormones, Brain Function and Behavior*. Ed. Hoagland, H. Academic Press. New York. 1957.

Hoffer A: Epinephrine derivatives as potential schizophrenic factors. *Journal of Clinical Experimental Psychopathology* 1957;18:27-60.

Hoffer A: Relation of epinephrine metabolites to schizophrenia. *Chemical Concepts of Psychiatry*. Eds. Rinkel M & Denber HGB. McDowell-Obolensky Inc., New York, 1958.

Hoffer A: Adrenochrome and adrenolutin and their relationship to mental disease. *Psychotropic Drugs*. Eds. Garattini S & Ghetti V. Elsevier Press, London 1957.

Hoffer A: The adrenochrome hypothesis of schizophrenia. Paper read to Proceedings Sixth Annual Psychiatric Institute, Princeton, September 1958. Published in *Proceedings*, 36-53.

Hoffer A: Mode of action of ergot hallucinogens. Brain Research Foundation, Jan 1958. In *Molecules and Mental Health*. Ed. FA Gibbs, JB Lippincott Co., Phil. 1959.

Hoffer A: Action of epinephrine breakdown products on cerebral function. Paper delivered at Society Biological Psychiatry, San Francisco, May 1958. *Biological Psychiatry*, Grune & Stratton, 1959.

Hoffer A & Osmond H: The adrenochrome model and schizophrenia. *J Nervous and Mental Disease* 1959;128:18-35.

Osmond H & Hoffer A: Schizophrenia: a new approach III. *Journal Mental Science* 1959;105:653-673.

Hoffer A & Callbeck MJ: Drug-induced schizophrenia. *Journal Mental Science*, 1960;106:138-159.

Hoffer A: Adrenaline metabolites and schizophrenia. *Diseases of the Nervous System* 1960; 21, Monograph Supplement, 79-86.

Hoffer A & Osmond H: The biochemistry of mental disease. *Canadian Medical Association Journal* 1961;85:1309-1311.

Hoffer A: The effect of adrenochrome and adrenolutin on the behavior of animals and the pyschology of man. *International Review Neurobiology* 1962;4:307-371.

Hoffer A & Osmond H: A comprehensive theory of schizophrenia. *Mind* 1963;1:119-121.

Hoffer A: The adrenochrome theory of schizophrenia: a review. *Diseases of the Nervous System* 1964; 25:173-178.

Osmond H & Hoffer A: A comprehensive theory of schizophrenia. *International Journal of Neuropsychiatry* 1965;2:302-309.

Hoffer A & Osmond H: *How To Live With Schizophrenia*. University Books, New York, NY, 1966. Also published by Johnson, London, 1966. Co-written by Fannie Kahan. New and Revised Ed. Citadel Press, New York, N.Y. 1992. Revised by Hoffer A and called *Healing Schizophrenia*, CCNM Press Toronto 2004.

Hoffer A & Osmond H: *The Hallucinogens*. Academic Press, New York, 1967. This book required three printings of 2,000 copies each in its first year. It was a scientific best seller (selling 2,000 copies alone would have made it so) and considered a classic by one reviewer. It is probably one of the most widely read and least referred to books in the literature.

Hoffer A: Biochemical aspects of schizophrenia. In *Schizophrenia: Current Concepts and Research*. Ed. DV Siva Sankar. P.J.D. Publications, Ltd., Hecksville, New York, 1969; 628-637.

Hoffer A: Hallucinogens. *Encyclopedia Britannica* 15th Ed., 1974; 557-560.

Hoffer A: The adrenochrome hypothesis of schizophrenia revisited. *Journal of Orthomolecular Psychiatry* 1981;10:98-118.

Hoffer A: Oxidation-reduction in the brain. *Journal of Orthomolecular Psychiatry* 1983;12:292-301.

Hoffer A: *Common Questions on Schizophrenia and Their Answers*. Keats Publishing, New Canaan, CT, 1988.

Hoffer A & Osmond H: The adrenochrome hypothesis and psychiatry. *Journal of Orthomolecular Medicine* 1990;5:32-45.

The treatment of schizophrenia

The adrenochrome hypothesis suggested that niacin and other nutrients might be of assistance to schizophrenics. We tested the idea in double-blind trials and in clinical practice and found we were correct.

Hoffer A & Parsons S: Histamine therapy for schizophrenia: a follow-up study. *Canadian Medical Association Journal* 1955;72:352-355.

Hoffer A, Osmond H, Callbeck MJ & Kahan I: Treatment of schizophrenia with nicotinic acid and nicotinamide. *Journal of Clinical Experimental Psychopathology* 1957;18:131-158.

Hoffer A: *Niacin Therapy in Psychiatry*. CC Thomas, Springfield, IL, 1962.

Hoffer A & Osmond H: Some schizophrenic recoveries. *Diseases Nervous System* 1962;23:204-210.

Osmond H & Hoffer A: Massive niacin treatment in schizophrenia. Review of a nine-year study. *Lancet* 1963;1:316-320.

Hoffer A: Nicotinic acid: an adjunct in the treatment of schizophrenia. *Am Journal of Psychiatry* 1963;120:171-173.

Hoffer A & Osmond H: Treatment of schizophrenia with nicotinic acid—a ten year follow-up. *Acta Psychiatrica Scandinavica* 1964;40:171-189.

Hoffer A: The effect of nicotinic acid on the frequency and duration of re-hospitalization of schizophrenic patients; A controlled comparison study. *International Journal of Neuropsychiatry* 1966; 2:234-240.

Hoffer A: Five California schizophrenics. *Journal of Schizophrenia* 1967;1:209-220.

Hoffer A: Treatment of schizophrenia with a therapeutic program based upon nicotinic acid as the main variable. *Molecular Basis of Some Aspects of Mental Activity, Vol II*; 435-456 Ed. O Walaas, Academic Press, New York, 1967.

Hoffer A: Nicotinamide adenine dinucleotide in the treatment of chronic schizophrenic patients. *British Journal of Psychiatry* 1968;114:915-917.

Hoffer A: A vitamin B-3 dependent family. *Schizophrenia* 1971;3:41-46.

Hoffer A: Megavitamin B-3 therapy for schizophrenia. *Canadian Psychiatric Association Journal* 1971;16:499-504.

Hoffer A: Orthomolecular treatment of schizophrenia. *Orthomolecular Psychiatry* 1972;1:46-55.

Hoffer A: Treatment of hyperkinetic children with nicotinamide and pyridoxine. *Canadian Medical Association Journal* 1972;107:111-112.

Hoffer A: Orthomolecular treatment for schizophrenia. *Medical Counterpart* 1973;4:10-20.

Hoffer A: Mechanism of action of nicotinic acid and nicotinamide in the treatment of schizophrenia. In *Orthomolecular Psychiatry*, Eds. DR Hawkins and Linus Pauling. WH Freeman and Co., San Francisco, 1973

Hoffer A: Treatment of schizophrenia. *Journal of Orthomolecular Psychiatry* 1974;3:280-290.

Hoffer A: Editorial. The Wittenborn study. *Journal of Orthomolecular Psychiatry* 1975;4:254-255.

Hoffer A: Natural history and treatment of thirteen pairs of identical twins, schizophrenic and schizophrenic-spectrum conditions. *Journal of Orthomolecular Psychiatry* 1976;5:101-122.

Hoffer A & Osmond H: Schizophrenia: another long term follow-up in Canada. *Journal of Orthomolecular Psychiatry* 1980;9:107-113.

Hoffer A: Chronic schizophrenic patients treated ten years or more. *Journal of Orthomolecular Medicine*, 1994;9:7-37.

Hoffer A: Treatment of Schizophrenia. *Townsend Letter for Doctors and Patients* #144, July 1995, 52-57.

Hoffer A: Orthomolecular: The optimum treatment for schizophrenia. *Journal of Orthomolecular Medicine* 1995;20:169-176

Hoffer A: Orthomolecular Treatment of Schizophrenia. *Complementary Medicine*. Offical Journal of the South African Complementary Medicine Association. 1998;4,9-14.

Hoffer A: Orthomolecular Treatment for Schizophrenia. *Integrative Medicine* 1:18-21,2002

Clinical observations of schizophrenia

Fogel S & Hoffer A: Perceptual changes induced by hypnotic suggestion for the posthypnotic state. *Journal of Clinical Experimental Psychopatholgy* 1962;23:24-35.

Fogel S & Hoffer A: The use of hypnosis to interrupt and to reproduce an LSD-25 experience. *Journal of Clinical Experimental Psychopathology* 1962;23:11-16.

Hoffer A & Osmond H: Olfactory changes in schizophrenia. *American Journal of Psychiatry* 1962;119:72-75.

Hoffer A & Osmond H: Abstraction and schizophrenia. *Canadian Psychiatric Association Journal* 1962;7:186-190.

Hoffer A & Osmond H. People are watching me. *Psychiatric Quarterly* 1963;37:7-18.

Hoffer A & Osmond H: A question of insight. *Diseases of the Nervous System* 1963;24.

Huxley J, Mayr E, Osmond H & Hoffer A: Schizophrenia as a genetic morphism. *Nature*, 1964;204:220-221.

Hoffer A & Osmond H: Some psychological consequences of perceptual disorder and schizophrenia. *International Journal of Neuropsychiatry* 1966;2:1-19.

Hoffer A & Osmond H: A perceptual hypothesis of schizophrenia. *Psychiatric Digest* 1967;28:47-53.

Osmond H & Hoffer A: Schizophrenia and suicide. *Journal of Schizophrenia* 1967;1:54-64.

Hoffer A: Inappropriate mood and schizophrenia. *Schizophrenia* 1970;2:116-118.

Hoffer A: Pellagra and schizophrenia. Academy of Psychosomatic Medicine, Buenos Aires, Jan. 12-18, 1970. *Psychosomatic II*, 1970;522-525.

Hoffer A: Schizophrenia: an evolutionary advance. *Journal of Orthomolecular Psychiatry* 1973;2:39-65.

Hoffer A: The prevention of tardive dyskinesia (tranquilizer induced illness). *Healthy Options*, 1990;127:17-20. P.O. Box 6041, Tauranga, New Zealand,

The mauve factor

Hoffer A & Mahon M: The presence of unidentified substances in the urine of psychiatric patients. *Journal of Neuropsychiatry* 1961;2:331-362.

Hoffer A & Osmond H: The relationship between an unknown factor (US) in the urine of subjects and HOD test results. *Journal of Neuropsychiatry* 1961;2:363-368.

Hoffer A: The presence of malvaria in some mentally retarded children. *American Journal of Mental Deficiency* 1963;67:730-732.

Hoffer A & Osmond H: Malvaria: a new psychiatric disease. *Acta Psychiatrica Scandinavica* 1963;39:335-366.

Hoffer A: Malvaria, schizophrenia and the HOD test. *Int. Journal of Neuropsychiatry* 1965;2:175-177.

Hoffer A: Malvaria and the law. *Psychosomatics* 1966;7:303-310.

Hoffer A: Families of malvarians. *Journal of Schizophrenia* 1967;1:77-89.

Diagnosing schizophrenia

To this day, schizophrenia is frequently misdiagnosed. The Hoffer-Osmond Diagnostic test (HOD) that Humphry and I developed proved accurate and invaluable in the diagnostic process. Our group also discovered a previously unknown substance in the urine of some schizophrenic patients.

Hoffer A: Objective criteria for the diagnosis of schizophrenia. *Confinia Neurologica* 1954;14:385-390.

Hoffer A & Osmond H: A card sorting test helpful in making psychiatric diagnosis. *Journal of Neuropsychiatry* 1961;2:306-330.

Hoffer A & Mahon M: The presence of unidentified substances in the urine of psychiatric patients. *Journal of Neuropsychiatry* 1961;2:331-362.

Hoffer A & Osmond H: The relationship between an unknown factor (US) in the urine of subjects and HOD test results. *Journal of Neuropsychiatry* 1961;2:363-368.

Hoffer A & Osmond H: A card sorting test helpful in establishing prognosis. *American Journal of Psychiatry* 1962;118:840-841.

Hoffer A & Osmond H: The association between schizophrenia and two objective tests. *Canadian Medical Association Journal* 1962;87:641-646.

Hoffer A: Reliability of the Hoffer-Osmond Diagnostic test. *Journal of Clinical Psychology* 1967;23:380-384.

Methodology

We were the first psychiatric group to conduct double-blind therapeutic trials, which are now considered the gold standard for treatment trials. I was also one of the first to point out the limitations of this technique.

Clancy J, Hoffer A, Lucy J, Osmond H, Smythies J & Stefaniak B: Design and planning in psychiatric research as illustrated by the Weyburn Chronic Nucleotide Project. *Bulletin Menninger Clinic*, 1954;18:147-153.

Osmond H & Hoffer A: On critics and research. *Psychosomatic Medicine* 1959;21:311-320.

Hoffer A & Osmond H: Double-blind clinical trials. *Journal of Neuropathology* 1961;2:221-227.

Hoffer A & Osmond H: Some problems of stochastic psychiatry. *Journal of Neuropsychiatry* 1963;5:97-11.

Hoffer A: Single case design and double-blind comparison studies for drug evaluation. *Mind*: Psychiatry in General Practice, 1964;2:119-120.

Hoffer A: Faith, hope and chemotherapy. *Chemotherapy* 1964;9:263-274.

Hoffer A: A theoretical examination of double-blind design. *Canadian Medical Association Journal* 1967;97:123-127.

Hoffer A: Symposium on statistical aspects of protocol design. Discussion. Cancer Clinical Investigation Review Committee, San Juan, Puerto Rico, 1970;224-229, Dec. 9-10.

Hoffer A: An examination of the double-blind method as it has been applied to megavitamin therapy. *Orthomolecular Psychiatry* 1973;2:107-114.

Hoffer A. The double-blind method. *Canadian Psychiatric Association Journal* 1976;6:449-450.

Hoffer A. Lies, Damn Lies and Statistics: The Statistics Game. *The Townsend Letter for Doctors & Patients*. #255 October 2004, 124-126

The treatment of alcoholism

Hoffer A, Chwelos N, Blewett DB & Smith CM: Use of d-lysergic acid diethylamide in the treatment of alcoholism. *Quarterly Journal of Studies in Alcoholism* 1959;20:577-590.

Hoffer A & Osmond H: Concerning an etiological factor in alcoholism. The possible role of adrenochrome metabolism. *Quarterly Journal of Studies in Alcoholism* 1959;20:750-756.

Hoffer A: Mode of action of ergot hallucinogens. Paper read at Scientific Conference of the Brain Research Foundation, Jan. 25, 1958, New York City, Published in *Molecules and Mental Health*, Ed. FA Gibbs, J.B. Lippincott Co Philadelphia, 1959.

Hoffer A: Enzymology of hallucinogens. Reprinted in *Enzymes in Mental Health*. Eds. JG Martin & B Kisch, J.B. Lippincott Co., 1966.

Hoffer A & Osmond H: *New Hope For Alcoholics*, University Books, New York, 1966. Co-written by Fannie Kahan.

Hoffer A: Treatment of alcoholism with psychedelic therapy. *Psychedelics: Their Uses and Implications*. Eds. BS Aaronson & H Osmond. Doubleday and Co., New York, 1967.

Hoffer A: A program for the treatment of alcoholism: LSD, malvaria and nicotinic acid. In *The Use of LSD in Psychotherapy and Alcoholism*. Ed. HA Abramson. Bobbs-Merrill, New York, 1967;343-402.

Hoffer A: Psychedelic experiences and the law. *Chitty's Law Journal* 1967;15:182-188.

Hoffer A: Treatment of alcoholism with psychedelic therapy. *Psychedelics*, Eds. B Aaronson & H Osmond. Anchor Books, Doubleday and Co. Inc., Garden City, NY, 1970.

Niacin and cholesterol

Altschul, Hoffer and Stephen discovered that niacin lowers cholesterol levels. Niacin today provides the gold standard by which all other cholesterol lowering compounds must be judged. It lowers total cholesterol, lowers triglycerides, lowers lipoprotein A and elevates high density lipoproteins (HDL). No other substance is known to be as beneficial. Since niacin is not patented, however, pharmaceutical firms insist on peddling anti-cholesterol drugs which have a whole range of potential dangerous side effects.

Altschul R, Hoffer A & Stephen JD: Influence of nicotinic acid on serum cholesterol in man. *Archives of Biochemical Biophysics* 1955;54:558-559.

Hoffer A & Callbeck MJ: The hypocholesterolemic effect of nicotinic acid and its relationship to the autonomic nervous system. *Journal of Mental Science* 1957;103:810-820.

Altschul R & Hoffer A: The effect of nicotinic acid upon serum cholesterol and upon basal metabolic rate of young normal adults. *Archives of Biochemistry and Biophysics* 1958;73:420-424.

Altschul R & Hoffer A: Effects of salts of nicotinic acid on serum cholesterol. *British Medical Journal* 1958;2:713-714.

Hoffer A, O'Reilly PO & Callbeck MJ: Specificity of the hypocholesterolemic activity of nicotinic acid. *Diseases of the Nervous System* 1959; 20:286-288.

O'Reilly PO, Callbeck MJ & Hoffer A: Sustained-release nicotinic acid (Nicospan). Effect on (1) cholesterol levels and (2) leukocytes. *Canadian Medical Association Journal* 1959;80:359-362.

Altschul R & Hoffer A: The effect of nicotinic acid on hypercholesterolemia. *Canadian Medical Association Journal* 1960;82:783-785.

Hoffer A: The relationship of nicotinic acid to cholesterol metabolism. *Journal of Clinical Experimental Psychopathology* 1961;22:165-179.

Hoffer A: Safety, side effects and relative lack of toxicity of nicotinic acid and nicotinamide. *Schizophrenia* 1969;1:78-87.

Hoffer A: Niacin, coronary disease and longevity. *Journal of Orthomolecular Medicine* 1989;4:211-220.

Hoffer A: *Vitamin B-3 (Niacin) Update. New Roles For a Key Nutrient in Diabetes, Cancer, Heart Disease and Other Major Health Problems.* Keats Publishing Inc., New Canaan, CT, 1990.

Hoffer A: Vitamin B-3: Niacin and its amide. *Townsend Letter for Doctors and Patients* #147, Oct 1995,30-39.

Hoffer, A. Vitamin B-3 Does Not Cure Tranquilizer Psychoses. *Townsend Letter for Doctors and Patients* 2001;88-91.# 213.

Niacin and arthritis

I wrote a book review of Dr. William Kaufman's two very important books, published around 1949 and totally ignored.

Hoffer A: Treatment of arthritis by nicotinic acid and nicotinamide. *Canadian Medical Association Journal* 1959;81:235-238.

Agnew N and Hoffer A: Nicotinic acid modified lysergic acid diethylamide psychosis. *Journal Mental Science* 1955;101;12-27.

Cancer

The following studies were published in order to promote interest in using vitamin C as a cancer treatment. Interest was generated, but mostly of a negative and hostile type.

Hoffer A & Pauling L: Hardin Jones biostatistical analysis of mortality data for cohorts of cancer patients with a large fraction surviving at the termination of the study and a comparison of survival times of cancer patients receiving large regular oral doses of vitamin C and other nutrients with similar patients not receiving those doses. *Journal of Orthomolecular Medicine* 1990;5: 143-154. Reprinted in *Cancer and Vitamin C*, Ed. Cameron and L Pauling, Camino Books, Inc. P.O. Box 59026, Phil. PA, 19102, 1993.

Hoffer A & Pauling L: Hardin Jones biostatistical analysis of mortality data for a second set of cohorts of cancer patients with a large fraction surviving at the termination of the study and a comparison of survival times of cancer patients receiving large regular oral doses of vitamin C and other nutrients with similar patients not receiving these doses. *Journal of Orthomolecular Medicine* 1993; 8:157-167.

Hoffer A: Orthomolecular Oncology. In *Adjuvant Nutrition in Cancer Treatment*, Ed. P Quillin & RM Williams. 1992 Symposium Proceedings, Sponsored by Cancer Treatment Research Foundation and American College of Nutrition. Cancer Treatment Research Foundation, 3455 Salt Creek Lane, Suite 200, Arlington Heights, IL 60005-1090, 1994.

Hoffer A: Orthomolecular Treatment of Cancer. In *Nutrients in Cancer Prevention and Treatment*. Ed. Prasad KN, Santamaria L & Williams RM. Pages 373-391,1995, Humana Press, Totowa, New Jersey.

Hoffer A: One Patient's Recovery From Lymphoma. *Townsend Letter for Doctors and Patients* #160,1996;50-51.

Hoffer, A. and Foster HD. Why Schizophrenics Smoke but Have Lower Incidence of Lung Cancer: Implications for the Treatment of Both Disorders. *Journal of Orthomolecular Medicine* 2000;15:141-144.

Criminal behaviour and nutrition

Hoffer A: The relation of crime to nutrition. *Humanist in Canada* 34:2-9, 1975.

Hoffer A: Some theoretical principles basic to orthomolecular psychiatric treatment. In *Ecologic-Biochemical Approaches to Treatment of Delinquents and Criminals*. Ed. LJ Hippchen. Van Nostrand-Reinhold Co, New York, 1978.

Hoffer A: Crime, punishment and treatment. *Journal of Orthomolecular Psychiatry* 1979;8:193-199.

Hoffer A: Nutrition and behavior. In *Medical Applications of Clinical Nutrition*. Ed. J Bland. Keats Pub, New Canaan CT, 1983.

Huntington's Disease

Hoffer A: Latent Huntington's disease—response to orthomolecular treatment. *Journal of Orthomolecular Psychiatry* 1983;12:44-47.

Hoffer A: Huntington's disease: a follow-up. *Journal of Orthomolecular Psychiatry* 1984;13:42-44.

Hoffer A: Huntington's Disease. *Townsend Letter for Doctors and Patients* #163/164, 1997;46-51.

General discussions of nutrition and disease

Hoffer A: Hong Kong veterans study. *Journal of Orthomolecular Psychiatry* 1973;3:34-36.

Hoffer A: Senility and chronic malnutrition. *Journal of Orthomolecular Psychiatry* 1974;3:2-19.

Hoffer A: Calories, protein, lipids, carbohydrates and the Saccharine Disease. *Journal of Orthomolecular Psychiatry* 1974;3:231-239.

Hoffer A: Nutrition and schizophrenia. *Canadian Family Physician* 1975;21:78-82.

Hoffer A & Walker M: *Orthomolecular Nutrition*. Keats Pub, New Canaan, CT, 1978.

Hoffer A: Nutrition and behavior. In *Medical Applications of Clinical Nutrition*. Ed. J Bland. Keats Pub, New Canaan CT, 222-251, 1983.

Hoffer A: Orthomolecular nutrition at the zoo. *Journal of Orthomolecular Psychiatry* 1983;12:116-128.

Hoffer A & Walker M: *Smart Nutrients: A Guide to Nutrients That Can Prevent and Reverse Senility*. Avery Publishing Group, Garden City Park, NY, 1994.

Hoffer A: *Hoffer's Law of Natural Nutrition*. Quarry Press, Kingston, ON, 1996.

Controversy

Hoffer A & Osmond H: *In Reply to The American Psychiatric Association Task Force Report on Megavitamin and Orthomolecular Therapy in Psychiatry*. Canadian Schizophrenia Foundation, Regina, Sask., now 16 Florence Ave., Toronto, ON, Canada M2N 1E9, August 1976. This rebuttal of the APA Task Force Report is available on www.Doctoryourself.com *http://www.iahf.com/orthomolecular/reply_to_apa_tfr_7.pdf.*

ABRAM HOFFER, M.D., PH.D. 50 YEARS OF MEGAVITAMIN RESEARCH, PRACTICE, AND PUBLICATION

BIBLIOGRAPHY OF THE NUTRITION-RELATED PUBLICATIONS OF ABRAM HOFFER, M.D.

Edited by Andrew W. Saul and Dr. Hoffer

Notes to the reader:

1) This bibliography is a shortened version of Dr. Hoffer's 550 scientific publications. This is a listing of his English language, nutrition-related books and articles only. Listings are oldest first. (Parenthetical comments are Dr. Hoffer's.)

2) "Orthomolecular" is essentially another word for "megavitamin".

3) "Nicotinic acid" is a chemical name for vitamin B-3, niacin. It is wholly unrelated to nicotine.

Books:

1. Hoffer A & Osmond H. *The Chemical Basis of Clinical Psychiatry.* CC Thomas, Springfield, IL, 1960.

2. Hoffer A. *Niacin Therapy in Psychiatry.* CC Thomas, Springfield, IL, 1962.

3. Hoffer A & Osmond H. *How To Live With Schizophrenia.* University Books, New York, NY, 1966. Also published by Johnson, London, 1966. New and Revised Ed. Citadel Press, New York, NY, 1992. Revised Ed. Quarry Press, Kingston, ON 1999 (Review). Co-written by Fannie Kahan.

4. Hoffer A & Osmond H. *New Hope For Alcoholics.* University Books, New York, 1966. Co-written by Fannie Kahan. (No known electronic link)

5. Kelm H, Hoffer A & Osmond H. *Hoffer-Osmond Diagnostic Manual.* Saskatoon, SK, 1967.

6. Hoffer A. *The Hallucinogens.* Academic Press (June, 1967)

7. Hoffer A & Osmond H. *Comment Vivre Avec la Schizophrenie.* Flammarion Editeur, 26 rue Racine, Paris, 1970.

8. Hoffer A, Kelm H & Osmond H. *The Hoffer-Osmond Diagnostic Test.* RE Krieger Pub. Co., Huntington, NY, 1975.

9. Hoffer A. *Megavitamin therapy: In reply to the American Psychiatric Association Task Force report on megavitamins and orthomolecular psychiatry.* Canadian Schizophrenia Foundation (1976) Full text posted at http://www.iahf.com/orthomolecular/reply_to_apa_tfr_7.pdf

10. Hoffer A & Walker M. *Orthomolecular Nutrition.* Keats Pub., New Canaan, CT, 1978.

11. Hoffer A. *Dr Abram Hoffer's Guide to the Identification and Treatment of Schizophrenia.* Keats Pub (June 1, 1980)

12. Hoffer A & Walker M. *Nutrients to Age Without Senility.* Keats Pub Inc, New Canaan, CT, 1980.

13. Hoffer A & Walker M. *Nutritione Ortomolecolare.* Translated by Crivelli & B. Dozzo, Edizioni Di red./studio redazionale, Via volla 43, 22100 Como. Italy, 1982.

14. Hoffer A. *Vitamin B3.* McFarland & Company (August 1, 1982)

15. Hoffer A. *Common questions on schizophrenia and their answers.* Keats Pub (1987), Keats Pub, New Canaan, CT, 1988, Reprinted by Quarry Press, Kingston, ON (1999)

16. Hoffer A. *Nutrition for the General Practitioner.* Keats Pub (November, 1988)

17. Hoffer A. *Orthomolecular Medicine for Physicians.* Keats Pub., New Canaan, CT, 1989. Translated into Korean, 2004.

18. Hoffer A. *Vitamin B3: Niacin: Update.* Keats Pub; Revised edition (April 1, 1990)

19. Hoffer A & Walker M. *Smart Nutrients—A Guide to Nutrients That Can Prevent and Reverse Senility.* Avery Publishing Group, Garden City Park, NY, 1994. Updated Version: *Smart Nutrients.* Avery, 2000.

20. Hoffer A. *Hoffer's Law of Natural Nutrition.* Quarry Press, Kingston, ON, 1996.

21. Hoffer A. *Vitamin B-3 and Schizophrenia. Discovery, Recovery, Controversy.* Quarry Press, Kingston, ON 1999. (Review)

22. Hoffer A. *Common Questions on Schizophrenia and Their Answers.* Keats Pub, New Canaan, CT, 1988. Reprinted Quarry Press, Kingston, ON 1999

23. Hoffer A & Walker M: *Putting It All Together: The New Orthomolecular Nutrition.* Keats Publishing Inc. New Canaan, Conn, 1996.

24. Hoffer A, Walker, M. *Putting It All Together: The New Orthomolecular Nutrition.* McGraw-Hill; 1 edition (October 11, 1998)

25. Hoffer A. *Dr. Hoffer's ABC of Natural Nutrition for Children.* Quarry Press. Kingston, ON 1999 (Review)

26. Hoffer A. *Orthomolecular Treatment for Schizophrenia.* Keats, 4255 West Touhy Avenue, Lincolnwood, Ill 60646-1975, 1999. (Review)

27. Hoffer A. *Vitamin C and Cancer: Discovery, Recovery, Controversy.* Quarry Press, Kingston, ON 2000 (Review)

28. Hoffer A. *Masks of Madness: Science of Healing, Orthomolecular Treatment of Mental Illness.* Sisyphus Comm. Ltd., documentary film (1998)

29. Hoffer A. *Healing Schizophrenia: Complementary Vitamin & Drug Treatments.* CCNM Press, Toronto, 2004.

30. Hoffer A. *Healing Children's Attention & Behavior Disorders: Complementary Nutritional & Psychological Treatments.* CCNM Press, Toronto, 2004.

31. Hoffer A & Pauling L. *Healing Cancer: Complementary Vitamin & Drug Treatments.* CCNM Press, Toronto, 2004.

32. Hoffer A & Challem J. *User's Guide to Natural therapies for Cancer Prevention & Control: Learn How Diet and Supplements Can Help Prevent and Treat Cancer.* Basic Health Publications (October, 2004)

33. Hoffer A & Foster H. *Feel Better, Live Longer With Vitamin B-3.* (In press, 2005.)

34. *Adventures in Psychiatry. The Scientific Memoirs of Dr. Abram Hoffer.* KOS Publishing, Toronto, 2005.

35. Hoffer A: *Mental Health Regained. Eighteen Stories of Recovery.* International Schizophrenia Foundation, Toronto, 2005.

36. Hoffer A: *Orthomolecular Treatment for Schizophrenia and Other Mental Illnesses: A Guide for Practitioners.* (In press, 2005.)

37. Hoffer A & Prousky JE. *Anxiety Disorders. The CCNM Grand Rounds.* CCNM Press Inc., Toronto, 2005.

38. Hoffer, A & Prousky JE. *Naturopathic Nutrition.* CCNM Press Inc., Toronto, 2005 (In press)

Papers and Articles:

1952

Hoffer A & Osmond H. Paper to Dementia Praecox Committee, Scottish Rites Masons, New York. Given at the Canada Room, The Waldorf Astoria, New York, 1952. (This was our first report on the adrenochrome hypothesis.) (No known electronic link)

Hoffer A, Osmond H & Smythies J: Schizophrenia: a new approach. II. Results of a year's research. J Ment Science 100:29-45, 1954. (No known electronic link)

Clancy J, Hoffer A, Lucy J, Osmond H, Smythies J & Stefaniak B: Design and planning in psychiatric research as illustrated by the Weyburn Chronic Nucleotide Project. Bull Men Clinic, 18:147-153, 1954. (No known electronic link)

Altschul R, Hoffer A & Stephen JD: Influence of nicotinic acid on serum cholesterol in man. Arch Biochem Biophys 54:558-559, 1955. (No known electronic link)

Szatmari A, Hoffer A & Schneider R: The effect of adrenochrome and niacin on the electroencephalogram of epileptics. Am J Psychiat 3:603-616, 1955. (No known electronic link)

Agnew N & Hoffer A. Nicotinic acid modified lysergic acid diethylamide psychosis. J Ment Science 101:12-27, 1955. (Abstract available here)

Hoffer A. Effect of niacin and nicotinamide on leukocytes and some urinary constituents. Can Med Assoc J 74:448-451, 1955. (No known electronic link)

Hoffer A, Osmond H, Callbeck MJ & Kahan I: Treatment of schizophrenia with nicotinic acid and nicotinamide. J Clin Exper Psychopathol 18:131-158, 1957. (No known electronic link)

Hoffer A & Callbeck MJ: The hypocholesterolemic effect of nicotinic acid and its relationship to the autonomic nervous system. J Ment Science 103:810-820, 1957. (No known electronic link)

Hoffer A. The relationship of nicotinic acid to thyroid function. Can Med Assoc J 77:965 only, 1957. (No known electronic link)

Hoffer A. Adrenochrome and adrenolutin and their relationship to mental disease. Psychotropic Drugs. Eds. Garattini S & Ghetti V. Elsevier Press, London, 10-20, 1957. (No known electronic link)

Hoffer A. Adrenochrome and blood plasma. Amer J Psychiatry 114:752-753, 1958. (No known electronic link)

Hoffer A. Relation of epinephrine metabolites to schizophrenia. In: Chemical Concepts of Psychiatry. Eds: Rinkel M & Denber HGB. McDowell-Obolensky Inc., New York, 1958. (No known electronic link)

Altschul R & Hoffer A. Effects of salts of nicotinic acid on serum cholesterol. Brit Med J 2:713-714, 1958. (No known electronic link)

Altschul R & Hoffer A. The effect of nicotinic acid upon serum cholesterol and upon basal metabolic rate of young normal adults. Arch Biochem Biophysics 73:420- 424, 1958. (No known electronic link)

Hoffer A & Osmond H. The adrenochrome model and schizophrenia. J Nerv Mental Dis 128:18-35, 1959. (No known electronic link)

Osmond H & Hoffer A. Schizophrenia: A new approach III. J Ment Science 105:653-673, 1959. (No known electronic link)

Hoffer A & Callbeck MJ: Effect of nicotinic acid on liver function and leukocytes. Can Med Assoc J 80:736-737, 1959. (No known electronic link)

Hoffer A, O'Reilly PO & Callbeck MJ: Specificity of the hypocholesterolemic activity of nicotinic acid. Dis Nerv Syst 20:286-288, 1959. (No known electronic link)

Osmond H & Hoffer A. On critics and research. Psychosomatic Med 21: 311-320, 1959. (No known electronic link)

Hoffer A. Treatment of arthritis by nicotinic acid and nicotinamide. Can Med Assoc J 81:235-238, 1959. (No known electronic link)

O'Reilly PO, Callbeck MJ & Hoffer A. Sustained-release nicotinic acid (Nicospan). Effect on (1) cholesterol levels and (2) leukocytes. Can Med Assoc J 80:359-362, 1959. (No known electronic link)

1960

Hoffer A & Osmond H. The Chemical Basis of Clinical Psychiatry. C. C. Thomas, Springfield, IL, 1960. (No known electronic link)

Hoffer A & Osmond H. Alcoholism and the researcher. AA Grapevine 1960. (No known electronic link)

Altschul R & Hoffer A. Letter to Editor Re: Nicotinic acid on hypercholesterolemia. Can Med Assoc J 83:36-37, 1960. (No known electronic link)

Hoffer A & Osmond H. Concerning an etiological factor in alcoholism. The possible role of adrenochrome metabolism. Quart J Stud Alcohol 20:750-756, 1959. (No known electronic link)

Hoffer A. The adrenochrome hypothesis of schizophrenia. Paper read to Proc Sixth Ann Psychiatric Institute, Princeton, September 1958. Pub in Proceedings, 36-53. (No known electronic link)

Hoffer A. Adrenaline metabolites and schizophrenia. Dis Nerv Syst 21, Monograph Supp, 79-86, 1960. (No known electronic link)

Altschul R & Hoffer A. The effect of nicotinic acid on hypercholesterolemia. Can Med Assoc J 82:783-785, 1960. (No known electronic link)

Hoffer A. The relationship of nicotinic acid to cholesterol metabolism. J Clin Exper Psychopath 22: 165-179, 1961. (No known electronic link)

Hoffer A & Osmond H. The biochemistry of mental disease. Can Med Assoc J 85:1309-1311, 1961. (No known electronic link)

Hoffer A & Osmond H. Double blind clinical trials. J Neuropath 2:221-227, 1961. (No known electronic link)

Hoffer A. Ascorbic acid and schizophrenia. B.M.J. 1:1342 only, 1962. (No known electronic link)

Hoffer A. The effect of adrenochrome and adrenolutin on the behavior of animals and the psychology of man. Int Rev Neurobiology 4:307-371, 1962. (No known electronic link)

Hoffer A. Niacin Therapy in Psychiatry. C. C. Thomas, Springfield, IL, 1962. (No known electronic link)

Hoffer A & Osmond H. A card sorting test helpful in establishing prognosis. Am J Psychiatry 118:840-841,1962. (No known electronic link)

Hoffer A & Osmond H. Some schizophrenic recoveries. Dis Nerv Syst 23: 204-210, 1962. (No known electronic link)

Hoffer A & Osmond H. Letter to Editor Re: Double blind clinical trials. J Neuropsychiatry 2:262-263, 1962. (No known electronic link)

Hoffer A & Osmond H. Letter to Editor: Adrenaline and schizophrenia. Lancet 1:643-644, 1962. (No known electronic link)

Hoffer A. Letter to Editor Re: Malnutrition and mental disease. Brit Med Assoc J 1:1342 only, 1962. (No known electronic link)

Hoffer A & Osmond H. Scurvy and schizophrenia. Dis Nerv Syst 24:273-285, 1963. (No known electronic link)

Hoffer A & Osmond H. A comprehensive theory of schizophrenia. Mind 1:119-121, 1963. (No known electronic link)

Hoffer A. What's new in psychiatric research. Introduction. Mind. Psychiatry in General Practice, 1:28 only, 1963. (No known electronic link)

Osmond H & Hoffer A. Massive niacin treatment in schizophrenia. Review of a nine-year study. Lancet 1:316-320, 1963. (No known electronic link)

Smith CM, Hoffer A, Dantow MD & McIntyre S: Nicotinic acid in old age. The placebo effect and other factors in the collection of valid data. J Amer Geriat Soc 11:580-585, 1963. (No known electronic link)

Hoffer A. Nicotinic acid: an adjunct in the treatment of schizophrenia. Am J Psychiat 120:171-173, 1963. (No known electronic link)

Hoffer A. The adrenochrome theory of schizophrenia. a review. Dis Nerv Syst 25:173-178, 1964. (No known electronic link)

Hoffer A. Single case design and double blind comparison studies for drug evaluation. Mind. Psychiatry in General Practice, 2:119-120, 1964. (No known electronic link)

Hoffer A & Osmond H. Treatment of schizophrenia with nicotinic acid—a ten year follow-up. Acta Psychiat Scand 40:171-189, 1964. (No known electronic link)

Hoffer A. Treatment of organic psychosis with nicotinic acid (a single case). Dis Nerv Syst 26: 358-360, 1965. (No known electronic link)

Hoffer A. Alcoholism Treatment and Research Center. The Can Forester, LXXXV, August 1965. (No known electronic link)

Hoffer A. Malvaria, schizophrenia and the HOD test. Int J Neuropsychiatry 2:175-177, 1965. (No known electronic link)

Osmond H & Hoffer A. A comprehensive theory of schizophrenia. Int J Neuropsychiatry 2:302-309, 1965. (No known electronic link)

Hoffer A. The effect of nicotinic acid on the frequency and duration of re-hospitalization of schizophrenic patients; A controlled comparison study. Int J Neuropsychiatry 2:234-240, 1966. (No known electronic link)

Hoffer A & Osmond H. How To Live With Schizophrenia. University Books, New York, NY, 1966. Also published by Johnson, London, 1966. Written by Fannie Kahan. New and Revised Ed. Citadel Press, New York, N.Y. 1992 (No known electronic link)

Hoffer A. Use of nicotinic acid and/or nicotinamide in high doses to treat schizophrenia. Can J Psychiatric Nursing 76:5-6, 1966. (No known electronic link)

Hoffer A. Enzymology of Hallucinogens. In, Enzymes in Mental Health, J.B. Lippincott, 43-55, 1966. (No known electronic link)

Hoffer A & Osmond H. New Hope For Alcoholics, University Books, New York, 1966. Co-written by Fannie Kahan. (No known electronic link)

Hoffer A. Biochemistry of nicotinic acid and nicotinamide. Psychosomatics 8:95-100, 1967. (No known electronic link)

Hoffer A & Osmond H. Nicotinamide adenine dinucleotide. J Psychopharm 1:79-95, 1967. (No known electronic link) (No known electronic link)

Kelm H, Hoffer A & Hall RW: Reliability of the Hoffer-Osmond Diagnostic test. J Clin Psychology 23:380-382, 1967. (No known electronic link)

Hoffer A. A theoretical examination of double-blind design. Can Med Assoc J 97:123-127, 1967. (No known electronic link)

Kelm H, Hoffer A & Osmond H. Hoffer-Osmond Diagnostic Manual. Saskatoon, 1967. (No known electronic link)

Hoffer A. Treatment of schizophrenia with a therapeutic program based upon nicotinic acid as the main variable. Molecular Basis of Some Aspects of Mental

Activity, Vol II. Ed. O Walaas, Academic Press, New York, 1967. (No known electronic link)

Kelm H, Callbeck MJ & Hoffer A. A short form of the Hoffer-Osmond Diagnostic test. Int J Neuropsychiatry 3:489-490, 1967. (No known electronic link)

Hoffer A. Nicotinamide adenine dinucleotide in the treatment of chronic schizophrenic patients. British J Psychiatry 114:915-917, 1968. (No known electronic link)

Hoffer A & MacLean JR: A brief history of the American Schizophrenia Foundation. Schizophrenia 1:10-12, 1969. (No known electronic link)

Hoffer A. Comparison of xanthine nicotinate and nicotinic acid as treatment for schizophrenia. Schizophrenia 1:24- 37, 1969. (No known electronic link)

Hoffer A. Safety, side effects and relative lack of toxicity of nicotinic acid and nicotinamide. Schizophrenia 1:78-87, 1969. (No known electronic link)

Hoffer A. Adverse effects of niacin in emergent psychosis. J Am Med Ass 207:1355 only, 1969. (Available here)

Hoffer A. Introduction to Mental Health Through Nutrition, by Judge Tom R. Blaine, The Citadel Press, New York, 1969. (No known electronic link)

1970

Hoffer A. Pellagra and schizophrenia. Academy of Psychosomatic Medicine, Buenos Aires, Jan. 12-18, 1970. Psychosomatic II, 522-525, 1970. (No known electronic link)

Hoffer A. Living with schizophrenia. Schizophrenia 2:80-86, 1970. (No known electronic link)

Hoffer A. Childhood schizophrenia. a case treated with nicotinic acid and nicotinamide. Schizophrenia 2:43-53,1970. (No known electronic link)

Hoffer A & Osmond H. Vitamin B-3 and Krebiozen—a polemic. Schizophrenia 2:161-165, 1970. (No known electronic link)

Hoffer A. Symposium on statistical aspects of protocol design. Discussion. Cancer Clinical Investigation Review Committee, San Juan, Puerto Rico, 224-229, Dec. 9-10, 1970. (No known electronic link)

Hoffer A. A vitamin B-3 dependent family. Schizophrenia 3:41-46, 1971. (No known electronic link)

Hoffer A. Megavitamins Can. Psychiatric Ass J. 19:124-5, 1971 (No known electronic link)

Hoffer A. Letter to Editor. Ascorbic acid and schizophrenia. C.M.C. News 2, May 1971. (No known electronic link)

Hoffer A. Letter to Editor. (Rebuttal of attack on Linus Pauling) Nutrition Today 6:34-35, 1971. (No known electronic link)

Hoffer A. Vitamin B-3 dependent child. Schizophrenia 3:107-113, 1971. (No known electronic link)

Hoffer A. Ascorbic acid and toxicity. New England J of Med 285:635-636, 1971. (No known electronic link)

Hoffer A. Vitamin C and the common cold. Can Med Assoc J 105:901-902, 1971. (No known electronic link)

Hoffer A. Megavitamin B-3 therapy for schizophrenia. Can Psychiatric Ass J 16:499-504, 1971. (No known electronic link)

Masters AB, Hoffer A, Nair NPV, Messer CJ, Zarzadias R & Moraes C: Care of chronic psychotics. Brit Med Ass J 4:489 only, 1971. (No known electronic link)

Hoffer A. Foreword to, Body Mind and the B Vitamins by R Adams & F Murray. Larchmont Books, New York, 1972. (No known electronic link)

Hoffer A. LSD-induced psychosis and vitamin B-3. Amer J Psychiatry 128:145 only, 1972. (No known electronic link)

Hoffer A. Orthomolecular treatment of schizophrenia. Orthomolecular Psychiatry 1:46-55, 1972. (No known electronic link)

Hoffer A. Treatment of hyperkinetic children with nicotinamide and pyridoxine. Can Med Assoc J 107:111-112, 1972. (No known electronic link)

Hoffer A. Orthomolecular treatment for schizophrenia. J Practical Nursing 22:16-19 and 20-22, 1972. (No known electronic link)

Hoffer A. LSD-induced psychosis and vitamin B-3 Amer J of Psychiatry. 128; 1155 only, 1972. (No known electronic link)

Hoffer A. Senility is a form of chronic malnutrition. Report of a National Conference on The Crisis in Health Care For The Aging, sponsored by the Huxley Institute of Biosocial Research, New York, Mar. 6, 1972. (No known electronic link)

Hoffer A. Clofibrate and nicotinic acid. Can Med Assoc J 107:488-489, 1972. (No known electronic link)

Hoffer A. Orthomolecular treatment for schizophrenia. Medical Counterpart 4:10-20, 1973. (No known electronic link)

Hoffer A. Mechanism of action of nicotinic acid and nicotinamide in the treatment of schizophrenia. In, Orthomolecular Psychiatry, Eds. David Hawkins and Linus Pauling. WH Freeman and Co., San Francisco, 1973. (No known electronic link)

Hoffer A. Orthomolecular therapy. Psychiatric Opinion 10:6-10, 1973. (No known electronic link)

Hoffer A. An examination of the double-blind method as it has been applied to megavitamin therapy. Orthomolecular Psychiatry 2:107-114, 1973. (No known electronic link)

Hoffer A. Orthomolecular treatment of schizophrenia. Can J Psychiat Nursing 14:11-14, 1973. (No known electronic link)

Hoffer A. Adverse effects of niacin in emergent psychosis. J.A.M.A. 207:1355 only, 1973. (No known electronic link)

Hoffer A. Learning disability. Can Med Assoc J 109:574 only, 1973. (No known electronic link)

Hoffer A. Vitamin C and infertility. The Lancet 2:1146 only, 1973. (No known electronic link)

Hoffer A. The great vitamin spree - pro and con. BC Med J 15:350 only, 1973. (No known electronic link)

Hoffer A. Orthomolecular psychiatry. BC Med J 16:137-140, 1974. (No known electronic link)

Hoffer A. Hallucinogens. Encyclopedia Britannica 15th Ed., 557-560, 1974. (No known electronic link)

Hoffer A. Double-blind studies. Can Med Assoc J 111:752 only, 1974. (No known electronic link)

Hoffer A. Treatment of choice. Saint Johns Edmonton Report, Volume 1, 1974. (No known electronic link)

Hoffer A. The megavitamin scene. The Lancet 2:908 only, 1974. (No known electronic link)

Hoffer A. Hyperactivity, allergy and megavitamins. Can Med Assoc J 111: 905-907, 1974. (No known electronic link)

Hoffer A. Senility and chronic malnutrition. J Orthomolecular Psychiatry 3: 2-19, 1974. (No known electronic link)

Hoffer A. The orthomolecular controversy. J Orthomolecular Psychiatry 3:164-166, 1974. (No known electronic link)

Hoffer A. History of orthomolecular psychiatry. J Orthomolecular Psychiatry 3:223-230, 1974. (No known electronic link)

Hoffer A. The drug addictions. The Answer. 11:2-5 & 38-40, 1974. (No known electronic link)

Hoffer A. Calories, protein, lipids, carbohydrates and the Saccharine Disease. J Orthomolecular Psychiatry 3:231-239, 1974. (No known electronic link)

Hoffer A. Treatment of schizophrenia. J Orthomolecular Psychiatry 3:280-290, 1974. (No known electronic link)

Hoffer A. The relation of crime to nutrition. Humanist in Canada 34:2-9, 1975. (No known electronic link)

Hoffer A. Nutrition and schizophrenia. Canadian Family Physician 21:78-82, 1975. (No known electronic link)

Hoffer A. Nutrition and Schizophrenia; the debate continues. Canadian Family Physician 21:15-16, 1975. (No known electronic link)

Hoffer A. A note on folklore and medical discovery. J Orthomolecular Psychiatry 4:211 only, 1975. (No known electronic link)

Hoffer A. Orthomolecular Medicine: What is it, How does it work. Impact of Science on Society 25:233-244, 1975. (No known electronic link)

Hoffer A, Kelm H & Osmond H. The Hoffer-Osmond Diagnostic Test. RE Krieger Pub Co. Huntington, New York, 1975. (No known electronic link)

Hoffer A. The orthomolecular controversy. J Orthomolecular Psychiatry 5: 54-67, 1976. (No known electronic link)

Hoffer A. Editorial. Establishment journal looks at orthomolecular psychiatry. J Orthomolecular Psychiatry 5:78-83, 1976. (No known electronic link)

Hoffer A. Natural history and treatment of thirteen pairs of identical twins, schizophrenic and schizophrenic-spectrum conditions. J Orthomolecular Psychiatry 5:101-122, 1976. (No known electronic link)

Hoffer A & Osmond H. Megavitamin Therapy. Can Schiz Foundation, Regina, 1976. PDF

Stone I & Hoffer A. The genesis of medical myths. J Orthomolecular Psychiatry 5:163-168, 1976.

Hoffer A. Megavitamin therapy for different cases. J Orthomolecular Psychiatry 5:169-182, 1976. (No known electronic link)

Hoffer A. Children with learning and behavioral disorders. J Orthomolecular Psychiatry 5:228-230, 1976. (No known electronic link)

Hoffer A & Osmond H. In Reply to The American Psychiatric Association Task Force Report on Megavitamin and Orthomolecular Therapy in Psychiatry. Canadian Schizophrenia Foundation, Regina, Sask., now 16 Florence Ave., Toronto, ON, Canada M2N 1E9, August 1976. Full text posted at http://www.iahf.com/orthomolecular/reply_to_apa_tfr_7.pdf

Hoffer A. The double blind method. Can Psych Ass Journal 6:449-450, 1976. (No known electronic link)

Hoffer A. Editorial. The medical model and mileau therapy. J Orthomolecular Psychiatry 5:246-252, 1976. (No known electronic link)

Hoffer A. Editorials. Does ascorbic acid destroy vitamin B-12? and Crime: the price of chemical tranquility. J Orthomolecular Psychiatry 6:2-7, 1977. (No known electronic link)

Hoffer A. Orthomolecular psychiatry in theory and practice. Drug Therapy 79-85, 1977.

Hoffer A. On evidence. Canadian Doctor 43:30 only, 1977. (No known electronic link)

Hoffer A. Evidence and belief. Can Med Assoc J 117:733-734, 1977. (No known electronic link)

Hoffer A. To the Editor. Tardive dyskinesia treated with manganese. Can Med Assoc J 117:859 only, 1977. (No known electronic link)

Hoffer A. An Interview. Ex-POW Bull Volume 34, Sept 30-33 and Oct 19-23, 1977. (No known electronic link)

Hoffer A. Editorial. Rules of inquiry. About the APA Task Force on Megavitamin Therapy and Orthomolecular Psychiatry. J Orthomolecular Psychiatry 7:82-85, 1978. (No known electronic link)

Hoffer A. Diagnosing depression. J Orthomolecular Psychiatry 7:177-179, 1978. (No known electronic link)

Hoffer A & Walker M. Orthomolecular Nutrition. Keats Pub, New Canaan, CT, 1978. (No known electronic link)

Hoffer A. Some theoretical principles basic to orthomolecular psychiatric treatment. In: Ecologic-Biochemical Approaches to Treatment of Delinquents and Criminals. Ed. LJ Hippchen. Van Nostrand-Reinhold Co, New York, 31-55, 1978. (No known electronic link)

Hoffer A. Letter to Editor. Megavitamins versus tranquilizer therapy. Canadian Family Physician 24:410 only, 1978. (No known electronic link)

Hoffer A. Orthomolecular psychiatry. Proc Section World Congress Biol Psychiatry, Barcelona, 1978. Elsevier North Holland Biomedical Press BV Amsterdam 1979. (No known electronic link)

Hoffer A. Obsessions and depression. J Orthomolecular Psychiatry 8:78-81, 1979. (No known electronic link)

Hoffer A. Behavioral nutrition. J Orthomolecular Psychiatry 8:169-175, 1979. (No known electronic link)

Hoffer A. Crime, punishment and treatment. J Orthomolecular Psychiatry 8:193-199, 1979. (No known electronic link)

1980

Hoffer A & Walker M: Nutrients to Age Without Senility. Keats Pub Inc, New Canaan, CT, 1980. (No known electronic link)

Hoffer A. Newer trends in orthomolecular medicine. Newsletter, Northwest Academy Preventive Med 7 pages 3 and 6, 1980. (No known electronic link)

Hoffer A & Osmond H. Schizophrenia. another long term follow-up in Canada. J Orthomolecular Psychiatry 9:107-113, 1980. (No known electronic link)

Hoffer A. To the Editor. Crime and delinquency. A reply to H Wagemaker, Biol Psychiatry 15:171-172, 1980. Biological Psychiatry 26:249-250, 1980. (No known electronic link)

Hoffer A. Mega amino acid therapy. J Orthomolecular Psychiatry 9:2-5, 1980. (No known electronic link)

Hoffer A. Allergy, depression and tricyclic anti-depressants. J Orthomolecular Psychiatry 9:164-170, 1980. (No known electronic link)

Hoffer A. Megavitamins. Biol Psychiatry 15:821-2, 1980. (No known electronic link)

Hoffer A. Letter to the Editor, re critique of Leonard Hippchen's book, Ecologic-Biochemical Approaches to Treatment of Delinquents and Criminals, by T. J. Gaensbauer. Crime and Delinquency 26:249-250, 1980. (No known electronic link)

Osmond H & Hoffer A. Naturally occurring endogenous major and minor tranquilizers. J Orthomolecular Psychiatry 9:198-206, 1980. (No known electronic link)

Hoffer A. Megavitamin Therapy. In: The Psychotherapy Handbook. 370-374, Ed.R Herink. New American Library, New York, 1980. (No known electronic link)

Hoffer A. The adrenochrome hypothesis of schizophrenia revisited. J Orthomolecular Psychiatry 10:98-118, 1981. (No known electronic link)

Hoffer A. Editorial. Mercury silver amalgams. J Orthomolecular Psychiatry 11:2 only, 1982. (No known electronic link)

Hoffer A. Why nicotinic acid lowers lipid levels. Can Med Assoc J 128:372 only, 1983. (No known electronic link)

Hoffer A. Nutrition and cancer. Anabolism. J Preventive Med 2:5-7, 1983. Ed. R Powell, La Jolla, CA. (No known electronic link)

Hoffer A. Nutrition and behavior. In, Medical Applications of Clinical Nutrition. Ed. J Bland. Keats Pub, New Canaan CT, 222-251, 1983. (No known electronic link)

Hoffer A. Latent Huntington's disease—response to orthomolecular treatment. J Orthomolecular Psychiatry 12:44-47, 1983. (No known electronic link)

Hoffer A. Update: (a) treatment of multiple sclerosis with hyperbaric oxygen. (b) Niacin hepatitis. J Orthomolecular Psychiatry 12:89-90, 1983. (No known electronic link)

Hoffer A. Orthomolecular nutrition at the zoo. J Orthomolecular Psychiatry 12:116-128, 1983. (No known electronic link)

Hoffer A. Editorial. Criticism. J Orthomolecular Psychiatry 12:252-259, 1983. (No known electronic link)

Hoffer A. Oxidation-reduction in the brain. J Orthomolecular Psychiatry 12:292-301, 1983. (No known electronic link)

Hoffer A. Comments on prevention. Canada's Mental Health 32:23 only, 1984. (No known electronic link)

Hoffer A. Megavitamin therapy. Times Colonist, Victoria, BC, March 29, 1984. (No known electronic link)

Hoffer A. Nutritional ignorance. B.C. Med J 26:345 only, 1984. (No known electronic link)

Hoffer A. Letter to Editor. Health Food Retailing, Australia, September 1984, page 25 only. (No known electronic link)

Hoffer A. Orthomolecular treatment of schizophrenia. Society for Environmental Therapy 4:3-6, 1984. (No known electronic link)

Hoffer A. Treating schizophrenia. Australasian Health and Healing 4:7-14, 1984. (No known electronic link)

Hoffer A. Gastric bypass surgery and nutrient deficiency. Can Med Assoc J 131:1019 only, 1984. (No known electronic link)

Hoffer A. Editorial. The Controversial Vitamins. J Orthomolecular Psychiatry 13:2-5, 1984. (No known electronic link)

Hoffer A. Vitamin B-3 (Niacin). Keats Pub, New Canaan CT, 1984. (No known electronic link)

Hoffer A. Editorial. The tomato effect. J Orthomolecular Psychiatry 13: 142-143, 1984. (No known electronic link)

Hoffer A. Editorial. On pain, developmental defects, and vitamin safety. J Orthomolecular Psychiatry 14:2-4, 1985. (No known electronic link)

Hoffer A. Foreword to Living With Schizophrenia. J Orthomolecular Psychiatry 14:39-41, 1985. (No known electronic link)

Hoffer A. Editorial. A basic flaw in modern medical research. J Orthomolecular Psychiatry 14:82-84, 1985. (No known electronic link)

Hoffer A. Thyroid and cancer. J Orthomolecular Psychiatry 14:85-87, 1985. (No known electronic link)

Hoffer A. Huntington's disease: a follow-up. J Orthomolecular Psychiatry 13:42-44, 1984. (No known electronic link)

Hoffer A. Letter to Editor. Nutrition Today, About Niacin 20:36 only, 1985. (No known electronic link)

Hoffer A. Dopamine, noradrenalin and adrenalin metabolism to methylated or chrome indole derivatives: two pathways or one? J Orthomolecular Psychiatry 14:262-272, 1985. (No known electronic link)

Hoffer A. Ascorbic acid and kidney stones. Can Med Assoc J 132:320 only, 1985. (No known electronic link)

Hoffer A. Children's Multiple Vitamin overuse lead to overdose CMAJ 133:13 only, 1985 (No known electronic link)

Hoffer A. Vitamin B-3. Can Med Assoc J 135:1250 only, 1986. (No known electronic link)

Hoffer A. Vitamin therapy for hyperactivity and schizophrenia. a family's struggle. J Orthomolecular Medicine 1:57-62, 1986. (No known electronic link)

Hoffer A. Editorial. The new debate in nutrition. J Orthomolecular Medicine 1:72 only, 1986. (No known electronic link)

Hoffer A. Editorial. Nutrition in institutions controlled by physicians. J Orthomolecular Medicine 1:216-218, 1986. (No known electronic link)

Hoffer A. Editorial. Seminar on orthomolecular medicine. Ben Gurion University Medical Center, May 21, 1987. J Orthomolecular Medicine 2:2 only, 1987. (No known electronic link)

Hoffer A. Editorial. Why flog a dead horse? J Orthomolecular Medicine 2: 74 only, 1987. (No known electronic link)

Hoffer A. Editorials: Schizophrenia and suicide, and, Let's help the FDA. J Orthomolecular Medicine 2:144-145, 1987. (No known electronic link)

Hoffer A. Is there a conspiracy? J Orthomolecular Medicine 2:158-165, 1987. (No known electronic link)

Hoffer A. Vitamin B-3 CMAJ 137:12 only, 1987 (No known electronic link)

Hoffer A. Linus Pauling honors the Canadian Schizophrenia Foundation. J Orthomolecular Medicine 2:183-184, 1987. (No known electronic link)

Hoffer A. How to study a controversial area in medicine. J Orthomolecular Medicine 3:207-210, 1987. (No known electronic link)

Hoffer A. Further report on a schizophrenic patient who had hyperasparaginemia 2:213-216, 1987. (No known electronic link)

Hoffer A. Editorial. Winds of change. J Orthomolecular Medicine 2:221-222, 1987. Editorial. (No known electronic link)

Hoffer A. Control of Huntington's disease by orthomolecular treatment. J Orthomolecular Medicine 2:229 only, 1987. (No known electronic link)

Hoffer A. Editorial. How can anything so simple help something so complicated? J Orthomolecular Medicine 3:2 only, 1988. (No known electronic link)

Hoffer A. Letter to Editor. Fluoridation: why is it not more widely adopted? Can Med Assoc J 138:11 only, 1988. (No known electronic link)

Hoffer A. Common Questions on Schizophrenia and Their Answers. Keats Pub, New Canaan, CT, 1988. (No known electronic link)

Hoffer A. Can alternative and conventional treatments of cancer co-exist? Health Sciences Program, University Extension and Community Relations, University of Victoria, Feb 8, 1989. (No known electronic link)

Hoffer A. Orthomolecular Medicine for Physicians. Keats Pub, New Canaan, CT, 1989. (No known electronic link)

Hoffer A. In memoriam: Carl C. Pfeiffer, B.A., Ph.D., M.D. 1908-1988. J Orthomolecular Medicine 4:3-5, 1989. (No known electronic link)

Hoffer A. The discovery of vitamin C: Albert Szent-Gyorgi, M.D. Ph.D. 1893-1986. J Orthomolecular Medicine 4:24-26, 1989. (No known electronic link)

Hoffer A. Editorial. This is what they said about medical mavericks. J Orthomolecular Medicine 4:54-57, 1989. (No known electronic link)

Hoffer A. The Bristol Regimen for Cancer Treatment CMAJ 144:411-412, 1989. (No known electronic link)

Hoffer A. The fluoride controversy—the first forty years. J Orthomolecular Medicine 4:119-122, 1989. (No known electronic link)

Hoffer A. Preface. In The Best of Health. The 101 Best Books. Sheldon Zerden, Four Walls Eight Windows, New York, xi-xii, 1989 (No known electronic link)

Hoffer A. Editorial. An historical note. J Orthomolecular Medicine 4:183-184, 1989. (No known electronic link)

Hoffer A. Niacin, Coronary Disease and Longevity. J Orthomolecular Medicine 4:211-220, 1989.

Hoffer A. Letter to Editor. Dr. Reading under fire in Australia. J Orthomolecular Medicine 4:234-235, 1989. (No known electronic link)

Hoffer A. Vitamin and mineral supplements increase intelligence. Nutrition Health Review, Fall 1989.

1990

Hoffer A. Editorial. Adrenochrome hypothesis revisited. J Orthomolecular Medicine 5:3 only, 1990. (No known electronic link)

Hoffer A & Osmond H. The adrenochrome hypothesis and psychiatry. J Orthomolecular Medicine 5:32-45, 1990. (No known electronic link)

Hoffer A. Cancer and Vitamin C. J Orthomolecular Medicine 5:123 only, 1990. (No known electronic link)

Hoffer A, Walker, M: Senility is not inevitable—history proves otherwise—notable historic figures accomplished great things at advanced ages. Nutrition Health Review, Winter 1990

Hoffer A & Pauling L: Hardin Jones biostatistical analysis of mortality data for cohorts of cancer patients with a large fraction surviving at the termination of the study and a comparison of survival times of cancer patients receiving large regular oral doses of vitamin C and other nutrients with similar patients not receiving those doses. J Orthomolecular Medicine 5:143-154, 1990. Reprinted in, Cancer and Vitamin C, E Cameron and L Pauling, Camino Books, Inc. P.O. Box 59026, Phil. PA, 19102, 1993. (No known electronic link)

Hoffer A. Editorial. More on fluoride, on mercury and teeth, and on Alaska Bill #146. J Orthomolecular Medicine 5:187-188, 1990. (No known electronic link)

Hoffer A. The prevention of tardive dyskinesia (tranquilizer induced illness). Open Forum for Health Information of New Zealand, Aug-Sept 1990, 17-20. (No known electronic link)

Hoffer A. Vitamin B-3 (Niacin) Update. New Roles For a Key Nutrient in Diabetes, Cancer, Heart Disease and Other Major Health Problems. Keats Pubs., Inc., New Canaan, CT, 1990. (No known electronic link)

Hoffer A. Letter to editor. Megavitamin and megamineral therapy in childhood. Reply to Appeltauer LC. Can Med Assoc J 145:105 only, 1991. (No known electronic link)

Hoffer A. Megavitamin and megamineral therapy in childhood. Can Med Assoc J 144:845-846, 1991. (No known electronic link)

Hoffer A. Editorials. Linus Pauling's 90th birthday. (and) National Cancer Institute and vitamin C. (and) In Memoriam: William Beebe, M.D. J Orthomolecular Medicine 6:3-4, 1991. (No known electronic link)

Hoffer A. Megavitamin and megamineral therapy in childhood. Can Med Assoc J, 144:845-846, 1991. (No known electronic link)

Hoffer A. Does decreasing cholesterol levels increase the death rate from accidents, homicides and suicide? J Orthomolecular Medicine 6:44-45, 1991. (No known electronic link)

Hoffer A. Editorial. Freedom of Choice Wins More Freedom. J Orthomolecular Medicine 6:55-56, 1991. (No known electronic link)

Hoffer A. Report of the Pharmaceutical Inquiry of Ontario on Alternative Therapies. J Orthomolecular Medicine 6:104-109, 1991. (No known electronic link)

Hoffer A. Orthomolecular Medicine. In: Molecules In Natural Science and Medicine, An Encomium for Linus Pauling. Ed ZB Maksic & M Eckert-Maksic, Ellis Horwood Ltd, Chichester, West Sussex, England, 1991. (No known electronic link)

Hoffer A. Double standard in the control of drugs and nutrients. Healthy Options, 11-13, April/May, New Zealand, 1991. (No known electronic link)

Hoffer A. Niacin Reaction. J of Family Practice, 34: 677 only, 1992. (No known electronic link)

Hoffer A. Protection against ultraviolet radiation. Can Med Ass J, 147:839-840, 1992. (No known electronic link)

Hoffer A. Re: Antioxidant vitamins. British Columbia Medical Association Journal, 35:148 only, 1993. (No known electronic link)

Hoffer A. Isoniazid and pyridoxine. Can Med Assoc J, 149:1232 only, 1993. (No known electronic link)

Hoffer A & Pauling L: Hardin Jones Biostatistical Analysis of Mortality Data for Cohorts of Cancer Patients with a Large Fraction Surviving at the Termination of the Study and a Comparison of Survival Times of Cancer Patients Receiving Large Regular Oral Doses of Vitamin C and Other Nutrients with Similar Patients not Receiving those Doses. J Orthomolecular Medicine 5:143-154, 1990. Reprinted in Cancer and Vitamin C, E. Cameron and L. Pauling, Camino Books, Inc. P.O. Box 59026, Phil. PA 19102, 1993. (No known electronic link)

Hoffer A. The True Cost of Cynicism. Why Vitamin E was Ignored as Heart Therapy for 40 Years. Journal of Orthomolecular Medicine Vol. 7, No. 4, 1992.

Hoffer A. Editorial: The Politics of Medical Research; Alternative Medicine Liberated in a Second State. J of Orthomolecular Medicine, 8:3-5, 1993. (No known electronic link)

Hoffer A. A case of Alzheimer's treated with nutrients and aspirin. J of Orthomolecular Medicine 8:43-44, 1993. (No known electronic link)

Letter. Hoffer A. Bill W. Cofounder of Alcoholics Anonymous and Vitamin B-3. J of Orthomolecular Medicine 8:57-58, 1993. (No known electronic link)

Hoffer A. Misconduct in High Places; Freedom to Practice Complementary Medicine Gaining Momentum. J of Orthomolecular Medicine, 8:67-68, 1993. (No known electronic link)

Hoffer A. Orthomolecular medicine advances into the mainstream. J of Orthomolecular Medicine, 8:99-103, 1993. (No known electronic link)

Hoffer A & Pauling L: Hardin Jones biostatistical analysis of mortality data for a second set of cohorts of cancer patients with a large fraction surviving at the termination of the study and a comparison of survival times of cancer patients receiving large regular oral doses of vitamin C and other nutrients with similar patients not receiving these doses. J of Orthomolecular Medicine, 8:157-167, 1993. (No known electronic link)

Hoffer A. Orthomolecular Oncology. In, Adjuvant Nutrition in Cancer Treatment, Ed. P Quillin & RM Williams. 1992 Symposium Proceedings, Sponsored by Cancer Treatment Research Foundation and American College of Nutrition. Cancer Treatment Research Foundation, 3455 Salt Creek Lane, Suite 200, Arlington Heights, IL 60005-1090, 331-362, 1994. (No known electronic link)

Hoffer A & Walker M: Smart Nutrients - A Guide to Nutrients That Can Prevent and Reverse Senility. Avery Publishing Group, Garden City Park, NY, 1994. (No known electronic link)

Hoffer A. Nutritional Relief for Schizophrenia. Health Naturally, 28-29, Dec 1993/Jan 1994. (No known electronic link)

Hoffer A. The Megavitamin Revolution. Health Counselor, 5:8-9, 1994.

Hoffer A. Chronic schizophrenic patients treated ten years or more. J of Orthomolecular Medicine, 9:7-37, 1994.

Hoffer A. Orthomolecular Oncology and Survival. 2nd International Symposium, Adjuvant Nutrition in Cancer Treatment, San Diego, Mar 17-19, 1994. (No known electronic link)

Hoffer A. Vitamin B-3 and Schizophrenia. Discovery, Recovery, Controversy. Quarry Press, Kingston, ON, 1995. (No known electronic link)

Hoffer A : Vitamin C and Cancer: Discovery, Recovery, Controversy. Quarry Press, Kingston, ON, 1995. (No known electronic link) Review

Hoffer A: The Discovery of Kryptopyrrole and its Importance in Diagnosis of Biochemical Imbalances in Schizophrenia and in Criminal Behavior. Journal of Orthomolecular Medicine, Volume 10, First Quarter, 1995, p 3.

Hoffer A. A dedication to Linus Pauling. The Health Guardian. Health Guard Distributing Corporation, Burnaby, BC, 1:2 only, 1995. (No known electronic link).

Hoffer A. Nutrition Therapy for Cancer Patients. 3rd International Symposium, Adjuvant Nutrition in Cancer Treatment. Tampa, Florida, Sept 28-30, 1995. (No known electronic link).

Hoffer A. Editorial: Double blind studies often the bane of health advancement; (and) Report on disciplinary proceeding: the State of New York against Warren Levin, M.D. J of Orthomolecular Medicine, 9:195-198, 1995. (No known electronic link).

Hoffer A. Another anecdote of schizophrenia. Psychological activity of nicotinamide adenine dinucleotide (NAD) J. Orthomolecular Medicine 10: 68-69, 1995.

Hoffer A. Vitamin B-3: Niacin and its amide. Townsend Letter for Doctors and Patients No. 147, Oct 1995, 30-39.

Hoffer A. Orthomolecular Treatment of Cancer. In, Nutrients in Cancer Prevention and Treatment. Ed. Prasad KN, Santamaria L & Williams RM. Pages 373-391, 1995, Humana Press, Totowa, New Jersey.

Hoffer A. Treatment of Schizophrenia. Townsend Letter for Doctors and Patients No. 144, July 1995, 52-57. (No known electronic link).

Hoffer A: Editorial—The Megavitamin Revolution. Journal Of Orthomolecular Medicine Vol. 7, No. 1, 1995.

Hoffer A. Schizophrenia. An Evolutionary Defense Against Severe Stress. Townsend Letter for Doctors and Patients No. 151/152, Feb/March 1996. (No known electronic link)

Hoffer A: Inside Schizophrenia: Before and After Treatment, Journal of Orthomolecular Medicine, Volume 11, First Quarter, 1996, p 45.

Hoffer A. Hoffer's Law of Natural Nutrition. Quarry Press, Kingston, ON, 1996. (No known electronic link)

Hoffer A. The Vitamin Paradigm Wars. Townsend Letter for Doctors and Patients No. 155, 56-60, 1996.

Hoffer A. Using Vitamins and Nutrition to Help Schizophrenics. An Orthomolecular Alternative. Schizophrenia Digest, 3:13-15, 1996. (No known electronic link)

Hoffer A. Epidermolysis Bullosa. A Zinc Dependent Condition? Townsend Letter for Doctors and Patients No.161, Dec 1996, 62-63. (No known electronic link)

Hoffer A; One Patient's Recovery from Lymphoma. Townsend Letter for Doctors and Patients No.160, 50-51, 1996.

Hoffer A. Interview by Dr. J. Wright. In Let's Live 64, 31-33, 1996. (No known electronic link)

Hoffer A. Schizophrenia. Interviewed by Linda Lazarides, Nutritional Therapy Today 6:6-8, 1996, with an addendum in a letter. (No known electronic link)

Hoffer A. How To Live Longer—Even With Cancer. Journal of Orthomolecular Medicine 11:147-167, 1996. (No known electronic link)

Hoffer A. Editorial: The Future of Psychiatry. Vol. 11, No. 1, 1996.

Hoffer A. Huntington's Disease. Townsend Letter for Doctors and Patients No.163/164, 46-51, 1997. (No known electronic link)

Hoffer A. Arthritis. Townsend Letter for Doctors and Patients. December, No. 173 104 to 106, 1997 (No known electronic link)

Hoffer A. Lupus Erythematosis. Townsend Letter for Doctors and Patients, No. 171, 74 to 75, 1997. Reprinted same journal No. 93/194, page 22-23, 1999. (No known electronic link)

Hoffer A. An anecdote describing the treatment of one case of schizophrenia. No. 168, page 76-79, 1997. (No known electronic link)

Hoffer A. Interview by Peter Barry Chowka On Orthomolecular Medicine, 1997.

Cover Story Amer J Natural Med June Gaining Control of Schizophrenia 5; 21-25, 1998. (No known electronic link)

Hoffer A. Editorial July/August (1998) Amer J Natural Med. Treatment of Children with Learning and/or Behavioral Disorders (No known electronic link)

Hoffer A. The niacin story: The first orthomolecular compound Amer J Natural Med, 5, 10-3, 1998. (No known electronic link)

Hoffer A. Treating Children with Learning and/or Behavior Disorders. Amer J of Natural Med Editorial 5; 7-9, 1998. (No known electronic link)

Hoffer A. Orthomolecular Psychiatry. The Whole Mind, Ed L. Bassman, New World Library, 14 Pamaron Way. Novato, Cal. 94949, Pages 423-432, 1998. (No known electronic link)

Hoffer A. Stress Busters. Great Life 1; 28-31, 1998. (No known electronic link)

Hoffer A. Orthomolecular Treatment of Schizophrenia. Complementary Medicine. Official Journal of the South African Complementary Medicine Association. 4, 9-14, 1998 (No known electronic link)

Hoffer A. Unproven cancer therapies 31, 160 only, 1998 (No known electronic link)

Hoffer A. Orthomolecular Psychiatry in Theory and Practice. Townsend Letter for Doctors and Patients No. 174, 107-111, 1998. (Morton Walker wrote an editorial to commemorate my 80th birthday on page 107.) (No known electronic link)

Hoffer A. Alzheimer's—An Anecdote (letter) Townsend Letter for Doctors and Patients, No.179, 107-109, 1998 (No known electronic link)

Hoffer A. Orthomolecular Treatment for Schizophrenia. Natural Med J, 2, 12-13, 1999 (No known electronic link)

Orthomolecular Medicine, An interview with Abram Hoffer Latitudes 3:6-10, 1998 (No known electronic link)

Hoffer A. Aging Without Senility . Reprint from Smart Nutrients Alive, No. 204, 16-17, 1999

Hoffer A. Vitamin B-3 and Schizophrenia. Discovery, Recovery, Controversy. Quarry Press, Kingston, ON, 1999. (No known electronic link)

2000

Hoffer A. Letter in Nutrition and Healing Newsletter, by Jonathan V Wright, March 2000, page 8. On Multiple sclerosis, niacin and histamine (No known electronic link)

Hoffer A. How Orthomolecular Medicine Can Help. Finding Care for Depression, December 2002 PDF

Hoffer A. Vitamin B-3 and Schizophrenia. Townsend Letter for Doctors and Patients; 4/1/2001

Hoffer A. Vitamin B-3 Does Not Cure Tranquilizer Psychoses. Townsend Letter for Doctors and Patients, April 2001

Hoffer A. Selenium and AIDS—Book Corners. Townsend Letter for Doctors and Patients, November 2001

Hoffer A. Editorial "Toxic" Vitamins. Journal of Orthomolecular Medicine, Vol. 18, Third and Fourth Quarters, 2003 from their Special Issue on The Safety and Efficacy of Vitamins.

Hoffer A. Comments on Comments on "Mega-Dose" Vitamins and Minerals in the Treatment of Nonmetastatic Breast Cancer. Integr Cancer Ther. 2003; 2: 155-157. (Available here)

Hoffer A. Schizophrenia and cancer: the adrenochrome balanced morphism, Medical Hypotheses, Volume 62, Issue 3, March 2004, Pages 415-419 (Abstract available here)

Hoffer A. Lies, damn lies and statistics: the statistics game. Townsend Letter for Doctors and Patients, October 2004

Hoffer A, Foster, HD: Schizophrenia and cancer: the adrenochrome balanced morphism, Med Hypotheses. 2004;62(3):415-9 (Abstract available here)

Hoffer A, Foster, HD: The two faces of L-DOPA. Benefits and adverse side effects in the treatment of Encephalitis lethargica, Parkinson's disease, multiple sclerosis and amyotrophic lateral sclerosis. Med Hypotheses. 2004;62(2): 177-81 (Abstract available here)

Hoffer A. High Doses of Antioxidants Including Vitamin C Do Not Decrease the Efficacy of Chemotherapy. Reprinted with permission of the author and the Townsend Letter for Doctors and Patients, 911 Tyler Street, Pt. Townsend WA 98368; (360) 385-6021

Hoffer A. The Journal of Orthomolecular Medicine and its Development 1967-1996. The Journal of Orthomolecular ("Megavitamin") Medicine

Hoffer A. FACTS AND FACTOIDS: An Information Sheet for Patients. Getting to the Facts.

INDEX

Books of Interest

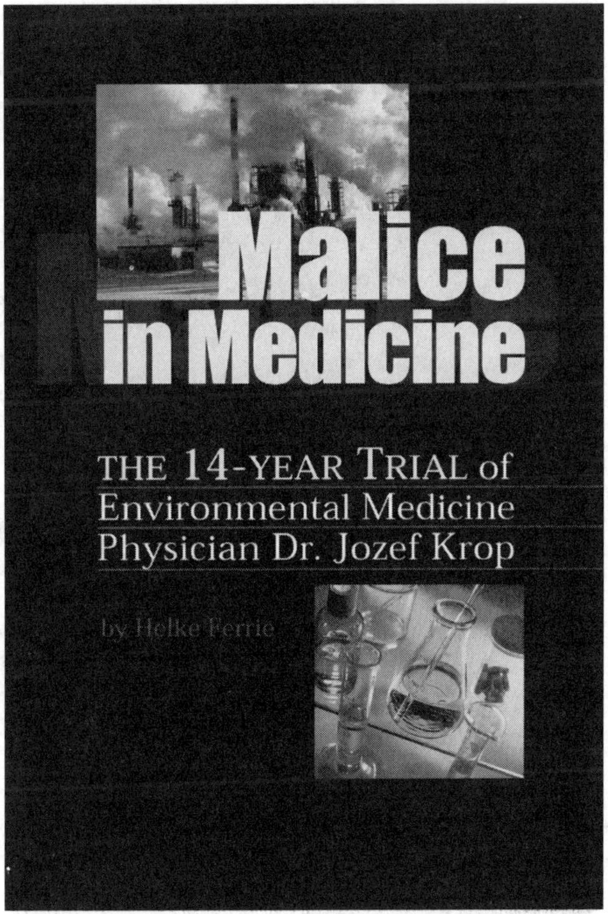

From 1988 to 2002 Dr. Jozef Krop fought for the legal right to practice state-of-the-art environmental medicine. Without patient complaint, the prosecuting College of Physicians and Surgeons of Ontario (mandated to control doctors' licenses) maintained that environmentally induced illness is at best a psychiatric disorder and ignored international medical consensus on Multiple Chemical Sensitivity, Sick Building Syndrome and related medical conditions. Dr. Krop's battle was supported by a stellar international panel of medical experts and by thousands of patients made ill by industrial chemicals and pesticides; legal costs exceeded 1 million dollars, all paid by public donations. This book tells the dramatic story of a physician's successful challenge of corruption in the medical regulatory system.

**6" × 9" | 400 pages | PB | $25.00
November 2005**

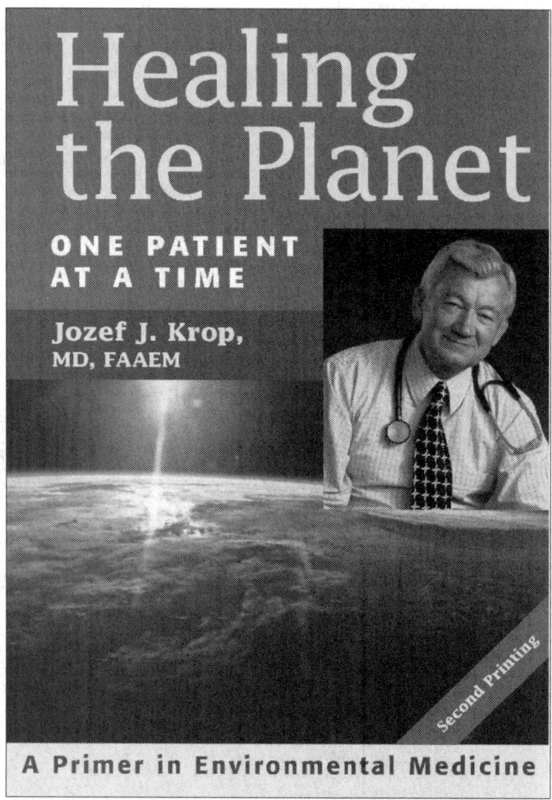

The general reader learns from his book to:

- identify health hazards in the home and work-place environments and what to do about them
- find help through a comprehensive resource section covering everything from pesticides to food allergies, electromagnetic fields, holistic dentistry, safe building materials, how to become a practitioner in environmental medicine and much more
- recognize warning signs that indicate probable environmental illness and how to find medically reliable help

Readers who are health professionals may use this book

- to find the references from the mainstream medical literature covering the field of environmental toxins and the treatment of environmental illness
- basic treatment and detoxification protocols for patients with environmental illness

ISBN 0-9731945-0-2
6" × 9" | 368 pages | PB | $25.00 | 2003

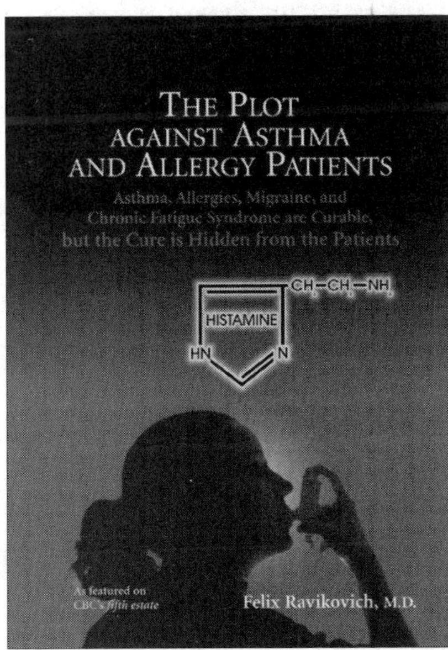

DR. FELIX RAVIKOVICH obtained his medical degree and specialized in Internal Medicine in the former Soviet Union. Since 1985, he has practiced in Toronto specializing in allergy and asthma. His presentations at international conferences on the effective treatment with histamine were published in leading medical journals. This is his first book for the general public and medical colleagues.

Dr. Ravikovich describes his clinical experience with histamine — a synthetic version of the body's substance that stimulates the body to heal itself. His histamine therapy freed hundreds of asthma, allergy and migraine sufferers from drugs that have disastrous effects on the patients' health and the course of the diseases for which these drugs are prescribed.

Unlike other books that concentrate on triggers, this book spells out the primary cellular and genetic defects in patients with allergies, asthma and related diseases and shows how to repair these defects. The author substantiates this through the theoretical works of the world's leading scientists.

Dr. Ravikovich undertook an extensive detective search of literature in molecular biology, immunopharmacology, genetics, and clinical medicine that led him to unprecedented revelations. The scientific foundation for the treatment that could save millions from suffering and dying has been concealed by the medical elite to enable the pharmaceutical industry to develop only those drugs that do not cure and ensure indefinite patient dependence.

Dr. Ravikovich tells the story of his own battle with the medical regulatory authorities which work actively to suppress good, scientifically grounded medicine and protect — not patients — but corporate interests.

ISBN 0-9731945-1-0 | 2003
6" × 9" | 432 pages | PB | $25.00

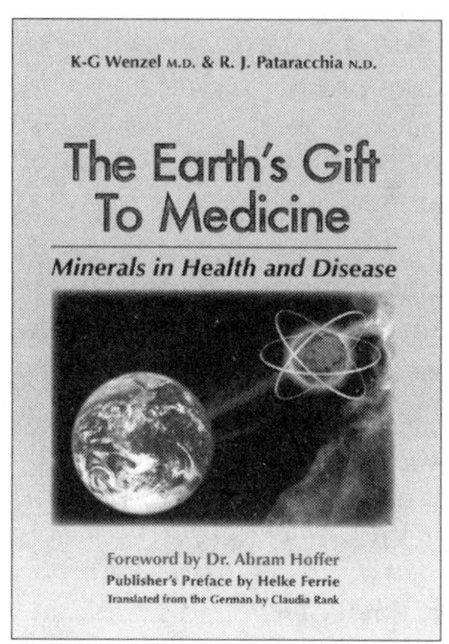

"Over the past 30 years, I have reviewed several hundred books in this new field of nutritional medicine. Of these, two dealing with minerals stand out. The first by Carl Pfeiffer called *Mental and Elemental Nutrients* published in 1975 — and this one. This book is well organized and reads well... I do recommend that every person dealing with health have this book in his or her library... Physicians who pay attention to the properties of these minerals and use them in their practice will be surprised and pleased at how much better their patients will be."

— From the Foreword to this book by Dr. A Hoffer, Prof. Emeritus (psychiatry) University of Saskatchewan, founder of the International Society for Orthomolecular Medicine. Editor-in-Chief of The Journal of Orthomolecular Medicine, author of many books.

"This book is as essential as the minerals it talks about. The word "trace" hides the enormous importance of these minerals that work in concert and are essential for maintaining health. This could not be further from the truth. Indeed, I would suggest, that this book should be understood as a most useful survey of all that is essential 'beyond calcium'.

We need all the minerals in sufficient quantities to replace what we no longer get in our food, which is grown on factory farms that do not use mineral fertilizers. Most plants may look fine, but they no longer provide all that we need for good health. Medical and nutritional research now shows that the current epidemic of chronic diseases is in large part due to chronic mineral deficiencies throughout the population. The list of diseases is as long as the list of minerals that are necessary for human functions: diabetes because of lack of chromium; cancer and AIDS for want of selenium; thyroid disease due to lack of iodine; immune deficiency because there is not enough zinc in the soil, and much more.

— Carolyn Dean, M.D., N.D., board member of the Canadian College of Naturopathy, author of *The Miracle of Magnesium*, Random, 2003.

ISBN 0-9731945-5-3

6" × 9" | 200 pages | PB | $25.00

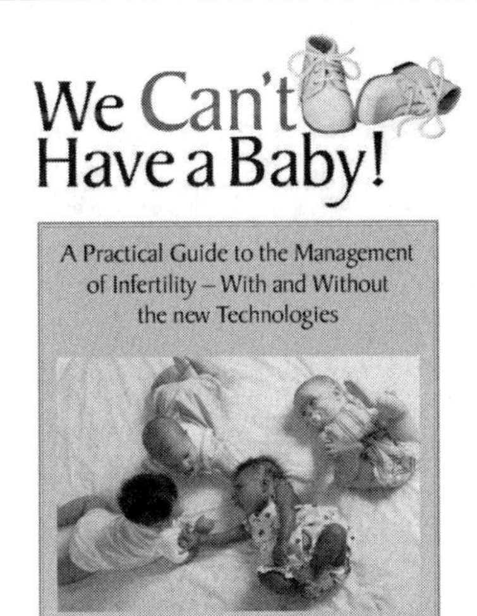

This book is intended to help those couples who find themselves confronted with their inability to have a baby.

Infertility is usually defined as "inability to conceive after twelve months of intercourse without contraception" but common sense is needed. If there is an obvious problem, for example related to a previous attack of pelvic infection and damage of the Fallopian tubes, then investigation and management should not be delayed. If the wife is in her late thirties or early forties, assessment should be done without waiting one year. In the absence of other factors, six months without contraception is long enough to wait before getting a professional opinion from your family doctor.

This book will guide you through the many problems you will encounter and will provide you with information to help you make informed decisions about the best management in your own personal situation. Some sections provide precise options for management and others provide more general information depending on the relevance of the information for the couple.

Probably the most important aspect of helping with the problem of infertility is to ensure that enough time and expertise are used to make rational decisions about management. It makes no sense to access the latest and most complicated technology just because you are seen in a high-technology unit and want the "latest treatment." Your management depends on sensible decisions being made with the help of competent professionals. Very simple changes may be all that is needed even in some couples with long-standing infertility. I have seen couples who have even been through in-vitro fertilization cycles when subsequent successful pregnancy followed simple advice about lifestyle changes or simple medical management of readily identifiable abnormalities.

ISBN 0-9731945-4-5 | 2005
6" × 9" | PB | $25.00

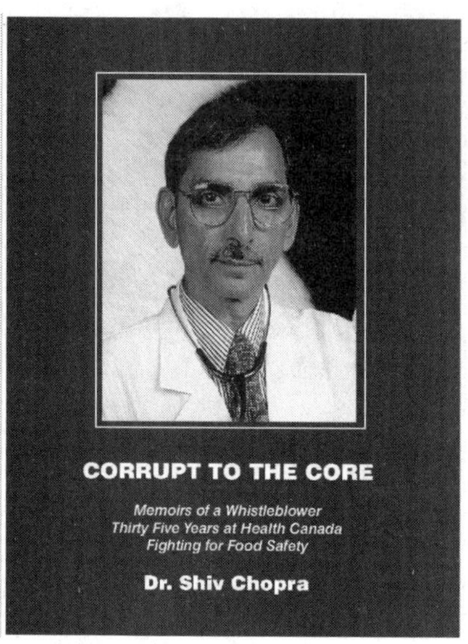

Dr. Shiv Chopra' s name has become synonymous with food safety. Dr. Chopra and some of his fellow scientists waged many battles over many years against a succession of Canadian federal ministries of health—theft employer.

With full support of The Professional Institute of the Public Service of Canada—a 50,000 member union of scientific and professional public service employees, Dr. Chopra and his colleagues refused to approve various harmful drugs to be used in meat and milk production. Despite the political pressures to do otherwise, and holding fast to sound science, they did better than the gambles that a series of prime ministers and health ministers played with public safety.

Time and again the federal courts supported Dr. Chopra and his fellow scientists and ruled against government attempts to shut them up. Also, time and again the government overruled these scientists to feed corporate greed and allowed dangerous drugs to enter food production. Yet, today, the dangers of these drugs are internationally recognized and many countries have forbidden their use for such purposes. In 1999, Bovine Growth Hormone was barred in Canada and in the European Union, which was due essentially to Dr. Chopra's negative findings on this drug going back to 1988. Since 2000, the United States government has been trying unsuccessfully to withdraw market approval for a very seriously hazardous antibiotic, Baytril for which regulatory compliance in Canada was rejected by Dr. Chopra in 1995.

Here is the full account of how government corruption endangers the public food supply and how Dr. Chopra and his colleagues fearlessly continue to "to speak truth to power." Here is also the story of how the elected representatives in both Canada and USA are more interested in protecting industrial profits and trade, instead of the public's health. The stories told here for the first time include products like Revalor-H, Baytril, Bovine Growth Hormone, Silicon Breast Implants, and slaughterhouse waste to cause the biggest ruin of health safety—Bovine Spongiform Encephalopathy (BSE) or "mad-cow disease."

Everybody who eats should read this book.

ISBN 0-9731945-7-X | 2005 | 6" × 9" | PB | $30.00

$40 w/CD which contains media interviews, government documents, federal court decisions, scientific bibliographies and more.

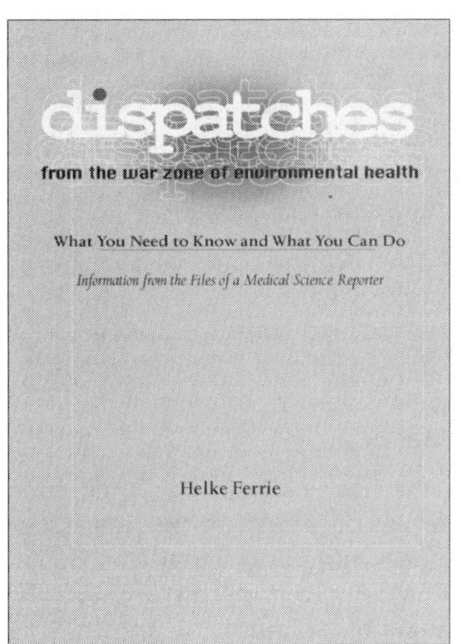

The weapons of mass destruction have been found, at least in medicine, and only we—the people, the consumers, the patients—can stop their proliferation by rouge corporations and their buddies in government. We have known about them for a long time actually, but their origins have been attributed to different sources over time. In antiquity, malevolent deities were thought responsible for the plagues that wiped out city-states and later caused economic disaster for the Roman Empire. In the Middle Ages, God was believed to be angry with sinful humanity and therefore visited epidemics on them, as he was believed to have done in the biblical stories about the Egypt at the time of Moses. In the mid-19th century, the poor of the vast slums associated with Europe's great cities were blamed for spreading mysterious diseases whose bacterial and viral causes were not yet understood by science.

Today, we know that the weapons of mass destruction are human-made chemicals, causing our current plague of chronic and degenerative diseases, and they are found in those substances intended to kill bugs, slugs, dandelions as well as in most of the drugs manufactured to fight cancer, impotence, heart disease, arthritis and other illnesses. These chemicals are the basis of an amoral economic system that sells toxic chemicals in all their forms with the promise of perfect lawns, perfect agricultural produce, perfectly hygienic kitchens, perfect white laundry, and perfect magic-bullet drugs. In fact, they harm us and are guaranteed to harm coming generations as well. Marketing techniques ensure that the whole truth is as carefully disguised as possible. That truth being, that our chemically saturated food, air, water, and soil are the sources of all our diseases—either directly, or by compromising our immune responses, or by giving pathogens the evolutionary advantage.

ISBN 0-9731945-3-7 | PB
336 pages | $25.00 CDN

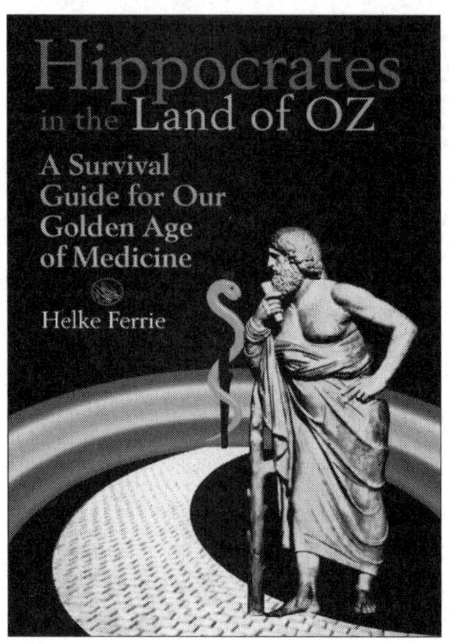

"There are no magic bullets. But miracles occur daily—if we accept illness as a teacher. The first doctor to be consulted is the one living in our hearts. Trusting that inner physician's advice is a political act of liberation for yourself and others."

"Why eat organic? The single most important health decision you can ever make is to protect your body from the witches' brew of money-science. Regaining the Garden of Eden is a task to be accomplished and we have the knowledge to re-create that garden."

"The requirements of human biology cannot be made to harmonize with the priorities of a world economy in which pesticides are of central importance."

"We have choices our ancestors never dreamed of. It takes an open mind and a fearless curiosity to benefit from what is available in medicine and the determination to protect that freedom of choice."

"Exploring how to have healthy children is a worthy meditation. They are not only our future, they are also the very incarnation of God's unfolding imagination. Paradoxically, it is up to us to protect and nurture this mystery."

ISBN 0-9731945-2-9

6" × 9" | 400 pages | PB | $25.00 | 2005

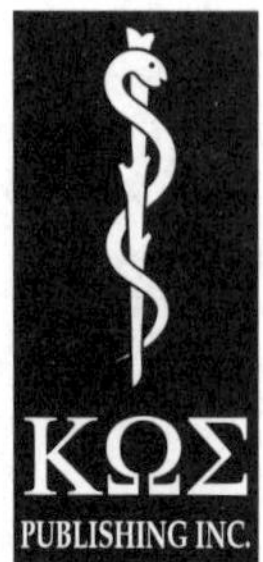

KOS Publishing Inc. is named after the Greek island where the father of modern medicine, Hippocrates, was born 2,500 years ago. Our books are dedicated to the hope that current developments in medicine will constitute a rebirth, in modern contexts, of ancient insights into the centrality of environment and nutrition. Our books hope to educate and empower readers in the politics of medicine and provide helpful information on non-toxic medicine based on basic science and clinical proof.

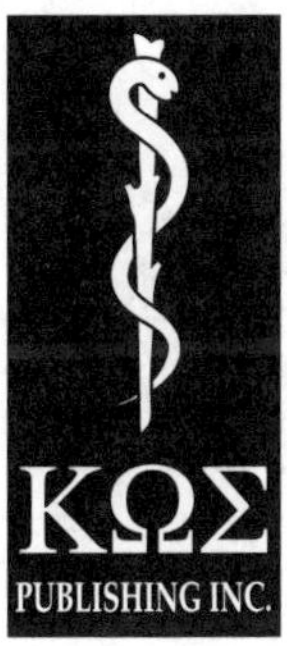

Order form

KOS can be contacted at the address given below to obtain more information or to place an order for any of our publications.

KOS PUBLISHING INC.

1997 Beechgrove Road,
Caledon, Ontario Canada L7K 0N3
Tel: (519) 927-1049 • Fax: (519) 927-9542
Email: helke@inetsonic.com • info@kospublishing.com

Name: _______________________________

Address: _____________________________

City: ________________________________

Prov./State: __________________________

Postal/Zip Code: ______________________

Telephone: ___________________________

Email:_______________________________

Date: _______________________________

Payment: ○ Cheque ○ Visa

　　　　　　○ Master Card

Name on Card: ________________________

Card #: ______________________________

Expiry Date: __________________________

Signature:____________________________

ISBN	TITLE	QTY.	PRICE	TOTAL
0-9731945-0-2	Healing the Planet		$25.00	
0-9731945-1-0	The Plot Against Asthma and Allergy Patients		$25.00	
0-9731945-2-9	Hippocrates in the Land of Oz		$25.00	
0-9731945-3-7	Dispatches From the War Zone of Environmental Health		$25.00	
0-9731945-4-5	We Can't Have a Baby!		$25.00	
0-9731945-6-1	Adventures in Psychiatry		$30.00	
0-9731945-5-3	The Gift of the Earth		$25.00	
0-9731945-7-X	Corrupt to the Core		$30.00	
0-9731945-7-X	Corrupt to the Core with CD		$40.00	

Shipping Charges: 1 title $6.00, for each additional title add $3 plus GST. Bulk orders of 10 copies or more of any *one title* receive a 50% discount on books only, regular shipping and taxes apply.

SUB-TOTAL	
TAXES	
TOTAL